Psychosocial Occupational Health

Psychosocial Occupational Health

An Interdisciplinary Textbook

Johannes Siegrist

*Professor Emeritus of Medical Sociology, Centre for Health
and Society, Heinrich-Heine-University Düsseldorf, Germany*

Jian Li

*Professor of Occupational Health, Department of Environmental
Health Sciences, Fielding School of Public Health, School for Nursing,
University of California Los Angeles, USA*

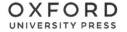

OXFORD
UNIVERSITY PRESS

OXFORD
UNIVERSITY PRESS

Great Clarendon Street, Oxford, OX2 6DP,
United Kingdom

Oxford University Press is a department of the University of Oxford.
It furthers the University's objective of excellence in research, scholarship,
and education by publishing worldwide. Oxford is a registered trade mark of
Oxford University Press in the UK and in certain other countries

© Oxford University Press 2024

The moral rights of the authors have been asserted

First Edition published in 2024

Published in the United States of America by Oxford University Press
198 Madison Avenue, New York, NY 10016, United States of America

British Library Cataloguing in Publication Data
Data available

Library of Congress Control Number: 2023950091

ISBN 978-0-19-288792-4

DOI: 10.1093/oso/9780192887924.001.0001

Printed in the UK by
Ashford Colour Press Ltd, Gosport, Hampshire

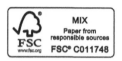

Preface

Textbooks are usually written for students, professionals, and other readers to get acquainted with an updated, systematic presentation of the state of knowledge on core topics within a scientific discipline. However, some topics of central interest transcend the boundaries of a single scientific discipline. 'Climate change' or 'demographic ageing' are examples where essential information derived from different scientific discourses needs to be integrated in an interdisciplinary approach. 'Modern work and health' is one such topic. The present text, arguing that modern work to a substantial extent is characterized by psychosocial features, aims to bring together essential information on this topic from several scientific fields. Occupational medicine, with its focus on epidemiological investigations, occupational health psychology, and medical or health-related sociology are the main evidence-producing disciplines to this end, supplemented by economics, safety sciences, occupational nursing, and rehabilitation sciences. While excellent textbooks are available for the main disciplines, an integrated and comprehensive analysis addressing crucial interactions between socioenvironmental, psychological, and biomedical aspects of modern work in association with working people's health has been largely absent so far. This textbook aims to fill in this gap. In a time of multiple societal challenges critical, systems-oriented thinking and acting is required to develop new solutions. The knowledge put together in this book is intended to support students, professionals, and decision-makers in the field of occupational health and safety in this process.

The textbook was written by two academic experts, a medical sociologist from Europe with several decades of scientific research experience in this field, and an occupational epidemiologist, trained as physician, with wide intercultural expertise derived from scientific collaboration in China, Europe, and the USA. The book evolved from a productive, long-lasting cooperation between the two authors. While the first author developed the main content of the book, the second author provided many essential additions and modifications. Every attempt towards providing an updated account of the state of art in a dynamic, rapidly growing field of scientific productivity is confronted with risks and shortcomings. Here, we focus mainly on research findings derived from epidemiological, quasi-experimental, and intervention studies performed on the basis of quantitative research methods during the past forty years. The majority of evidence comes from investigations in Europe and North America, and in part from Asia-Pacific. It reflects topics that were of mainstream interest during this time, and therefore may not do justice to important, more re- cent themes, such as nonstandard and precarious work, work-life interface, gender, and diversity. Moreover, with its reference to research conducted in high-income countries, it neglects burning issues of work and health in the Global South. We invite colleagues to fill in these gaps with complementary publications.

The book serves as a source of reference, summarizing accumulated knowledge on an broad range of content in eleven chapters. Each chapter can also be read on its own, and information presented in boxes, tables, and figures, as well as Relevant Questions, Recommended Readings, and Useful Websites help readers to become acquainted with this knowledge. We hope that this new, interdisciplinary introduction into a field of research with high relevance to science and policy stimulates, enriches, and motiv- ates readers to contribute, within their contexts, to a further promotion of healthy work.

Acknowledgements

The development and publication of the book was substantially supported by a grant from the German Research Foundation provided to the first author (DFG; No. 470515295). This support is gratefully acknowledged. The Faculty of Medicine, Heinrich-Heine-University, offered an ideal work environment to the first author. Both authors are deeply grateful to Pia Schneider who with her excellent skills contributed to the preparation of the manuscript during several stages of development. Draft versions of chapters were sent to colleagues for informal review, and their comments were highly appreciated. Our special thanks go to Peter Angerer, Chantal Brisson, Nico Dragano, Christine Fekete, Siegfried Geyer, Timothy A. Matthews, Mariann Rigó, Wendie Robbins, Reiner Rugulies, Andrew Steptoe, Töres Theorell, Pablo Verde, and Morten Wahrendorf. Furthermore, we thank the team at Oxford University Press, in particular Rachel Goldsworthy and Janine Fisher, for a most productive collaboration.

Düsseldorf and Los Angeles
Johannes Siegrist and Jian Li

Contents

PART I
GENERAL BACKGROUND

1

Psychosocial occupational health

A new perspective

1.1 The psychosocial dimension of work and its relationship with health

In the twenty-first century, paid work performed by humans continues to play a crucial role. Despite far-reaching technological progress, large parts of the adult population globally are engaged in recurrent economic activity by participating in the labour market. While pronounced levels of long-term unemployment and informal employment are still a serious concern, especially so in low- and middle-income countries, formal employment involving an occupational position or job is the predominant pattern in economically advanced and some rapidly developing countries. For instance, in OECD countries, around seventy-seven per cent of the work age population (15–64 years) were participating in the labour market in 2020 (OECD 2021). Overall, access to an occupational position mainly depends on qualification and training. The primary significance of paid work is due to its capacity of producing a double benefit. For the working person, participation in the labour market offers a continuous income and basic social protection: it confers social status; it promotes the development of skills and achievements; and despite its strenuous demands, it often generates experiences of control, reward, meaning, and satisfaction. Notably, these benefits vary substantially according to the quality of work and employment. For society, the benefits of work consist in a general advancement of welfare and social progress, economic growth, and improvement in tangible living conditions. Again, these benefits vary substantially and most markedly according to the degree of wealth distribution across society. It is this combination of personal and societal benefit that accords a unique *primacy* to the work role in modern societies, thus structuring and determining the adult life-course over several decades. Given their significant role and long-term

Psychosocial Occupational Health. Johannes Siegrist and Jian Li, Oxford University Press.
© Oxford University Press 2024. DOI: 10.1093/oso/9780192887924.003.0001

impact, work and employment matter for human health and well-being in rather substantial ways. To analyse the associations of modern work with the health of working people and to discuss the practical implications of this knowledge is the main aim of this book.

1.1.1 The impact of work and employment on health

It is not easy to determine the impact of work and employment on health. One reason of this difficulty concerns the fact that the occupational sphere and the broader environmental sphere are intimately intertwined. Take for example the case of climate change and global warming. This broader environmental challenge can affect the health of workers by increasing exposure to heat at work with related adverse consequences. It can also contribute to reduced health by causing redundancy and forced occupational mobility due to climate-induced migration and dislocation of companies and organizations (Kjellstrøm et al. 2020). Or remember the huge burden on workers' health due to the COVID-19 pandemic, whereby infection risks at the workplace increased, resulting in an elevated burden of morbidity and mortality. In addition, poor mental health resulted from job loss and income reduction, social isolation, and distant work induced by lockdown measures and the pandemic's economic consequences (International Labour Organization 2022).

To disentangle these intimate links of the broader environment with the work environment and their impact on health, three different levels of analysis can be distinguished and examined: the macro-, meso-, and micro-level. At the macro-level of analysis, a broad range of large-scale, distant structural conditions is identified that exert their impact on intermediary factors operating in people's more proximate living and working environments. Macro-level factors are generally defined in geographical, economic, epidemiologic, legal, or policy terms. Examples include climate change (geography), global financial crisis (economics), epidemic health risks (epidemiology), international trade agreements (law), or national labour market programmes (policy). Rather than acting directly on individuals' behaviour, health, and well-being, they influence intermediate, proximate contextual conditions to which individuals are exposed. These conditions are located at the meso-level of analysis. Work environments, as defined by organizations, enterprises, other work settings or distinct employment groups, are the main category of meso-level conditions in our approach, and exposure to these conditions defines the main pathway to workers' health risks and health gains. Indirect effects of macro-level factors on health via meso-level conditions were already illustrated in case of climate change and COVID-19. Similarly, the global financial crisis did not directly affect workers' health, but it had deleterious effects on employment opportunities, increasing downsizing, redundancy, and income loss, and these latter factors increased workers' risk of poor health (Riumallo-Herl et al. 2014). Or take the case of transnational supply chains. Improved legal regulations exert their beneficial effects on workers primarily through strengthening safety at work, reducing the number of unhealthy workplaces, or limiting excessive workload (Labonté et al. 2011). In conclusion, macro-level factors originating from the broader environment are important for health by exerting their adverse effects on intermediary, proximate conditions. These conditions are located at the meso-level of work environments within organizations, where they operate as risk factors or protective conditions of workers' health. Conceptually, a micro-level aspect can be distinguished from meso-level work environments, focusing on individual workplaces with their specific features. However, research dealing with health effects on working populations is mainly concerned with macro- and meso-level environments. Importantly, these work environments are experienced as exposures by working people, and their ways of dealing with work tasks and job conditions, their coping efforts, and cognitive, affective and behavioural responses exert a substantial impact on health outcomes (see 1.1.2.2., Fig. 1.1. and Chapter 3). While the analysis of individual differences in outcomes is of considerable interest for disciplines such as psychology (Cunningham and Black 2021) and genetics (Conley and Fletcher 2017), it has been less extensively addressed in occupational epidemiology, sociology, demography, or economics, where downstream effects of macro- and meso-level conditions on population health risks define the main focus.

A further difficulty of determining the impact of work and employment on health relates to the multi-faceted nature of work environments. Traditionally, their material dimensions received main attention in occupational medical research as well as in safety sciences. Material determinants of health are mainly transmitted via physical, chemical, and biological pathways ('material work environment'). On one hand, the work environment or workplace contains toxic substances, such as asbestos, cadmium, benzene, and particulate matters. It produces gases or fumes, and workers are exposed to heat or cold temperature. Dangerous and risky work

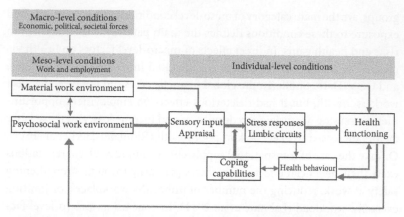

Figure 1.1 Psychosocial work environment and health: A conceptual framework developed and extended based on a model proposed by Rugulies (2019).

Source: Adapted with permission from Rugulies, R. (2019), 'What is a psychosocial work environment?', *Scand J Work Environ Health,* 45 (1), 1–6 [Figure 1, p. 2] (Creative Commons Attribution 4.0 International License, https://creativecommons.org/licenses/by/4.0/).

increases the occurrence of injuries. These hazards are analysed by toxicology and related basic sciences of occupational medicine. Experimental evidence, supported by epidemiological findings, shows that these hazards exert causal effects on workers' health. Physical work environments additionally contribute to the burden of occupational diseases by job tasks that require repetitive movements or heavy lifting, stressing the musculoskeletal and cardiovascular systems. Large parts of today's workforce are required to exert repetitive movements, and even with improved work settings (e.g. computer work) these demands increase the risk of musculoskeletal and cardiovascular complaints and disorders in the long run. The same holds true for excessive sedentary work with adverse consequences for cardiovascular functioning. On the other hand, there are occupational conditions with adverse effects on health whose direct causal pathways are either still under examination or act in concert with other work-related circumstances. Noise is one such hazard that affects health via excessive auditory stimulation, but also via psychological, autonomic nervous system-mediated factors of irritation or anger. Shift work is another example, where health effects are partly due to disturbed circadian biological rhythms, partly due to the impact of conflicts of adapting changed work time patterns to the individual living conditions (e.g. disturbances with family life) (for literature reviews on these work hazards for health, see Bültmann and Siegrist 2020; Theorell 2020). Equally so, long working hours, a main occupation health risk factors in todays' world of work, can impair health by the length and intensity of time exposed to adverse working conditions as well as by an impact on reduced recovery and relaxation opportunities (World Health Organization and International Labour Organization 2021).

Importantly, exposure to occupational factors is not restricted to the material work environment, but it extends to the psychosocial work environment. Here, health is negatively affected via sensory input of signals emanating from work situations that are perceived and appraised as challenging or threatening, triggering negative emotions of irritation, anger, anxiety, or helplessness, and stimulating psychobiological stress responses. These psychosocial work environments and their non-material effects on health, mediated by psychobiological processes, are of central importance to our analysis and will be dealt with extensively throughout this book. The spectrum of psychosocial aspects at work is very broad. It includes features of job tasks that are positively evaluated by workers, given their importance, meaning, interest, and challenge, but that may overtax workers' efforts due to their intensity and duration, or due to recurrent interruptions and adaptive changes. Health-care work is an example where chronic work overload in a professional activity that is performed by workers who are strongly motivated and highly appreciated often results in feelings of exhaustion and burnout. Monotonous jobs are another example where the task profile per se is not unhealthy, but where the working person's awareness of lack of stimulation, control, and personal agency provokes feelings of powerlessness, frustration, and stressful tension. Yet, many work situations produce conflicts between superiors and subordinates, and between co-workers and colleagues. Competition, aggression, unfair behaviour, as well as lack of trust, support, and solidarity are just some of the many manifestations of conflicts at work causing tension, anger, disappointment, and stressful arousal. As will be detailed in later chapters, difficulties and failures of organizational and human resource management contribute to work overload, unbalanced work division, poor work performance, and job dissatisfaction. Another source of stressful experiences at work concerns contextual economic and labour market-related conditions, such as high risks of downsizing, redundancy, and job loss, or lack of promotion prospects. In all these cases, an adverse psychosocial work environment threatens basic psychological needs of the working person, such as the need for security, autonomy, and self-direction; the need for successful agency and self-esteem; the need for trust, belonging, and support; and the need for appreciation, respect, and fair treatment. Need frustration is associated with pronounced negative emotions and psychobiological stress responses (see Chapter 3). Despite the complexity of its manifestations the psychosocial work environment displays an essential common feature in all types of job: distinct from the material work environment that exerts its direct health effects on the working person's organism, in all instances of a psychosocial work environment, it is the working person with his or her perceptions, appraisals, emotions, motivations, and behavioural responses that influences the final stress response that matters for health. This process is termed 'coping' (see 1.1.2.2and Chapter 3). Therefore, despite an overriding impact of situational ('extrinsic') factors, person characteristics (as 'intrinsic' factors) contribute to the health effects at individual level.

Summing up the arguments, we can state that analysing the impact of work and employment on health is a challenging task, given the difficulty of separating the work environment from the broader environment, and given the multifaceted nature of work environments. The former challenge is addressed by applying a multilevel approach where conditions operating at the macro-, meso-, and micro-level are distinguished. To tackle the second challenge, an interdisciplinary perspective is required that enables a combined study of material (physical, chemical, biological) and psychosocial (psychological, social) aspects of work environments. As health is the central outcome of interest, this interdisciplinary perspective is best realized in the frame of a biopsychosocial model of health and disease (Engel 1977). In this model, the three spheres of organism (molecules, genes, receptors, organs), individual person (emotions, cognitions, motivations), and social environment (macro-, meso-, micro-level conditions) are assumed to be interconnected by bi-directional pathways, reflecting the systemic nature of dynamic interactions between person and environment. Importantly, a main pathway is assumed to lead from the social environment (work demands) to the individual person (coping with these demands), whose action affects the health of the organism (through duration and intensity of psychobiological stress responses). This pathway will be of main interest in this book (see Part III). Yet, an alternative pathway is of interest as well. Impaired health at the level of the organism (e.g. reduced physical functioning) can affect the cognitions, emotions, and motivations of individual persons (e.g. depressed mood, reduced achievement motivation), and can impair the opportunities of working and being employed (e.g. inability to return to work). Obviously, this alternative pathway deserves primary attention as well, particularly in view of an aging workforce where chronic disorders are prevalent and exert huge effects on work performance and employability (see Part IV).

1.1.2 The psychosocial work environment

1.1.2.1 Historical development

The term 'psychosocial work environment' was proposed some fifty years ago as an umbrella concept representing the complexity of non-material working conditions with potential relevance for health (Levi 1971). It was not by chance that this occurred in Sweden as this country, and in particular Stockholm University and the Karolinska Institute, had been conducting pioneering occupational health research since the late 1960s. One aspect of research, led by psychiatrists and psychologists, focused on health effects of piecework and time pressure at work. Probably for the first time, effects of underload and overload on stress hormones and cardiovascular function were analysed in experimental studies (Frankenhaeuser and Gardell 1976). Another aspect was concerned with the impact of low control and other organizational constraints on workers' attitudes and behaviour, applying concepts from work and organizational psychology (Gardell 1971). In a third aspect, epidemiologists included questions on life events and working conditions in cohort studies on risk factors for coronary heart disease and demonstrated the first evidence on their association (Theorell et al. 1975). A couple of years later, Robert A. Karasek, an American sociologist, went to Stockholm to collaborate with this epidemiological research team, led by cardiologist Töres Theorell. This was the first opportunity to test a theoretical model of a stressful psychosocial work environment, termed 'demand-control', developed by Karasek, with regard to its ability to explain elevated health risks. This model assumes that job tasks characterized by high psychological demands in combination with low control and decision latitude generate health-adverse stress reactions (Karasek 1979; see Chapter 3). As a result of this collaboration, preliminary evidence of the model's contribution towards explaining elevated risks of cardiovascular disease was obtained (Alfredsson et al. 1982; Karasek et al. 1981). These are prominent examples of early research on psychosocial work environments and health in Sweden and other Scandinavian countries that had a significant impact on the shape of this field of research, as will be documented in later chapters of the book.

Yet, this does not mean that Scandinavian researchers were the only pioneers in this domain. In fact, several far-reaching discoveries were made by scientists in the US and in the United Kingdom, even if the term 'psychosocial work environment' was not used. One of the first landmark studies was published as early as 1958 by cardiologists Meyer Friedman and Ray Rosenman as first authors. They documented a striking association between a period of excessive psycho-mental workload, called 'occupational stress', among tax accountants and increased levels of cholesterol as well as altered blood clotting (Friedman et al. 1958). Another study revealed changes in blood lipids among workers who lost their job (Kasl et al. 1968). It is of interest to note that the cardiovascular system was the main target of analysis in these studies. In the 1960s, extensive animal experimental research laid scientific ground for the pathogenic role of chronic stress in the development of high blood pressure, atherogenic lipids, and other determinants of coronary atherosclerosis, the main risk factor of ischaemic heart disease (IHD) (Henry and Cassel 1969; Henry and Stephens 1977). At the same time, epidemiological studies documented elevated risks of IHD in population groups characterized by stressful circumstances, such as frequent occupational change (Syme et al. 1964), occupational mobility (Kaplan et al. 1971), inconsistency of occupational and educational status (Shekelle et al. 1969), and low occupational position (Cassel et al. 1971). These pioneer studies preceded a stage of substantial scientific progress starting in the final decades of the twentieth century that will be documented in later parts of the book.

However, one of the most influential contributions to the development of psychosocial occupational health originates from Great Britain, and more specifically from the Whitehall II study inaugurated by epidemiologist Michael Marmot (Marmot et al. 1991). Based on data obtained from an earlier occupational cohort, the Whitehall I study of civil servants, Marmot and colleagues documented a consistent, steep social gradient of morbidity and mortality, most pronounced in case of IHD, according to the civil servants' occupational position (Marmot et al. 1978). The Whitehall II study was set up to explain this fundamental pattern of social inequality in health. In fact, over the past three decades, the research consortium of the Whitehall II study produced a unique wealth of outstanding innovative research that promoted evidence on the psychosocial work environment as an important determinant of health to the forefront of international science. Several parts of this book capitalize on this rich collection of new knowledge.

Taken together, these research findings from different disciplines contributed to the construction of a biopsychosocial model of cardiovascular disease, as they were able to link factors related to the social environment (and in particular the work environment) to the individual person experiencing stressful encounters, and to biomedical indicators of elevated risk of cardiovascular disease (see Chapters 3, 6, 7). For a long time, cardiovascular disease (and more specifically IHD) was the prototype of an evidence-based biopsychosocial human disorder, but more recently, metabolic disorders, mental disorders, and different physiological systems (inflammation, immune competence) contributing to these disorders were integrated into this analysis. Against this background, we now ask how the notion of 'psychosocial work environment' can be elaborated in a more convincing way.

1.1.2.2 Proposed model

Proposing a model that specifies levels and pathways of analysis is one way of depicting the complex notion of 'psychosocial work environment'. **Figure 1.1** represents one such model. It integrates the core arguments mentioned above, and it adds precision using arrows indicating the direction of proposed effects. In detail, factors located at the macro-level are assumed to influence the work and employment contexts and settings located at the meso-level. These contexts and settings contain the multifaceted material and psychosocial work environments, and they are considered the main exposures to workers' health outcomes. As can be seen, at the individual level, effects on health are transduced to the organism by different channels, partly via physical, chemical, and biological hazards, and partly via sensory input. This latter pathway is crucial in case of psychosocial work environments, where sensory input is cognitively appraised and emotionally evaluated, and where the individual worker's coping activity impacts on the physiological and behavioural stress response. Two qualifying statements are important at this stage. Firstly, the way individual workers experience a psychosocial work environment varies according to their learning history, their coping capabilities, and their genetic and personality profile. Therefore, the cognitive and affective appraisal of an identical exposure by a group of workers is likely to reveal considerable individual differences. This means that individual appraisals of psychosocial work environments represent a mixture of 'objective', situation-related, and 'subjective', person-related information. This fact points to a central methodological challenge in view of a widely established research approach that assesses exposure to a psychosocial work environment via self-rated information reflecting workers' experiences as subjective evaluations. A discussion will be devoted to this methodological problem in later parts of the book (see Chapters 4 and 5). A second argument concerns the question of whether sensory input of environmental information always reaches the level of consciousness, as proposed by cognitive stress theory (Lazarus and Folkman 1984), or whether this input bypasses conscious appraisal under certain conditions, by directly affecting limbic structures and the hypothalamus that transduces afferent neocortical input into signals of the autonomic nervous system. Neuroscientific evidence on the brain's information processing supports this latter assumption (LeDoux 1996). Only a limited proportion of the total amount of information input reaching the brain every second is subjected to cognitive awareness, and this input is prioritized according to novelty and threat. Redundant information confirming previous experience more easily bypasses the threshold of conscious awareness. Thus, repeated, routinized experience of a psychosocial work environment is more likely to bypass this threshold than new, threatening sensory input that interrupts the stock of habituated previous knowledge (see Chapter 3).

The core link from stress responses to health functioning depicted in Figure 1.1 is hypothesized to involve a direct and an indirect pathway. The direct pathway from sensory input to an activated stress response matters most, and research has devoted its major interest to unravelling this crucial process. Importantly, the quality and intensity of a stress response is modified by the working person's coping capability. Yet, extrinsic and intrinsic constraints often limit successful coping efforts. Under these latter circumstances, an indirect pathway is often mobilized. Here, people tend to reduce their emotional strain by the consumption of stress-relieving substances. This consumption may offer an instantaneous relief but, as it does not target the sources of stressful experience, there is a considerable risk of chronic use resulting in addictive health-damaging behaviour (smoking, alcohol or drug consumption; unhealthy food; physical inactivity; sedentary behaviour) (see Chapter 3). Ultimately, these direct and indirect pathways result in altered health functioning (see Chapter 6).

The explanation of this notion of a psychosocial work environment with relevance for health deserves a further comment. In line with a biopsychosocial approach to health and disease, a reverse pathway from health to the social environment is operating as well. Impaired health can have a severe impact on a person's coping capability, his or her health-related behaviour, cognitive appraisal, and emotional state (see reverse arrow in Fig. 1.1). For instance, substantive research documented increased levels of depression following the manifestation of a variety of chronic diseases, where depressed mood in turn weakens cognitive and motivational coping capabilities. Moreover, these afflictions reduce the opportunities of returning to work after rehabilitation and to participate in productive activity (Bültmann and Siegrist 2020; see reverse arrow in Fig. 1.1). To demonstrate the importance of this reverse pathway in analysing relationships between psychosocial work environments and health, a special part of this book is devoted to its elaboration (Part IV).

So far, few attempts have been made to elaborate and visualize the different pathways linking the psychosocial work environment with health. A remarkable model depicted by Reiner Rugulies (2019) has inspired us to conceptualize these links in a slightly different way, as depicted in Figure 1.1. The figure indicates the main directions of assumed causes and effects of interest in this book, but it does not represent an empirically validated causal model.

1.1.2.3 Dimensions of health

'Health functioning' is the outcome of central interest in our analysis of effects of psychosocial work environments. Although the term can be applied to places, geographical regions, or even the planet, it is conventionally limited to the individual person. Importantly, when discussing this notion, it is obvious that health can be improved or harmed, thus providing a positive and a negative dimension. Traditionally, for compelling reasons, its negative dimension has been investigated and tackled much more intensely than its positive dimension. Absence of health is more visible and urges more attention than its presence. This absence of health is dealt with in three different systems of reference, termed 'disease', 'illness', and 'sickness'. 'Disease' reflects the professional system of reference where signs of reduced health are analysed in a biomedical framework of pathophysiological developments of organs and organ systems. Based on scientific evidence and clinical knowledge, the International Classification of Diseases (ICD) (World Health Organization 2022a) has identified and classified a large number of physical and mental disorders. Each disease is identified via a set of symptoms, biochemical and physiological data obtained through laboratory or functional tests, imaging techniques, and medical history information. Ideally, each disease is explained by one or several causal factors, and specific medical treatment approaches are available to restore health or to reduce disease severity. To a certain extent, due to insufficient knowledge, the causes of disease are not yet established. In these cases, at least distinct risk factors are known whose manifestations increase the probability of disease occurrence. As many diseases have multiple causes derived from socio-environmental and personal (psychological, behavioural, genetic) factors, they are best analysed and tackled in a systemic, interdisciplinary, and inter-professional approach, as proposed by the biopsychosocial model. 'Illness' represents the system of reference of lay persons experiencing their personal health state. Due to the subjective interpretation and differential knowledge of symptoms and bodily signs, people's definitions of illness vary widely according to socio-cultural, educational, ethnic, age- and gender-related circumstances. In view of the significance of illness behaviour (e.g. to seek medical aid, to comply with treatment obligations), these wide variations of defining illness and of responding to related needs can be problematic as they may diverge from the health needs induced by distinct diseases. For instance, symptoms of a severe disease (cancer, stroke, IHD) may remain unobserved or misinterpreted, causing delay of treatment or premature mortality. Alternatively, over-utilization of health services may occur due to inappropriate illness behaviour. 'Sickness' delineates the society's system of reference. As many disorders largely prevent economically active people from participation in paid work and from contributing to economic productivity, and as the treatment and prevention of diseases induce substantial financial costs, every society is obliged to establish systems of cost control and compensation. Sickness funds, regulations of health-care utilization, and cash transfer systems are examples of how the reference system of sickness is working.

In today's aging societies, physical and mental disabilities are of growing concern from a public health perspective, in addition to acute and chronic diseases mentioned above. Their main general feature is the restriction of functioning. Accordingly, to supplement the ICD, an International Classification of Functioning, Disability and Health (ICF) has been developed (World Health Organization 2001). This classification contains the three dimensions of bodily functions and structures (impairment), activity (limitations), and participation in social life (restrictions), and these dimensions are influenced not only by type and extent of the disabling condition, but also by environmental and personal factors. Thus, compared to the ICD, the ICF has incorporated distinct personal and social factors into a biomedical paradigm of disease and disability.

In conclusion, the negative dimension of health is addressed as a high priority and by multiple activities of scientific research, medical and paramedical professional agency, health-care delivery, and structural measures of health and social policy. The terms 'disease', 'disability', 'illness', and 'sickness' illustrate this priority. In contrast, the positive dimension of health has received less prominence within the professional systems of medicine and health care, and within the priority agendas of governments. It is true that health promotion and prevention of disease have been recognized as relevant health policy goals more recently, not least by several initiatives from the World Health Organization (2008). Yet, there is still a huge imbalance in terms of investments and concerns between the two dimensions. Furthermore, from a scientific point of view, it seems difficult to find a consensual definition of 'positive health' other than 'absence of disease or illness'. A variety of biological markers was proposed as indicators of positive health, but this debate is ongoing. Internationally, there is a strong emphasis on defining positive health in terms of subjective well-being (Diener 1984). 'Subjective well-being' is considered a three-dimensional construct, incorporating an evaluative component of cognitive judgment about one's personal situation ('life satisfaction', 'purpose in life'), an experiential component of emotional state ('positive and negative affect'), and a eudaemonic component of positive functioning (in terms of self-realization, agency, and social relatedness) (Ryan and Deci 2018). These components are assessed by self-rated scales indicating the amount and comprehensiveness of subjective well-being. There is no doubt that subjective well-being promotes mental and physical health, thus being a relevant outcome criterion in research on work and health. However, mainstream occupational health research has largely focused on indicators of 'disease', 'disability', or 'illness' to measure work-related outcomes. This mainstream approach will be documented in later chapters dealing with empirical evidence in this field of research.

In summary, Figure 1.1 and the explanatory text may offer an instructive introduction into the complex, yet intriguing and relevant matter of this book. Research on psychosocial work environments and health represents a new, rapidly expanding field of knowledge accumulation that is still debated at theoretical, methodological, and empirical levels (for discussion, see Kivimäki et al. 2018). This book is one of the first attempts to synthesize this knowledge and to advance the state of art by critical discussions and proposed suggestions.

1.2 Scientific disciplines and challenges of psychosocial occupational health

We have seen that knowledge of psychosocial work environment and its relationship with health comes from different scientific disciplines. Here, a short description of the main disciplines, their specific contributions, and their relevance for the practice of occupational health is given. The focus on five core disciplines does not claim to be exhaustive, but it covers essential developments. This section will be followed by an introductory illustration of some prominent challenges of the world of modern work and employment for psychosocial occupational health, where the useful role of knowledge and competences evolving from the study of this new field becomes evident.

1.2.1 Main scientific disciplines

In very general terms, science is considered a controlled collective activity which searches for truth and new knowledge. The notion of control refers to common criteria of the quality of knowledge acquisition, and collective activity indicates that expertise from different people and different areas is required, and that findings from individual scientists require independent replication and collective approval. The development of scientific expertise follows a process of division of labour, where different disciplines are established, often resulting in sub-disciplines and innovative cross-disciplinary specializations. A scientific discipline is best characterized as a field of expertise that describes and explains a specific area, aspect, or phenomenon of the living or non-living world by a structured process of knowledge acquisition. To this end, a common language of description, common methods of information collection, and a common set of explanatory theoretical models are required. Scientific disciplines stand out by high levels of expertise, shared standards of training, and procedures of quality control, and by their impact on society through professional associations and organizations. The following scientific disciplines have contributed most significantly to the development of the field of occupational health in its current shape (see Box 1.1).

1.2.1.1 Occupational medicine
Occupational Medicine is the primary, most established, and oldest discipline dealing with our topic. As a specialty field of medicine, this

Box 1.1 **Main scientific disciplines**

- Occupational Medicine: As a specialty field of medicine, this discipline is concerned with the detection, surveillance, prevention, and rehabilitation of occupational hazards and occupational diseases. Main activities are research, teaching, preventive, and consulting activities, and to some extent clinical work. Close links were developed with Environmental Medicine and Occupational Health Nursing.
- Epidemiology: A discipline concerned with the distribution and the determinants of health conditions in populations, using quantitative methods. Its descriptive, analytic, and interventional approaches enable the application of research results to prevention, public health, and health care. Occupational epidemiology is a crosscutting interdisciplinary field, rather than a sub-discipline.
- Psychology: The main discipline of behavioural sciences concerned with perceptions, cognitions, emotions, motivations, and behaviours of individual persons and of groups of individuals. It offers a broad spectrum of methods, including tests and experiments, and a variety of theoretical models. Practical applications refer to individual counselling and therapy, and to monitoring and intervention activities.
- Sociology: This discipline is concerned with the analysis of structures and processes of societies at macro-, meso-, and micro-level of social life, applying theories and methods developed in social sciences. With close links to social epidemiology and to the subdiscipline of medical or health sociology, it explores occupational determinants and consequences of health.
- Economics: A discipline applying the analysis of two important pathways between economy and health to the field of occupational research: the impact of economic conditions (e.g. unemployment) on people's health, and the economic consequences (financial costs) of healthy or unhealthy work. Its advanced quantitative methods are considered a particular strength.

discipline is concerned with the detection, surveillance, and prevention of occupational hazards and occupational diseases, and with processes of rehabilitation and return to work of disabled workers. Its focus is on research, teaching, and on preventive and consulting activities, and with certified qualifications it also addresses clinical work. Close links exist with the discipline of Environmental Medicine (Lance 2019). Traditionally, occupational medicine was developed as a scientific discipline in the area of industrialization during the nineteenth century, when toxicology, physics, biochemistry, biology, and clinical medicine shaped its scientific profile. With its search for specific substances and conditions at work that cause certain diseases, occupational medicine combined two methodological approaches from the very beginning: experimental studies using basic science methods, and epidemiological investigations of working populations. More recently, with substantial changes of employment sectors, technologies, and work environments, the discipline was gradually enlarged to include environmental medicine, and, in part, ergonomics and industrial hygiene. In some countries, the academic institutionalization of occupational medicine includes preventive and social medicine. Moreover, on many sites, collaborative links were developed with the fields of industrial-organizational psychology and occupational health psychology (see 1.2.1.3). As a distinction, occupational physicians are an internationally established professional group with legally defined tasks, in addition to strong boundaries with research and teaching in tertiary institutions. Guidelines for training and practice strengthen the professionalization process, and beyond associations at local and national level, a strong international professional organization was developed, the International Commission on Occupational Health (ICOH). Founded in 1906, this worldwide non-governmental professional society exerts an influential role in occupational health policy, not least in collaboration with the World Health Organization and the International Labour Organization. Although significant research input to psychosocial occupational health comes now from social and behavioural sciences, occupational medicine contributes substantially to the biomedical foundation of analyses linking the psychosocial work environment with health. In addition, occupational medicine has an important role in translating scientific evidence into practice in terms of screening and surveillance, expert opinions, guidelines, and implementation of preventive measures at worksites. One important extension is Occupational Health Nursing, which is a specialty within the nursing discipline to train occupational health nurses. In the US, such training is mainly supported by the National Institute for Occupational Safety and Health (NIOSH) through the Education and Research Centres. Modern roles and responsibilities of occupational health nurses have expanded immensely to include case management, counselling and crisis intervention, health promotion and risk reduction, legal and regulatory compliance, worker and workplace hazard detection. Particularly, 'psychosocial needs/concerns' and 'stress management' are clearly highlighted by the American Association of Occupational Health Nurses (see 'Useful websites').

1.2.1.2 Epidemiology

Epidemiology represents the discipline with the major methodological impact on the field of occupational health. Epidemiology is commonly defined as the discipline concerned with the distribution and the determinants of health conditions (usually diseases) in populations, using quantitative methods. Its descriptive, analytic, and interventional approaches enable the application of research results to prevention, public health, and health care (Lash et al. 2021).

Historically, several ground-breaking epidemiological investigations on the burden of work-related disease promoted the academic development of occupational medicine as well as the establishment of occupational safety and health legislation and occupational health-care services. Most famous in this regard was the study by Louis-René Villermé, a French physician, who, among others, revealed and criticized the noxious working conditions in cotton, linen, and silk industry in 1840 (Julia and Valleron 2011). Rather than being a distinct sub-discipline, occupational epidemiology is a crosscutting field of scientific inquiry, reaching from genetics, environmental sciences, clinical medicine, to social epidemiology. During the twentieth century, occupational epidemiologists made many relevant discoveries. To mention just two examples related to different diseases: In the 1960s, prospective evidence of a causal role of asbestos fibres for the development of lung cancer and a formerly unknown disease, mesothelioma, was obtained (Selikoff 1990). As a practical consequence, a range of countries banned the use of asbestos, but more developed than developing countries. Around the same time, a landmark study of London bus drivers showed a clear link between sedentary work and elevated risk of IHD (Morris et al. 1966). Although this study could not rule out all relevant confounding factors and although excessive physical activity at work can also increase this risk, findings had far-reaching implications for worksite health prevention programmes of compensating physical activity among sedentary jobs. It is, by the way, of interest to observe that leisure-time physical activity exerts beneficial effects on cardiovascular health (Holtermann et al. 2020).

The sub-discipline of social epidemiology is concerned with the analysis of social determinants of health, where social inequalities of working and employment conditions are of major interest. This was most convincingly demonstrated in the classic British Whitehall study of civil servants mentioned above, documenting a social gradient of cardiovascular mortality according to occupational grade: the lower the grade, the higher the mortality risk (Marmot et al. 1978). More recently, a further characteristic of this sub-discipline was suggested by the term 'psychosocial epidemiology', where the close links between social and psychological factors are at stake. Clearly, research on psychosocial work environments and health is one of the core areas in this regard (Kivimäki et al. 2018). Yet, when it comes to explanations of observed statistical associations, social and psychosocial epidemiologists often depend on input from other disciplines, and in particular from psychology and sociology, as will now be described.

1.2.1.3 Psychology

Psychology is the main discipline of behavioural sciences as it is concerned with perceptions, cognitions, emotions, motivations, and behaviours of individual persons and of groups of individuals. It uses systematic observations, tests, experiments, and surveys to explore these phenomena, and it applies theories to their explanation. Psychology has a strong connection with practical applications, either in terms of individual counselling and therapy, or in terms of monitoring and intervention activities. As a mature academic discipline with a long history, this field has developed a number of sub-disciplines where two specializations have put their main focus on work. Industrial-organizational psychology analyses the interface of working persons with organizational contexts, with a broad spectrum of interest, including work motivation and performance, recruitment and training, leadership and teamwork, or organizational and personnel development. While many concepts in this research are useful when applied to relationships between work and health, health is not an explicit priority of this sub-discipline. Rather, this is the case for occupational health psychology. Evolving during the 1990s, this field has put its main emphasis 'on the ways in which experiences at work, exposures to work tasks, and associated environmental factors impact worker health, safety, and well-being', as defined in an excellent recent textbook (Cunningham and Black 2021, p. 2).

Occupational health psychology owes its rapid growth not least to the influential *Journal of Occupational Health Psychology*, to special training and promotion activities of the American Psychological Association, to innovative scientific associations, and to a series of handbooks under the leadership of British psychologist Cary L. Cooper (Cooper and Quick 2017). Throughout this book, several chapters will draw quite substantially on research findings derived from this field. At the same time, it should be noted that essential theoretical input to this sub-discipline comes from the general field of psychology. To cite just two classic examples, one of the fundamentals of this research is provided by psychological stress theory (Lazarus 1966), and one of the core concepts of coping with work applied to occupational health psychology concerns Bandura's theory of self-efficacy (Bandura 1977). Moreover, concept such as 'conservation of resources' (Hobfoll 1989), 'equity' (Adams 1965), and 'organizational injustice' (Greenberg and Cohen 1982) were integrated in respective investigations. Chapter 3 will discuss some leading current concepts of occupational health psychology in more detail. Last not least, the psychological notion and assessment of 'burnout' had a major impact on empirical research in this field (Maslach 1982).

1.2.1.4 Sociology

Sociology is the discipline concerned with the analysis of structures and processes of societies. Over the course of their evolution, humans evolved as social animals, developing groups, norms, social roles, social differentiations, and social institutions. The interplay of individual and society is at the core of sociological analysis, and this interaction is analysed at different levels, the macro-, meso-, and micro-level. The societal structure of work and employment and the organization of work with its impact on workers' behaviour were main topics in the founding period of sociology, as documented by the seminal work on alienated labour by Karl Marx (Marx 1984). However, the application of leading sociological concepts to the analysis of work and health occurred much later, mainly during the second half of the twentieth century. Examples of relevant concepts are 'social support' (Durkheim 1897, 1951), 'social status' (Merton 1968), 'control and self-direction' (Kohn and Schooler 1973), and 'social exchange and reciprocity' (Gouldner 1960). Social support was shown to be a protective factor in associations of work stress with coronary heart disease (House 1981), while social (or occupational) status was identified as an important determinant of life expectancy and overall mortality (Antonovsky 1967). Social status was also linked to mental illness (Hollingshead and Redlich 1958) and, in combination with critical life events, to the onset of depression (Brown and Harris 1978). How leading sociological models of a psychosocial work environment with relevance to health and disease were influenced by classical theoretical concepts in sociology will be discussed in Chapter 3. Of interest, among the sub-disciplines of sociology, medical (or health) sociology is a field of research with an extensive interest in relationships of work and health.

1.2.1.5 Economics

The discipline of economics enriched the field of occupational health in two different directions. One direction deals with the impact of economic conditions (unemployment, low income, income inequality) on people's health, whereas the other direction is concerned with the analysis of economic consequences (financial costs) of healthy or unhealthy work. Based on large datasets from the USA that were subjected to ecological analysis, Harvey M. Brenner discovered a significant increase of indicators of mental pathology, including suicide and homicide, within a year of heightened unemployment rates (Brenner 1973). Subsequently, this approach was applied to chronic diseases, such as IHD, where a time lag of two to three years following job loss was observed, and it was extended to explore the impact of economic business cycles on morbidity, using time-series analyses (Brenner and Mooney 1982). Although innovative and intriguing, the validity of these results was restricted, given the methodological problem of ecological fallacy. Thus, individual-level cohort studies corroborated an association of unemployment with morbidity and mortality (e.g. Dupre et al. 2012; J. K. Morris et al. 1994; Moser et al. 1987). A further line of research investigated the links between income, income inequality, and health. Many studies documented higher morbidity and mortality among people with low income, but research identified a reciprocal association between these two factors, such that poor health also results in low income (Mackenbach 2019). In a similar way, the causality of a prominent role of augmented income inequality in explaining high morbidity and mortality across different countries is still debated (Wilkinson and Pickett 2009). The second direction of economic research with relevance to occupational health focuses on evaluating and estimating the costs of the burden of work-related diseases (Goetzel et al. 2004), and the benefits of health-promoting worksite interventions (Johanson and Aboagye 2020).

These remarks on relevant disciplines serve as an introductory orientation to readers, and they are by no means exhaustive. Yet, cumulative research conducted in the frame of these five scientific disciplines laid the ground for essential knowledge on psychosocial occupational health. How useful this knowledge can be in tackling dominant challenges to occupational health is illustrated in the next section. Three such challenges are selected as instructive examples.

1.2.2 Some current challenges

1.2.2.1 The COVID-19 pandemic

The outbreak of the COVID-19 pandemic early in 2020 with its subsequent worldwide surges of infection was an unpredicted and threatening event to humanity. According to the WHO Coronavirus (COVID-19) Dashboard, more than 6.8 million deaths and more than 700 million cases were recorded by March 2023 (World Health Organization 2023). In addition, evidence on adverse long-term effects of this infection became evident, with a syndrome of symptoms defined as 'long COVID'. Thanks to rapid, successful development of vaccines, the deleterious effects of this pandemic could be substantially reduced, but large parts of populations in less developed countries had no or very limited access to these vaccines. Moreover, considerable parts of the population even in highly developed countries rejected vaccination, thus reinforcing the outbreak and expansion of new waves of infection.

The associations between the COVID-19 pandemic and the world of work are particularly worrying as they involve at least two different aspects of working people's health. Firstly, specific occupational groups were—and continue to be—at high risk of infection due to the nature of their work. These occupations include medical and paramedical professions dealing with victims of infection, most often in the context of treatment in intensive care units of hospitals. Through this direct pathway, the demands of their work, further occupational groups were continuously exposed to the wider public, thus suffering from elevated rates of viral infection (e.g. delivery of services; taxi drivers; police, military service; teachers, social workers). Many factories and organizations failed to protect workers from infectious risks, in particular those with less developed occupational health services, and those with a less skilled or even precarious workforce (e.g. construction workers, cleaners; Mutambudzi et al. 2020). As a result, social inequalities of mortality due to the COVID-19 epidemic were reported from several national reports, with highest levels among those in lowest socioeconomic positions (as an early document, see Wise 2020).

What does the psychosocial dimension of occupational health add to these observations? Obviously, the recurrent threat of being infected in one's daily work aggravated an already high burden of workload in these occupations. Signs of exhaustion, burnout, and physiological breakdown were observed to be more frequent, calling for measures of mitigation. Improving mental health among occupational and professional groups exposed to the pandemic has become an internationally acknowledged high priority for workplace intervention efforts (World Health Organization 2022b). During the COVID-19 pandemic, many workers were asked to work from home, which was one of the public health measures of prevention at macro-level. Indeed, research evidence indicated that working from home was associated with reduced risk of infection, in this unexpected natural experiment (Alipour et al. 2021). However, essential workers (including health-care workers) had to work onsite, and they suffered from high levels of stress and mental symptoms. An intervention study among health-care workers in Canada, using online cognitive-behavioural therapy techniques at micro-level, demonstrated significant improvements in symptoms of anxiety, depression, and post-traumatic stress disorder (Trottier et al. 2022).

The second aspect of how this pandemic affects workers' health concerns indirect rather than direct pathways. Widespread and long-lasting 'lockdown' measures resulted in substantial reductions of employment. For instance, according to an estimate of the International Labour Organization, total hours worked globally in 2022 remained almost two per cent below the pre-pandemic level, resulting in a deficit of some fifty-two million full-time equivalent jobs (International Labour Organization 2022). Thus, reduced working time resulting in income loss has become a major concern, specifically in the absence of national social policy measures. Furthermore, the COVID-19 pandemic threatened the economic survival of several branches of the economy, such as travel enterprises, gastronomy, hotels, and arts and culture. In addition, a global recession dampened the labour market. These developments increased the risks of experiencing job instability and job loss, conditions that are associated with an elevated occurrence of anxiety and depression (Dragano et al. 2022). During the pandemic, job loss hit primarily those with less protected employment contracts (e.g. temporary or short-term contracts), those with low skill levels or in precarious jobs, and those engaged as 'own account' workers, specifically in the 'gig' economy. It became also more frequent among younger employees, among women, among people of colour, and among less skilled and less privileged people (International Labour Organization 2022).

To conclude, this new pandemic exerted a far-reaching impact on the world of work and employment, accelerating technological change as well as deepening inequalities and threats to less privileged parts of the workforce (Peters et al. 2022; see Chapter 11). For decision makers in governments and enterprises, the pandemic revealed the high significance of comprehensive efforts of primary prevention at work, ensuring material and psychosocial safety for all workers.

1.2.2.2 Mental disorders and addiction

According to a global estimate more than a billion people are affected by mental disorders and addiction (Rehm and Shield 2019). Mental disorders, and specifically depression, are more prevalent among women, whereas addiction is more prevalent among men. Given a pronounced onset of these conditions in early and middle adulthood, working-age populations are exposed to a high respective burden of disease. In high-income countries, the age-standardized incidence of depression seems to have grown from 1990 to 2017 (Liu et al. 2020). With an estimated twelve-month prevalence of about six per cent of the population, and a lifetime prevalence that may exceed twenty per cent (Mikkelsen et al. 2021), the scale of the problem of reduced mental health becomes evident, even more so, if anxiety disorders and states of burnout are added to this burden (Salvagioni et al. 2017). As will be demonstrated, a considerable part of increased risks of reduced mental health is attributed to poor working and employment conditions, thus pointing to a high need for preventive efforts in occupational public health. Unfortunately, reduced mental health is often combined with additional health risks. Among these risks, addictive disorders including drug misuse are prevalent in a variety of occupational groups. Two such drugs deserve attention, given their long-term adverse effects on health: opioids and benzodiazepines. In the USA, a recent excess mortality due to opioid misuse has significantly reduced life expectancy among middle-aged white men, and its use has been associated with the despair experienced under threatening socioeconomic living and working conditions (Case and Deaton 2020). More specifically, direct associations of opioid use with high levels of stressful psychosocial work were observed (see Chapter 6). Although less prevalent and less dangerous, the recurrent consumption of benzodiazepines has negative effects on health, promoting dependency and cognitive impairment. Given their anxiolytic properties, their continued use is enforced by stressful conditions. Again, close links with stressful work were reported (see Chapter 6).

Taken together, different adverse work and employment conditions are likely to increase the risk of poor mental health, as indicated by depression and anxiety, exhaustion and burnout, and addictive disorders, in particular drug misuse. In part, these conditions are located at the macro-level of labour market and economic development; in part, they evolve from stressful material and psychosocial work environments located at the meso-level of analysis. As will be shown in subsequent parts, empirical evidence on this latter level of analysis is particularly rich. For instance, leading theoretical models of an adverse psychosocial work environment were tested with regard to their capacity to explain depressive symptoms in prospective cohort studies in a variety of developed and rapidly developing countries (Chapter 6). Notably, in a majority of cases, significant associations were observed, and in a review of European studies, it was concluded that these exposures account for about one third of all cases of depressive symptoms in working-age populations (Niedhammer et al. 2022). If further substantiated, the association between stressful psychosocial work and poor mental health must be considered a major occupational public health challenge that deserves attention from responsible stakeholders. Unfortunately, several conditions of poor mental health are long-lasting, with considerable risks of relapse or recurrence, and therapeutic treatment successes are often limited. A European report concluded that about half of those workers with mental health problems who have taken a period of sick leave encounter difficulties of returning to work (Nielsen et al. 2020). Therefore, special efforts are needed to enable a vulnerable workforce to continue productive employment. As a priority, comprehensive programmes of reintegration into paid work need to be implemented that strengthen personal capabilities as well as support from organizations and from health-care providers (see Chapters 8 and 9). Such programmes will be successful to the extent that they are reinforced by distinct integrative labour market policies at the national level that offer training opportunities, part-time positions, and economic resources to secure sufficient living standards and sustainable participation in societal life.

1.2.2.3 Social inequalities in health

The COVID-19 pandemic and the wide prevalence of mental health problems among working populations are two important challenges to occupational health requiring interventional activities and policies that take into consideration core psychosocial aspects at work. Yet, there is another challenge that points to an even more fundamental way of how work affects health. The following three statements best describe this challenge. Firstly, the lower the socioeconomic position of working populations in terms of educational level, income, and occupational standing, the higher is their risk of suffering from a wide spectrum of diseases, from disability, and from premature mortality. Secondly, the lower the socioeconomic position of working populations in terms of educational level, income, and occupational class, the higher is their risk of exposure to adverse material and psychosocial work environments. Thirdly, exposure to adverse work environments contributes to social inequalities in health in these populations.

In a nutshell, these three statements summarize several decades of socioepidemiological research that demonstrate a highly worrying fact: despite economic welfare, technological progress, and advances in health care and medical therapy, substantial social inequalities in health persist in modern societies. These inequalities are best described as a social gradient of morbidity and mortality across the whole of a society, with best health among those at the top and worst health among those at the bottom (Marmot 2004). As an illustration of the scope of this gradient, In European countries, differences in life expectancy between those at the top and those at the bottom of a societal structure vary between seven and ten years among men, and between four and six years among women (Mackenbach 2019). Although some exceptions were observed, a majority of highly prevalent chronic diseases and disorders follow this social gradient. Examples are cardiovascular diseases, type 2 diabetes, lung cancer, respiratory diseases, accidents, depression, and infectious diseases, such as HIV and COVID-19. Research on social inequalities in midlife health often uses indicators of occupational class, mirroring working people's position in a hierarchy of privileged or disadvantaged job conditions. Consistent occupational gradients of morbidity and mortality were documented (d'Errico et al. 2017; Mackenbach 2019; Marmot et al. 1978).

The British Whitehall II study mentioned earlier was not only a major research initiative to promote new knowledge on health effects of psychosocial work environments; in addition, it contributed significantly to the description and explanation of health inequalities according to socioeconomic and occupational conditions (Marmot 2004; see also Chapters 5, 6, 7). In one of the major cohort studies of ageing populations, the English Longitudinal Study of Ageing (Marmot et al. 2003), the focus on health inequalities according to occupational position was extended to a life-course perspective, documenting steep social gradients of cardiovascular disease mortality in relation to two complementary indicators of socioeconomic status (SES) that included a transgenerational aspect (paternal occupational position) and pre-employment conditions (educational level) (Stringhini et al. 2018). The first indicator, termed 'SES trajectory' (see Fig. 1.2A), was measured by four categories of social stability/mobility, ranging from 'stable high' (high paternal and own position) to 'stable low' (low paternal and own position). In the second indicator, termed 'Life-course SES score' (see Fig. 1.2B), a summary index of cumulative career advantage/disadvantage was based on four criteria (paternal occupational status, own occupational status, educational degree, wealth in early adulthood). Figure 1.2 demonstrates the social/occupational gradient of cardiovascular disease mortality for both indicators of this cohort. Compared to those in the privileged reference category, elderly men and women exposed to cumulative disadvantage in their occupational career suffered from a twofold-elevated risk of cardiovascular mortality during the observation period. Results were based on multivariable logistic regression analysis adjusted for a range of relevant confounders (Stringhini et al. 2018).

The findings displayed in Figure 1.2 are just one piece of extended evidence on SES-related morbidity and mortality risks, where indicators of occupational advantages/disadvantages demonstrate a consistent association with morbidity and mortality risks (d'Errico et al. 2017; Hoffmann 2023; Landsbergis et al. 2018; Mackenbach 2019). Importantly,

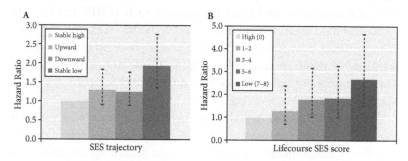

Figure 1.2 Association of two indicators of cumulative social/occupational advantage/disadvantage over the life course with cardiovascular disease mortality risk in the ELSA cohort (N= 7,846 men and women >50 years; mean 8.4 year follow-up). For further explanation see text.

Source: Reproduced with permission from Stringhini, S., Zaninotto, P., Kumari, M., et al. (2018), 'Socio-economic trajectories and cardiovascular disease mortality in older people: the English Longitudinal Study of Ageing', Int J Epidemiol, 47 (1), 36–46 [Figure 1, p. 42]; license no.: 5493601175491.

subsequent research revealed that these associations are mediated, in part, by exposure to adverse material and psychosocial working conditions (see Chapter 6). Moreover, people employed in low occupational positions have fewer chances of receiving adequate secondary and tertiary prevention measures, have more difficulties of returning to work after disease onset, and are more often forced to leave paid work prematurely (see Chapters 8 and 9). Coverage by protective labour and social policies is less extended among socially disadvantaged groups, not only in low- and middle-income countries, but also in modern Western societies (see Chapter 11). Thus, the existence of socially unequal health and its determination by adverse working and employment conditions represents a major challenge for occupational health policy, as will be illustrated in several parts of the book.

In summary, the three selected challenges of the COVID-19 pandemic, the widespread occurrence of mental disorders and addictive behaviours in working populations, and the differential work-related burden of disease with its impact on social inequalities in health point to the urgent need for strengthening preventive efforts at work. In all these cases, new insights into a prominent role of psychosocial features of work and employment may offer innovative approaches to tackle these challenges.

1.3 Summary

As a response to far-reaching changes of the world of modern work and employment new research developments covered under the umbrella of 'psychosocial occupational health' are emerging. They address social and psychological aspects of occupational conditions with relevance to health, and they analyse new challenges in the context of economic globalization and vast technological changes. The knowledge derived from these developments is expected to enrich and strengthen the expertise, skills, and attitudes of students and professionals committed to occupational health.

1.4 Relevant questions

- What are the essential features of a psychosocial work environment? Why is it useful to apply them to the analysis of associations of modern work with health?

- What are the main reasons that research so far focused much more on the negative than the positive effects of psychosocial work environments on health?
- Can you identify other challenges in addition to the three worrying current challenges of modern work mentioned that impair workers' health? To what extent is it important to study their potential psychosocial aspects?

Recommended reading

❖   Cooper, C. L., and Quick, J. C. (eds.) (2017), *The handbook of stress and health*. Chichester: Wiley Blackwell.

❖   Cunningham, C. J. L., and Black, K. J. (2021), *Essentials of occupational health psychology*. New York, NY: Routledge.

❖   International Labour Organization (2022), *World employment and social outloo—trends 2022*. Geneva: ILO.

❖   Marmot, M. G. (2004), *Status syndrome: how social standing affects our health and longevity*. London: Bloomsbury.

❖   Theorell, T. (ed.) (2020), *Handbook of socioeconomic determinants of occupational health*. Cham: Springer.

Useful websites

❖   World Health Organization (WHO): Mental health in the workplace. https://www.who.int/news-room/commentaries/detail/mental-health-in-the-workplace

❖   International Labour Organization (ILO): Decent work. https://www.ilo.org/global/topics/decent-work/lang--en/index.htm

❖   European Foundation for the Improvement of Living and Working Conditions (Eurofound): European Working Conditions Surveys (EWCS). https://www.eurofound.europa.eu/surveys/european-working-conditions-surveys-ewcs

❖   US National Institute for Occupational Safety and Health (NIOSH): Stress at work. https://www.cdc.gov/niosh/topics/stress/default.html

❖   Asia Pacific Academy for Psychosocial Factors at Work (APA PFAW). https://www.apapfaw.org/

References

Adams, J. S. (1965), 'Inequity in social exchange'. In B. Leonard (ed.), *Advances in experimental social psychology*, vol. 2. New York: Academic, 267–99.

Alfredsson, L., Karasek, R. A., and Theorell, T. (1982), 'Myocardial infarction risk and psychosocial work environment: an analysis of the male Swedish working force', *Soc Sci Med*, 16 (4), 463–7.

Alipour, J.-V., Fadinger, H., and Schymik, J. (2021), 'My home is my castle—the benefits of working from home during a pandemic crisis', *J Publ Econ*, 196, 104373.

Antonovsky, A. (1967), 'Social class, life expectancy and overall mortality', *Milbank Mem Fund Q*, 45 (2), 31–73.

Bandura, A. (1977), *Self-efficacy: the exercise of control*. New York: Freeman.

Brenner, M. H. (1973), *Mental illness and the economy*. Cambridge, MA: Harvard University Press.

Brenner, M. H., and Mooney, A. (1982), 'Economic change and sex-specific cardiovascular mortality in Britain 1955–1976', *Soc Sci Med*, 16 (4), 431–42.

Brown, G. W., and Harris, T. (1978), *Social origins of depression. A study of psychiatric disorder in women*. London: Tavistock.

Bültmann, U., and Siegrist, J. (eds.) (2020), *Handbook of disability, work and health*. Cham: Springer.

Case, A., and Deaton, A. (2020), *Deaths of despair and the future of capitalism*. Princeton: Princeton University Press.

Cassel, J., Heyen, S., Bartel, A. G., et al. (1971), 'Incidence of coronary heart disease by ethnic group, social class, and sex', *Arch Intern Med*, 128 (6), 901–6.

Conley, D., and Fletcher, J. (2017), *The genome factor. What the social genomics revolution reveals about ourselves, our history and the future*. Princeton: Princeton University Press.

Cooper, C. L., and Quick, J. C. (eds.) (2017), *The handbook of stress and health*. Chichester: Wiley Blackwell.

Cunningham, C. J. L., and Black, K. J. (2021), *Essentials of occupational health psychology*. New York, NY: Routledge.

d'Errico, A., Ricceri, F., Stringhini, S., et al. (2017), 'Socioeconomic indicators in epidemiologic research: A practical example from the LIFEPATH study', *PLoS One*, 12 (5), e0178071.

Diener, E. (1984), 'Subjective well-being', *Psychol Bull*, 95 (3), 542–75.

Dragano, N., Reuter, M., Peters, A., et al. (2022), 'Increase in mental disorders during the COVID-19 pandemic—the role of occupational and financial strains', *Dtsch Arztebl Int*, 119 (11), 179–87.

Dupre, M. E., George, L. K., Liu, G., et al. (2012), 'The cumulative effect of unemployment on risks for acute myocardial infarction', *Arch Intern Med*, 172 (22), 1731–7.

Durkheim, E. (1897, 1951), *Suicide: A study in sociology*. Glencoe, IL: Free Press.

Engel, G. L. (1977), 'The need for a new medical model: a challenge for biomedicine', *Science*, 196 (4286), 129–36.

Frankenhaeuser, M., and Gardell, B. (1976), 'Underload and overload in working life: outline of a multidisciplinary approach', *J Human Stress*, 2 (3), 35–46.

Friedman, M., Rosenman, R. H., and Carroll, V. (1958), 'Changes in the serum cholesterol and blood clotting time in men subjected to cyclic variation of occupational stress', *Circulation*, 17 (5), 852–61.

Gardell, B. (1971), 'Alienation and mental health in the modern industrial environment'. In L. Levi (ed.), *Society, stress and disease*, vol. 1. Oxford: Oxford University press, 148–80.

Goetzel, R. Z., Long, S. R., Ozminkowski, R. J., et al. (2004), 'Health, absence, disability, and presenteeism cost estimates of certain physical and mental health conditions affecting U.S. employers', *J Occup Environ Med*, 46 (4), 398–412.

Gouldner, A. W. (1960), 'The norm of reciprocity: a preliminary statement', *Am Soc Rev*, 25 (2), 161–78.

Greenberg, J., and Cohen, J. R. (eds.) (1982), *Equity and justice in social behaviour*. New York: Academic.

Henry, J. P., and Cassel, J. C. (1969), 'Psychosocial factors in essential hypertension. Recent epidemiologic and animal experimental evidence', *Am J Epidemiol*, 90 (3), 171–200.

Henry, J. P., and Stephens, P. A. (1977), *Stress, health, and the social environment*. New York: Springer.

Hobfoll, S. E. (1989), 'Conservation of resources. A new attempt at conceptualizing stress', *Am Psychol*, 44 (3), 513–24.

Hoffmann, R. (ed.) (2023), *Handbook of health inequalities across the life course*. Cheltenham: Edward Elgar.

Hollingshead, A. B., and Redlich, F. C. (1958), *Social class and mental illness: A community study*. New York: John Wiley & Sons.

Holtermann, A., Coenen, P., and Krause, N. (2020), 'The paradoxical health effects of occupational versus leisure-time physical activity'. In T. Theorell (ed.), *Handbook of socioeconomic determinants of occupational health: from macro-level to micro-level evidence*. Cham: Springer, 241–67.

House, J. S. (1981), *Work stress and social support*. Reading, MA: Addison Wesley.

International Labour Organization (2022), *World employment and social outlook—trends 2022*. Geneva: ILO.

Johanson, U., and Aboagye, E. (2020), 'Financial gains, possibilities, and limitations of improving occupational health at the company level'. In T. Theorell (ed.), *Handbook of socioeconomic determinants of occupational health: from macro-level to micro-level evidence*. Cham: Springer, 537–53.

Julia, C., and Valleron, A. J. (2011), 'Louis-Rene Villerme (1782–1863), a pioneer in social epidemiology: re-analysis of his data on comparative mortality in Paris in the early 19th century', *J Epidemiol Community Health*, 65 (8), 666–70.

Kaplan, B. H., Cassel, J. C., Tyroler, H. A., et al. (1971), 'Occupational mobility and coronary heart disease', *Arch Intern Med*, 128 (6), 938–42.

Karasek, R. A. (1979), 'Job demands, job decision latitude, and mental strain: implications for job redesign', *Adm Sci Q*, 285–308.

Karasek, R. A., Baker, D., Marxer, F., et al. (1981), 'Job decision latitude, job demands, and cardiovascular disease: a prospective study of Swedish men', *Am J Public Health*, 71 (7), 694–705.

Kasl, S. V., Cobb, S., and Brooks, G. W. (1968), 'Changes in serum uric acid and cholesterol levels in men undergoing job loss', *JAMA*, 206 (7), 1500–7.

Kivimäki, M., Batty, G. D., Kawachi, I., et al. (2018), *The Routledge international handbook of psychosocial epidemiology*. Abingdon, New York, NY: Routledge/Taylor & Francis Group.

Kjellstrøm, T., Oppermann, E., and Lee, J. K. W. (2020), 'Climate change, occupational heat stress, human health, and socioeconomic factors'. In T. Theorell (ed.),

Handbook of socioeconomic determinants of occupational health: from macro-level to micro-level evidence. Cham: Springer, 71–89.

Kohn, M. L., and Schooler, C. (1973), 'Occupational experience and psychological functioning: an assessment of reciprocal effects', *Am Soc Rev*, 38 (1), 97–118.

Kuh, D., Ben-Shlomo, Y., and Ezra, S. (eds.) (2004), *A life course approach to chronic disease epidemiology* (2nd edn). Oxford: Oxford University Press.

Labonté, R., Mohindra, K., and Schrecker, T. (2011), 'The growing impact of globalization for health and public health practice', *Annu Rev Public Health*, 32, 263–83.

Lance, C. (2019), *Occupational and environmental medicine*. Forest Hills, NY: Foster Academics.

Landsbergis, P. A., Choi, B., Dobson, M., et al. (2018), 'The key role of work in population health inequities', *Am J Public Health*, 108 (3), 296–7.

Lash, T., VanderWeele, T. J., Haneause, S., et al. (2021), *Modern epidemiology* (4th edn). Alphen aan den Rijn: Wolter Kluwer Health.

Lazarus, R. S. (1966), *Psychological stress and the coping process*. New York, NY: McGraw-Hill.

Lazarus, R. S., and Folkman, S. (1984), *Stress, appraisal and coping*. New York, NY: Springer.

LeDoux, J. E. (ed.) (1996), *The emotional brain*. New York, NY: Simon & Schuster.

Levi, L. (ed.) (1971), *The psychosocial environment and psychosomatic diseases* 1: Society, stress and disease. Oxford: Oxford University Press.

Liu, Q., He, H., Yang, J., et al. (2020), 'Changes in the global burden of depression from 1990 to 2017: findings from the Global Burden of Disease study', *J Psychiatr Res*, 126, 134–40.

Mackenbach, J. P. (2019), *Health inequalities*. Oxford: Oxford University Press.

Marmot, M. G. (2004), *Status syndrome: how social standing affects our health and longevity*. London: Bloomsbury.

Marmot, M. G., Rose, G., Shipley, M., et al. (1978), 'Employment grade and coronary heart disease in British civil servants', *J Epidemiol Community Health (1978)*, 32 (4), 244–9.

Marmot, M. G., Stansfeld, S., Patel, C., et al. (1991), 'Health inequalities among British civil servants: the Whitehall II study', *The Lancet*, 337 (8754), 1387–93.

Marmot, M. G–, Banks, J., Blundell, R., et al. (eds.) (2003), *Health, wealth, and lifestyles of the older population in England: the 2002 English Longitudinal Study of Aging*. London: Institute for Fiscal Studies.

Marx, K. (1984), *Das Kapital. Buch III: Der Gesammtprocess der kapitalistischen Produktion*. Hamburg: Otto Meissner.

Maslach, C. (1982), *Burnout. The cost of caring*. Englewood Cliffs, NJ: Prentice Hall.

Merton, R. K. (1968), *Social theory and social structure*. New York, NY: The Free Press.

Mikkelsen, S., Coggon, D., Andersen, J. H., et al. (2021), 'Are depressive disorders caused by psychosocial stressors at work? A systematic review with metaanalysis', *Eur J Epidemiol*, 36 (5), 479–96.

Morris, J. K., Cook, D. G., and Shaper, A. G. (1994), 'Loss of employment and mortality', *BMJ*, 308 (6937), 1135–9.

Morris, J. N., Kagan, A., Pattison, D. C., et al. (1966), 'Incidence and prediction of ischaemic heart-disease in London busmen', *Lancet*, 2 (7463), 553–9.

Moser, K. A., Goldblatt, P. O., Fox, A. J., et al. (1987), 'Unemployment and mortality: comparison of the 1971 and 1981 longitudinal study census samples', *Br Med J (Clin Res Ed)*, 294 (6564), 86–90.

Mutambudzi, M., Niedwiedz, C., Macdonald, E. B., et al. (2020), 'Occupation and risk of severe COVID-19: prospective cohort study of 120 075 UK Biobank participants', *Occup Environ Med*, 78 (5), 307–14.

Niedhammer, I., Sultan-Taieb, H., Parent-Thirion, A., et al. (2022), 'Update of the fractions of cardiovascular diseases and mental disorders attributable to psychosocial work factors in Europe', *Int Arch Occup Environ Health*, 95 (1), 233–47.

Nielsen, K., Yarker, J., Munir, F., et al. (2020), 'IGLOO: a framework for return to work among workers with mental health problems'. In U. Bültmann and J. Siegrist (eds.), *Handbook of disability, work and health*. Cham: Springer, 615–32.

OECD (2021), *OECD employment outlook 2021*. Paris: OECD.

Peters, S. E., Dennerlein, J. T., Wagner, G. R., et al. (2022), 'Work and worker health in the post-pandemic world: a public health perspective', *Lancet Public Health*, 7 (2), e188–94.

Rehm, J., and Shield, K. D. (2019), 'Global burden of disease and the impact of mental and addictive disorders', *Curr Psychiatry Rep*, 21 (2), 1–7.

Riumallo-Herl, C., Basu, S., Stuckler, D., et al. (2014), 'Job loss, wealth and depression during the Great Recession in the USA and Europe', *Int J Epidemiol*, 43 (5), 1508–17.

Rugulies, R. (2019), 'What is a psychosocial work environment?', *Scand J Work Environ Health*, 45 (1), 1–6.

Ryan, M. R., and Deci, E. L. (2018), *Self-determination theory. Basic psychological needs in motivation, development, and wellness*. New York, NY: Guilford Press.

Salvagioni, D. A. J., Melanda, F. N., Mesas, A. E., et al. (2017), 'Physical, psychological and occupational consequences of job burnout: a systematic review of prospective studies', *PLoS One*, 12 (10), e0185781.

Selikoff, I. J. (1990), 'Historical developments and perspectives in inorganic fiber toxicity in man', *Environ Health Perspect*, 88, 269–76.

Shekelle, R. B., Ostfeld, A. M., and Paul, O. (1969), 'Social status and incidence of coronary heart disease', *J Chronic Dis*, 22 (6), 381–94.

Stringhini, S., Zaninotto, P., Kumari, M., et al. (2018), 'Socio-economic trajectories and cardiovascular disease mortality in older people: the English Longitudinal Study of Ageing', *Int J Epidemiol*, 47 (1), 36–46.

Syme, S. L., Hyman, M. M., and Enterline, P. E. (1964), 'Some social and cultural factors associated with the occurrence of coronary heart disease', *J Chronic Dis*, 17 (3), 277–89.

Theorell, T. (ed.), (2020), *Handbook of socioeconomic determinants of occupational health: from macro-level to micro-level evidence*. Cham: Springer.

Theorell, T., Lind, E., and Floderus, B. (1975), 'The relationship of disturbing life-changes and emotions to the early development of myocardial infarction and other serious illnesses', *Int J Epidemiol*, 4 (4), 281–93.

Trottier, K., Monson, C. M., Kaysen, D., et al. (2022), 'Initial findings on RESTORE for healthcare workers: an internet-delivered intervention for COVID-19-related mental health symptoms', *Transl Psychiatry*, 12 (1), 222.

Wilkinson, R. G., and Pickett, K. E. (2009), *The spirit level. Why equality is better for everyone*. London: Penguin.

Wise, J. (2020), 'Covid-19: low skilled men have highest death rate of working age adults', *BMJ*, 369, m1906.

World Health Organization (2001), *International Classification of Functioning, Disability and Health (ICF)*. Geneva: WHO.

World Health Organization (2008), 'Closing the gap in a generation: health equity though action on the social determinants of health. Final report of the Commission on Social Determinants of Health', Geneva: WHO.

World Health Organization (2022a), *ICD-11. International classification of diseases for mortality and morbidity statistics. 11th revision*. Geneva: WHO.

World Health Organization (2022b), *WHO guidelines on mental health at work*. Geneva: WHO.

World Health Organization (2023), 'WHO Coronavirus (COVID-19) Dashboard', https://covid19.who.int/, accessed 05 April 2023.

World Health Organization and International Labour Organization (2021), 'WHO/ILO joint estimate of the work-related burden of disease and injury. 2000–2016', (Geneva: WHO, ILO).

2
The changing nature of work and employment in modern societies

2.1 Historical background

Can we identify distinct conditions that shaped today's modern world of work? Historians agree that the process of modernization of the Western world started several centuries ago, with major roots in the European Middle Ages. Yet, two developments during the second half of the eighteenth century are considered decisive turning points in history, the industrial revolution starting in England, and the political revolution in France. Despite their independent origin, they jointly prepared the way of transforming traditional societies through unprecedented economic, social, and political progress (Hobsbawm 1968). With the industrial revolution, machine-based mass production of goods, starting with cotton, created new markets, strengthened import and export, and stimulated the application of technical innovations to metal processing, with far-reaching implications for energy production, transport, industrial growth, but equally so for a destructive transformation of natural environments. It was not until the second half of the nineteenth century that the misery and poverty of an exploited labour class was mitigated. Supported by state reforms, basic social security, safety, and measures to protect workers were implemented, and the welfare and health of working populations were gradually improved. This development was favoured by political movements inaugurated by the French revolution, which not only transferred the political power from aristocracy to citizens, but which, for the first time in history, declared the legal equality of all individuals, independent of their social standing. Equality rights and individual liberty initiated a long-lasting societal transformation where people's life chances increasingly depended on their personal achievement rather than on their social background. To the extent that democracy replaced aristocratic rule, the right of equality was transferred to people's opportunities to participate in political decision-making. Yet, it still took a long time until all citizens enjoyed an equal right

Psychosocial Occupational Health. Johannes Siegrist and Jian Li, Oxford University Press.
© Oxford University Press 2024. DOI: 10.1093/oso/9780192887924.003.0002

to vote. Even more difficult were the political attempts towards reducing social and economic inequalities within societies. An influential interpretation of the historical process of expanding the principle of equality across populations—a process lasting for centuries—claimed that, starting in Europe and the US, the eighteenth century gave birth to legal equality, the nineteenth century promoted political equality, and the twentieth century set out to extend social equality (Marshall 1965). Right now, at the beginning of the twenty-first century, we are still struggling with the challenge of reducing social and economic inequalities within and between countries, as several chapters of this book will document.

Returning to the early stage of industrialization, the conditions of work and employment were critically poor and unjust. At the start of this process, an agrarian population migrating from rural to urban areas formed the unskilled, powerless labour force, exploited by capitalist owners urging women, men, and children to perform machine-paced work in their factories or in mining facilities. These manifestations of alienated, dangerous, and coercive work were analysed and criticized most convincingly in the writings of Karl Marx (1984), giving rise to the powerful political movement of communism. The sharp antagonism between two classes of capital owners and powerless workers produced recurrent social tension and political upheaval, urging national governments to enforce legal restrictions and to inaugurate labour and social policies, in order to improve employees' working and living conditions. Restriction of child labour and reduction of daily working hours are examples of such regulations. Importantly, more progressive socio-political measures at the state level were implemented for the first time by Bismarck's policy in Germany at the end of the nineteenth century. Blue-collar workers were covered by health, disability, and accident insurance, and a comprehensive pension system was established. This reform was the result of considerable social and political pressure from trade unions and the social democratic party. As a pioneering development, it laid ground to the so-called 'social state', one of the future European welfare state regimes (Esping-Andersen 1990).

The nineteenth century witnessed rapid technological and economic progress in Western and Northern Europe and in North America. As job tasks became more demanding, increased skill levels were required from workers, resulting in a growing stratification of the blue-collar workforce into skilled, semi-skilled, and unskilled groups. Skill level was becoming a dominant criterion of quality of work, amount of earnings, and job security. By the turn of the century, the largest part of the labour force in modern societies was still employed in the industrial sector, where exploitation of fossil energies (coal, oil) and steel production laid the ground for, among others, an unprecedented expansion of traffic (cars, railways, ships, airplanes). In the early twentieth century, the stage of economic development required raising levels of productivity within industrial production. To this end, the principles of Taylorism and Fordism, originating from the US, were widely applied. These principles reshaped the organization of work in profound ways. According to Taylor, job tasks had to be divided into small, highly repetitive units that could easily and routinely be handled by low-skilled workers. These tasks were designed by trained industrial engineers who implemented a respective division of labour among employees. By controlling the production process, these engineers increased the pace of work and the degree of productivity, and as an incentive, productivity-related wages were offered. This transformation of work was further intensified by the mechanically controlled auto assembly line, introduced by Henry Ford. While piecework with predefined tasks determined the job profiles of large working populations, the resulting lack of control and skill discretion, and a high degree of monotony and powerlessness triggered adverse reactions, such as dissatisfaction, boredom, disengagement, obstructive behaviour, and absenteeism. These reactions urged managers to improve the production processes, at least in advanced parts of the industrial sector, where approaches such as 'human relations', job enrichment, job variety, or job rotation as well as the development of autonomous work groups were implemented (Karasek and Theorell 1990; Piore and Sabel 1984).

Since the end of World War Two, several far-reaching developments transformed the world of work and employment. One such development concerns the shift of employment sectors. The share of workers employed in industry was continuously shrinking in many places, while the proportion of people working in the service sector or dealing with information and communication technology (ICT) was growing, shifting the workforce from a manufacturing-based industrial towards an information-based economy (Piore and Sabel 1984). Given its significance, this trend deserves a short description. According to classic labour market analysis, employment sectors follow a pattern of compensation over time. When the primary sector, agriculture, lost substantial parts of its workforce, due to technological advances, in the late eighteenth and early nineteenth century, the secondary sector, industry, by and large absorbed the jobless workers. During the second half of the twentieth century, again with the advent of technological progress, blue-collar workers increasingly moved from the industrial to the service sector. In other words, technological developments are the driving force behind these substantial shifts. Currently, as a result of the shift from the secondary to the tertiary sector, we observe that a large majority of employed people are working in the service and ICT sector. Data from Germany illustrate this general trend over the past few decades (see Fig. 2.1).

The spectrum of tertiary jobs is quite broad as it includes white-collar office and administrative employees, clerks, traders, people engaged in business, technicians, educators, health professionals, social workers, and jobs in catering, accommodation, and transport, among others. The major difference from industrial blue-collar work concerns the paucity of work environments containing physical, chemical, and biological hazards or requiring heavy physical workload, while many tertiary jobs are characterized by sedentary work with tasks of handling information, communication, and control, and of coping with psycho-mental and socio-emotional demands. Many tertiary jobs deal with people rather than with machines or computers, and these person-focused jobs need to be performed with a high degree of responsibility, concentration, competence, and empathy, as well as emotional detachment, thus requiring professionals who can deliver a high level of effort and personal engagement.

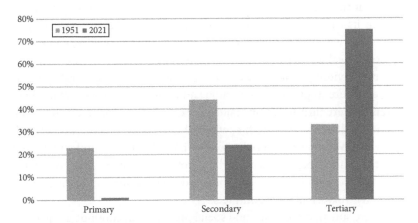

Figure 2.1 Percentage of employed population in agriculture (primary sector), industry (secondary sector), and service (tertiary sector) in Germany 1951 and 2021.

Source: Data from German Federal Statistical Office (2022), 'Erwerbstätige im Inland nach Wirtschaftssektoren.' (https://www.destatis.de/DE/Themen/Wirtschaft/Konjunkturindikatoren/Lange-Reihen/Arbeitsmarkt/lrerw13a.html, accessed February 21, 2023).

It is important to stress that, despite a shrinking industrial workforce, industrial production continues to be a powerful determinant of economic progress worldwide, and that the production of energy, food, goods, machines, vehicles, and all types of devices provides a major input to global markets in modern societies. Equally important, the transformation of work and employment during recent decades has not been restricted to a major shift in employment sectors, but it was mainly shaped by the process of economic globalization, in conjunction with microelectronic breakthroughs of digitization, automation, and artificial intelligence (AI). It seems justified to consider the last quarter of the twentieth century as a turning point towards these developments (see the following sections).

Although it may be premature to classify the recent historical development of modern societies into an industrial and a 'post-industrial' period (Bell 1973), there is no doubt that the industrial revolution, starting in the second half of the eighteenth century, transformed human societies in unprecedented ways. By expanding production and consumption in a period of rapid population growth, it promoted urbanization, technological and scientific progress, and it offered opportunities for social mobility, extended education, and improved living conditions. In the long run, economic progress and welfare were achieved, but this progress occurred at the expense of far-reaching exploitation of working people, at least in its early stage, and of precious natural resources. Gradually, an expanding world of industrialization improved the working conditions of economically active populations, by implementing regulation and control, by providing social protection, safety, and health care, and by reducing exposure to physically strenuous and dangerous work. While these advances were threatened by major political and economic crises during the first half of the twentieth century, the decades of economic growth following World War Two reduced the risks of mass unemployment and poverty. Rather, large parts of the blue-collar and white-collar workforce were offered better quality of work and continuous employment prospects within formal work contracts.

Are we sure that economic and social progress can continue along these lines? What are the consequences of the new challenges of economic globalization and technological transformation? How do the pressing issues of climate change and environmental destruction affect economy and society? These questions point to the emergence of a global stage of development that is no longer 'industrial' in its essence.

2.2 The process of economic globalization

The socio-political and economic development of the twentieth century was largely dominated by two antagonistic movements within the global north. In Europe, North America, and Japan, economic progress was based on the strategy of private capitalism with its free-market principles supported by democratic governments. Under the hegemony of the former Soviet Union, Central and Eastern European countries implemented a centrally planned economy, and this latter approach was also established under communist rule in China. These two 'Western' and 'Eastern' regimes expanded their influence in many developing countries in the Global South, striving towards worldwide superiority by a very turbulent process of political and economic competition. With the fall of the Soviet Union and the decline and transformation of its economy in the early 1990s, the economic paradigm of Western private capitalism seemed to have achieved its global superiority. In fact, the dynamic power inherent in this system had triggered economic growth and technological advances already in the 1970s and 1980s, ahead of the breakdown of the Soviet Union and its economic system, in a process that is labelled 'economic globalization'.

Economic globalization is an umbrella term that describes a process of increasing transnational trade liberalization and the growing impact of financial markets, supported by ground-breaking innovations in ICT. Further characteristics of this process are an increased deregulation of labour market rules, an accelerated privatization of public services, and a dominant role of transnational corporations that expand their operations in developing countries. At the institutional level, this process was promoted by international organizations, most importantly the World Bank (WB), the International Monetary Fund (IMF), and the World Trade Organization (WTO). At the ideological level, the paradigm of 'neoliberalism' set the agenda for far-reaching decisions on the direction of economic development. It is hardly possible to give a convincing description of the initiation of this process as its distinct elements did not appear simultaneously and did not originate in a single country or region. However, the deregulation of national financial markets played a decisive role. Initiated in an era of financial recession in the 1970s and early 1980s, neoliberal principles dominated political decision-making, resulting in an end of fixed currency exchange rates. As early as in 1971, the conjunction of the US dollar with the gold standard was abandoned. This decision reinforced the predominant role of the US dollar as standard currency, but at the same time favoured transnational currency speculation. The deregulation also affected measures of control of transnational capital flow, thus stimulating the growth of financial markets operating worldwide. The process of inter-governmental trade liberalization was promoted by the international organizations mentioned. Importantly, this development enabled leading, rapidly growing transnational corporations, mainly those located in the US, in Japan, and in Northern-Western European countries, to expand their market strategies to emerging economies and developing countries. The growing transnational exchange was not restricted to capital and trade, but it included the labour force. Myriads of new jobs were created in developing countries as multinational companies increasingly transferred their workplaces from high-income countries to others offering lower wages and salaries. Moreover, poorly developed standards of occupational safety and health in these countries enabled productivity at low cost but high risk of occupational injury and disease. At the same time, transnational labour force migration resulted in the entrance of millions of working people from developed countries into the global labour pool, thus aggravating economic competition and increasing work pressure.

One may ask why neoliberalism was able to exert a high impact on the direction of economic development. One reason points to the consequences of the oil crisis in the early 1970s, when production costs sharply rose, and when risks of economic recession increased. Opening free market competition by removing national barriers and by extending deregulation was assumed to encourage economic growth. Moreover, gains in economic efficiency were expected from increased privatization of public services, including those concerned with health, traffic, housing, education, and supply of essential goods like energy and water. The number and influence of transnational corporations multiplied during the past four decades, and their expansion was supported by trade agreements influenced by the WTO and other agencies that incorporated the principles of neoliberalism (Labonté 2015). In fact, on a global scale, economic growth was achieved during this period, and the number of people living in extreme poverty was significantly reduced. Yet, this growth was unequally distributed across the world's regions, and it clearly favoured the richest societies and, above all, the wealthiest capital-owner groups (Piketty 2014).

Economic growth corresponded with an expanded financial industry that advanced to a worldwide leading business sector. Unlike commerce with goods, commerce with money is largely based on exchange of capital between banks, where financial transactions in essence aim at optimizing the profit of share capital and other financial resources. Increasingly, these financial operations instigated speculations and risky operations among stakeholders of capital markets, including irresponsible mortgage lending, invalid credit rating, and excessive bonuses of bankers, thus precipitating their volatility. The Global Financial Crisis initiated in 2008 by a breakdown of credits in some internationally operating US banks was the most dramatic outcome of these uncontrolled, highly risky, and irresponsible activities. This crisis not only stopped and reversed economic growth for a couple of years, with substantial impact on labour market development, but it threatened the legitimacy of the dominant economic model as governments were forced to use public money in order to save the banking system, a largely privatized sector of the economy. Bailing out banks at the expense of public welfare, and implementing austerity programmes with substantial cuts of public spending has produced lasting damage to the credibility of free market capitalism and to the political institutions that were responsible for these decisions. Austerity measures included reductions in social protection spending, freezing of salaries and promotion prospects, and further economy measures towards reducing public deficits. Taken together, the Global Financial Crisis has caused one of the most threatening interruptions of social, political, and economic progress, and has severely impaired the welfare and health of large parts of populations on a global scale (Backhaus et al. 2022; Baum 2016).

The process of economic globalization described so far is not well explained without considering the role of technological innovations. Groundbreaking advances in microelectronic ICT promoted the global diffusion of knowledge through computers, internet use, smartphones, and satellites. The availability of computer power grew exponentially during a very short period of time, with continuous improvement of processor speed and storage capacity, reducing communication costs and extending interaction opportunities on a global scale. Tourism, transcontinental traffic, international supply chains using worldwide containerization, and continuous use of electronic financial transactions developed multiple dense webs of virtual and real interconnectivity and interdependence across countries and continents. This development changed the world in many significant ways. The worldwide availability of internet and smartphones offered billions of people new opportunities for rapid communication, information flow, and social contacts, with unexpected far-reaching consequences for changes in lifestyles, consumption, cultural and religious habits and beliefs, societal norms and institutions, political attitudes, and social movements.

While improvements in people's education, knowledge, and competencies are welcome as signs of progress in human development, new dangers emerged as well, enabling the spread of radical ideologies and cybercrime, the distortion of reality by fake news, and growing media-directed supervision and control of individual behaviour. Perhaps, we can state that no other aspect of modern life has been transformed by the new technological developments as deeply as the world of work and employment. Here, two major innovations matter most, the impact of digitization, automation, and AI on human labour, and the disruption of established employment relationships by the growth of nonstandard employment. The next two sections describe these trends emanating from economic globalization in more detail. However, the contribution of globalization to economic development and growth need to be critically evaluated against the increasing danger and threat of ecological damage and climate change. Therefore, this chapter ends with a section dealing with the tensions between economy and ecology and the evolving challenges (see also Box 2.1).

2.3 Digitization, automation, and artificial intelligence

These three terms are often used as labels to describe a global technological trend in current societies with large transformational impact on working and living conditions. Originally, 'digitization' was used to define any transformation of analogous information into digital information. Digital data are discrete entities that can be stored and processed electronically by microprocessors. More recently, the term 'digitization' was extended to point to an increased impact of digital information on production systems and on the provision of services. For instance, in industry, computers and software algorithms are integrated in the production process, thus enhancing efficacy and flexibility. These processes are either still controlled by working people, or they are fully automated, where these technologies 'allow for a direct and automated communication between different parts of the value chain such that workers only need to intervene in case of failures' (Arntz et al. 2019, p. 7).

Progress in digitization is closely linked to progress in 'artificial intelligence'. This term describes the capacity of a machine to develop new decisions based on automated data processing (machine learning). Developing new decisions based on available input in machines is considered an

Box 2.1 **Core features of economic globalization**

- Economic globalisation is a process of increasing transnational trade liberalisation and growing impact of financial markets, supported by ground-breaking innovations in ICT. Global supply chains are an essential link between developed and developing countries.
- It initiated a deregulation of labour market rules, weakening the influence of state governance on the economy while strengthening privatisation of organisations and services.
- International organisations, in particular WB, IMF, and WTO, promoted the neoliberal paradigm of free market expansion that helped transnational corporations to enlarge their dominance in global oligopolistic markets.
- With the surge of an influential financial industry, economic progress was threatened by uncontrolled, risky, and irresponsible financial transactions resulting in the Global Financial Crisis in 2008, with its long-lasting negative effects on human welfare and well-being.
- The crucial ambivalence of economic globalization is best illustrated by the impact of new technologies on the nature of work and employment. Whereas new options of freedom, autonomy and progress become available, increased risks of dependency and of losing control, social status and welfare are experienced.
- Less visible, but even more threatening in the long run, economic globalization is endangering the survival on this planet by destroying its natural resources and by promoting dangerous climate change.

imitation of human intelligence as this process applies expertise on decision-making from mathematics and informatics. AI and machine learning have a far-reaching range of applications as they support human performance and provide instantaneous new, rapidly disseminated information. Increasingly, robots equipped with AI replace humans in performing jobs with routine or dangerous tasks, but equally so in providing services to customers, using artificial language. Another area of AI-application relates to computation and analysis of knowledge. Search engines, expert systems, techniques of data control and data mining, language translation, and text production do not only support the daily workflow of a knowledge-based workforce, but they result in a decrease of its size and impact. It seems difficult to identify occupations and professions that are not affected by these technological advances, at least to a certain extent. We have already seen a substantial loss of jobs in industrial production, specifically among low-skilled manual workers. In addition, many routine jobs in the service sector have been replaced by computers and automated devices, such as robots. As illustrated in Figure 2.2, the degree of automation of jobs heavily depends on the level of educational attainment required to perform them. However, often, occupational profiles are only partially affected by new technologies as their application improves the speed and/or quality of distinct tasks, without replacing human skills. The use of AI in medicine is an example of beneficial effects of this latter process. In other areas, such as automated driving of vehicles, the essence of professional activity is threatened as it has been transferred to intelligent machines.

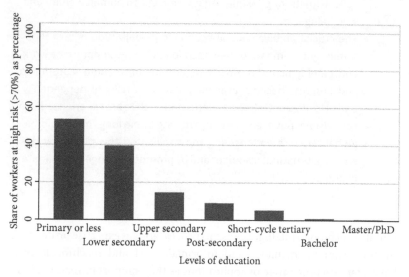

Figure 2.2 Share of workers with high risk (> 70%) of job loss due to education.

Source: Reproduced with permission from Arntz, M., Gregory, T., and Zierahn, U. (2016), *The risk of automation for jobs in OECD countries: A comparative analysis*, OECD Social, Employment and Migration Working Papers, No. 189. Paris: OECD Publishing [Figure 6, p. 20]; license ID: 1335957-1.

At present, the impact of digitization, automation, and AI on the development of labour markets within and beyond industrialized societies can barely be estimated. Yet, labour market researchers set out to develop prognostic scenarios, based on expert judgments, survey data, and time trend analyses. Interestingly, their results differ in rather significant ways. It is instructive to consider two such scenarios. In their now famous report, Frey and Osborne (2017) used task and job descriptions from an extensive US database to assess the degree to which a task can be performed by computer-controlled equipment. Applying a set of variables characterizing job tasks, they estimated the technical potential of automation within each one of a series of jobs subjected to in-depth analysis. Subsequently, these findings instructed a machine learning algorithm that classified occupations with regard to their potential of technical automation. The extent of this algorithm was expressed in a range between zero and one hundred per cent, where values of seventy per cent and more were considered as 'at high risk'. The authors applied their algorithm to several hundred job descriptions within this US database. As a review of the results of this analysis concludes, 'finally, they combine this with occupational employment data to compute that 47% of workers in the U.S. are currently working in 'high risk' or automatable occupations' (Arntz et al. 2019, p. 3).

This high amount of potential technological unemployment projected for the next one or two decades, due to the expansion of computerized, machine-learning based work, has raised controversial debates about the future of human labour. Some proponents predicted the 'end of work' (Rifkin 1995), while others emphasized the creation of new jobs resulting from digitization (Autor 2015). To inform this debate, additional empirical analyses were performed. One such approach differs in its methodology from the Frey and Osborne study as it takes the variety of tasks within occupations into account (Arntz et al. 2019). It is evident that many occupations and professions require an accomplishment of different tasks, where some, but not all can easily be automated. Relying on individual-level data from a survey containing an assessment of job-related competencies, this study compared these new, more nuanced ratings of technological automation risk with the ratings based on occupation classifications applied in the former study. As a result, less than ten per cent of occupations were found to be susceptible to technological job loss, compared to the forty-seven per cent of the former study (Arntz et al. 2019).

How can this discrepancy be explained? Do the former findings reflect an overestimation and the latter findings an underestimation of the employment effect of automation? Arntz et al. (2019) discussed two important reasons in addition to those attributed to a different methodology. Firstly, although digitization may lower costs and increase profits for enterprises, its implementation is costly and time-consuming. Gains differ according to type and size of businesses, and it is therefore unlikely that a rapid and radical change will occur within a short time, as suggested by the Frey and Osborne study. A second argument maintains that automation goes along with adaptive responses developed by those whose jobs are threatened. New tasks are created, and intensified training offers options of enriching task profiles among those who were formerly exposed to the automated jobs. Although some studies conclude that job loss due to digitization is compensated by the creation of new jobs (Autor 2015), we need to stress that job polarization is enhanced and that workers with lower socio-economic positions are most severely hit by job loss due to their restricted skill resources. On the other hand, a highly qualified workforce will be able to perform irreplaceable tasks and to complement machine-controlled processes, perhaps even enjoying new privileges at work. Viewed from a global perspective, the impact of macro-economic forces on the availability of jobs is probably stronger than the impact of digitization. Recent figures support this notion as the global labour force grew from 2.2 to 3.3 billion from 1991 to 2016, and within the European Union, the number of employed people grew by fifteen million following the Great Financial Crisis, from 2013 to 2018 (Abrahamsson and Larsson 2021).

In the context of this book, the health consequences of recent technological breakthroughs at work deserve special attention. They concern the stress levels associated with job instability, job insecurity, and job loss, the emotional, cognitive, and physiological costs of adaptation to new technologies, and the exposure to new stressors at work, in particular the challenges of human–robot interaction and coping with mental overload and underload in a variety of onscreen activities at computers. Often, opportunities of autonomy at work, including control over tasks, are restricted, evoking feelings of alienation at work. In terms of occupational safety and health, health-protective standards and norms are difficult to establish and to control, given the high flexibility and instability of work environments and the rapid technological change (Cockburn 2021). Yet, there are also health-enhancing effects resulting from technological innovations, most importantly a decrease of physically demanding job tasks as well as improved physical work environments. Moreover, more options of return to work among people with physical disabilities are provided by computer-assisted and automated jobs. These aspects are discussed in later chapters of the book.

2.4 The growth of nonstandard employment

Economic growth is one of the key features of the globalization process. Yet, this growth occurred unequally across countries, with rapid progress in some large emerging economies like China and India, and with a rather moderate development in the Global North. The reduction of trade barriers between countries gave rise to a transnational labour force, and in these rapidly growing economies, millions of new jobs resulted from cheap labour costs. China is the most important case in this respect. A rapid, unprecedented growth of real income reduced in-work poverty to a substantial extent, fuelled by export-oriented industrial development. However, the impact of this growth on the quality of work and employment was ambivalent. Opportunities of formal employment in organizations of the industrial and service sector were widening, specifically those in urban areas and in regions with a rapidly improved infrastructure, and standards of safety and health at work were gradually improved. Yet, a majority of jobs were of low quality, often characterized as precarious, insecure, and stressful. The largest proportion of these jobs was located in the service sector with its continuous expansion. For instance, in the period from 1991 to 2017, the relative size of the service sector workforce in China increased from seventeen per cent to fifty-six per cent, with a rapidly shrinking proportion in the agricultural sector and a stagnant industrial sector (International Labour Organization 2018). Overall, in emerging and developing countries, informal employment prevailed. As estimated by the International Labour Organization (ILO), more than two-thirds of the employed population in developing countries are in informal employment (Hyde et al. 2020). This form of employment is not protected by national labour laws and related regulations that offer some social security as well as minimum standards of working conditions and pay.

Against this background, international organizations have called for coordinated transnational regulatory improvements of global working conditions. The ILO's 'Social Protection Floor Initiative' is one such important achievement (International Labour Organization 2013). It recommends, among others, the introduction of minimum wages, of health and unemployment insurance, and of reliable pension systems. Moreover, it calls for labour market programmes to tackle unemployment, and transnational corporations are asked to apply identical employment standards along all steps of the supply chain, from low-income to high-income countries. A similar initiative was launched by the World Health Organization's (WHO) Commission on Social Determinants of Health Final Report (Box 2.2).

More recently, the United Nation's Sustainable Development Goals were endorsed by the Member States in an attempt to ensure the world's viable future. These recommendations include the goal to 'promote sustained, inclusive and sustainable economic growth, full and productive employment, and decent work for all' (United Nations 2015).

While the majority of informal employment is concentrated in low-income countries and in rapidly emerging nations, the developed parts of the world offer formal employment to large parts of their workforce, and

---

Box 2.2 Core recommendations of the WHO's Commission on Social Determinants of Health

- Full and fair employment and decent work be made a shared objective of international institutions and a central part of national policy agendas and development strategies;
- National governments develop and implement economic and social policies that provide secure work and a living wage that takes into account the real and current cost of living for health;
- Public capacity be strengthened to implement regulatory mechanisms to promote and enforce fair employment and decent work standards for all workers;
- Governments reduce insecurity among people in precarious work arrangements;
- Occupational Health and Safety (OHS) policy and programs be applied to all workers ... and include work-related stressors and behaviours as well as exposure to material hazards' (World Health Organization 2008, p. 76ff).

Source: Data from World Health Organization (2008), 'Closing the gap in a generation: health equity though action on the social determinants of health. Final report of the Commission on Social Determinants of Health.', (Geneva: WHO). Available at http://apps.who.int/iris/bitstream/handle/10665/43943/9789241563703_eng.pdf

programmes of social and labour policies as well as laws were implemented to protect employees from basic threats and hazards. However, this development varied substantially across countries, with well-developed arrangements in the northern European Scandinavian countries, and with much less-inclusive measures in 'liberal welfare states', such as the US (Esping-Andersen, 1990). It is important to understand how employment relationships and their welfare support in high-income countries were affected by economic globalization. This process is best explained by introducing the concept of nonstandard employment and by describing its causes and its main forms of manifestation.

A brief look at the history of employment in Western industrialized societies after World War Two demonstrates that the following period, encompassing some three to four decades, was characterized by economic growth and augmented welfare of populations. During this time, the so-called 'standard employment relationship' was implemented and extended as a dominant way of organizing the contractual arrangements between employers and employees (Kalleberg 2009). Supported by low unemployment figures, by an increasingly skilled workforce with strong trade unions, and by marked state investments in labour and social policies, this relation marked definite progress over long-lasting conditions of insecurity, disadvantage, and precariousness among employed people (Box 2.3).

Employment relationships based on formal work contracts are assumed to function through compliance with these explicitly stated norms, but they are reinforced by additional implicit normative expectations. These expectations include employees' commitment towards meeting quality standards of their work, refraining from deviance and fraud, whereas employers are expected to guarantee fair treatment and job security. Ideally, this type of formal work enables employed people to pursue a steady, uninterrupted occupational trajectory within a fixed organizational setting. In many cases, such trajectories offer options of training and career advancement, with access to some privileges of seniority. Given these criteria, the implementation of standard employment relations among large parts of the workforce in high-income countries, mainly during the decades following World War Two, represents major progress in a long-standing history of power and conflict relationships between employers and employees. Stable, continuous employment as a key feature of decent work is a primary goal of active labour market policies, considered an important prerequisite for working people's health and well-being. Yet, one should remember that

Box 2.3 **Core features of standard employment relations**

- A formal work contract is completed between an employer and an employee, often guaranteeing continued, permanent employment in terms of a fulltime job;
- Important rights and duties are defined in the contract, and they are valid within the employer's scope of responsibility for work;
- These rights include employees' protection by social insurance, pension, occupational safety and health laws and services, and collective bargaining;
- Main duties concern employees' regular achievement of job tasks within defined conditions as well as basic loyalty towards the employer;
- Work-time arrangements and conditions of leave are often defined, with options of negotiating reconciliation of work and extra-work demands.

this construct reflects a male-dominated labour market where men are expected to act as breadwinner husbands in family arrangements with wives caring primarily for children and home duties. Although this construct does not do justice to the fact of an increasingly gendered workforce, it has reinforced—and continues to reinforce—women's social and economic disadvantages on a grand scale. To date, this normative construct is losing its predominance, and is being replaced by a new paradigm of increased career flexibility and gender equity (Tomlinson et al. 2018).

Why and how did economic globalization challenge the standard employment relationship? An important reason relates to the growth of transnational markets of goods, services, capital, and workforce. For instance, with an increasing labour market in emerging economies producing goods and services with low labour costs, employers in high-income countries were forced to reduce labour costs within a context of fierce competition. Strategies of restructuring businesses by downsizing and outsourcing their employees were widely applied, resulting in substantial amounts of lay-offs of formerly protected employees. At the same time, new personnel were hired with fixed-term contracts, temporary employment, or part-time jobs. Moreover, extended privatization opened up opportunities for more flexible contracting. These trends contributed to the polarization of the labour market into a privileged, well trained workforce preserving its stable employment conditions, and a disadvantaged, low-skilled workforce exposed to unstable, flexible, and discontinuous occupational trajectories.

Technological advances of production, dissemination, information, and communication define a second powerful determinant of enhanced flexibility of working conditions and of expanding nonstandard employment relations. This latter term was introduced to identify less secure, short-term contracts with reduced social protection. These contracts cover different types of employment arrangements, such as self-employed independent contracting, temporary agency-based work, involuntary part-time work, or freelancing in digitalized jobs using platform business with customers ('gig work'; Kalleberg 2018). In many such arrangements workers are exposed to precariousness in short-lived, highly insecure work environments (see 2.4.1). However, technological advances also offer a high amount of flexibility and de-standardization in better-paid, more secure jobs. For instance, with the ubiquitous availability of smartphones and internet access, workers can perform their tasks at spatially distant places from enterprises or factories, and at times independent from a standard eight-hour workday. Home office and other forms of remote work have increasingly weakened the predominant form of accomplishing work with regular physical presence of employees in an organization (e.g., factory, administration) that is under direct control of an employer or manager. It goes unsaid that technical progress resulting in 'just-in-time' and online delivery or in producing and handling customer-specific products requires increased flexibility of work and employment arrangements. Equally, shortened life cycles of products, rapidly changing market preferences of customers, and fluctuations of supply and demand support this trend.

In addition to the economic and technological reasons, the growth of flexibility and nonstandard employment was precipitated by significant changes at the political level. Influential international organizations, mainly WB, IMF, and WTO, as well as some important conservative governments, such as in the US and Great Britain, adopted the neoliberal economic policy of extending free markets, and of reducing structural barriers against rapid growth. These barriers were once introduced by national laws and by measures of social and labour policies with the aim of strengthening the rights of workers and of limiting an uncontrolled amount of power on the side of employers and their organizations. Within this context, trade unions offered options of collective bargaining, dealing mainly with terms of employment, minimal wages, occupational safety and health, extended social protection, working time, and protection of migrants and other vulnerable employment groups. Increasingly, neoliberal policies cast doubt on these achievements. Around 1980, the density of trade unions started to decline in Europe and elsewhere, and several national laws and regulations were eased or withdrawn. In Europe, the conservative UK government was the first to turn down multi-employer bargaining and to reduce union power. Given growing economic competition, weakening trade unions, and thereby reducing earnings, was an obvious strategy of economic liberalization (Eichhorst and Portela de Souza 2018). A direct link between economic globalization and declining power of trade unions as well as a weakening of national social and labour policies became again obvious after the Global Financial Crisis of 2008. National austerity policies urged governments to cut public spending and to relax regulations that prevented the transnational flow of capital, goods, and labour force. Despite these drawbacks, social democratic governments within Western democracies generally were not strengthened. Rather, neoliberalism seems to be supported by a majority of governments and by influential institutions and organizations.

All three trends—economic constraints of a globally competitive business world, technological advances calling for flexible ways of accomplishing work and of staying employed, and shrinking political power of national policies and trade unions—contribute to the growth of nonstandard employment in modern economics. Though affected in different ways, high-income countries as well as emerging economies are facing this challenge. It is therefore important to explore core features of nonstandard employment, for instance by considering two particular manifestations, precariousness and gig work. These manifestations shed light on developments that are of growing interest in the frame of a digitalized economy.

2.4.1 Precarious employment and 'gig work'

In current research the terms 'nonstandard employment', 'contingent work', and 'precarious employment' are not clearly distinguished despite the fact that they point to a phenomenon of growing interest and concern, both in scientific analysis and in labour policy debates. The latter term is somewhat more general than the former ones as it includes the main consequences of a critical employment condition for the working person's living situation. Related empirical studies, therefore, have conceptualized 'precariousness' as a multi-dimensional construct. Two attempts were made to describe the construct more precisely, and their conclusions are a useful contribution towards achieving conceptual clarification. In a systematic review of sixty-three papers originating from research dealing with precarious work in quantitative and qualitative studies conducted in four continents, Kreshpaj et al. (2020) identified three overarching dimensions of precarious employment. The first dimension relates to employment insecurity. Here, aspects of contractual insecurity, temporariness, and underemployment matter, as well as being forced to hold a second or even a third job. The second dimension emphasizes income inadequacy in terms of a critically low level of earning or of high volatility and insecurity of income. The third dimension concerns a lack of rights and protection at work. This lack becomes manifest as poor coverage by standard non-wage employment benefits (e.g. health care, sick leave) and regulatory support (e.g. pensions), as restricted access to workplace rights (e.g. protection against discrimination, sexual harassment), and as a lack of unionization, giving voice to workers' demands and concerns.

In a related discussion paper (Bodin et al. 2020), an expert panel proposed a similar model of precarious employment with the following three core dimensions: instability (e.g. temporary job), lack of power and rights (e.g. restricted option to exert rights), and poor terms (e.g. low income). Their adverse effects on health are attributable in part to exposure to hazardous or stressful work environments, in part to material deprivation. The model is enriched by the introduction of two sets of variables that moderate the effects of precariousness on health. With the first set of variables, distinct macroeconomic and policy-related conditions are identified, whereas the second set of moderators includes main sociodemographic features of individual workers (e.g. education, occupational position, gender, age). Once these two similar analytical frameworks are assessed in a consistent way in epidemiologic studies, a new body of empirical evidence is expected to evolve. This knowledge can then enrich the state of art summarized below (see Chapter 6).

Precariousness in terms of unstructured work environment, work schedule, and contractual arrangement is nowhere as visible as in the case of gig work. This form of employment is often delivering services via a platform, based on short-term assignments between providers and customers. Providers are either hired by companies or self-employed, and the nature of performed work and recompense is typically paid at a piece rate (Wood et al. 2019). In times of growing convergence between information technology and telecommunication, a broad spectrum of gig workers is evolving. A proposed typology classifies this spectrum into three over-arching types: (1) on-demand physical services; (2) crowd work; (3) online freelancing (Bérastégui 2021).

- **On-demand physical services:** These services are defined as 'location-based applications which distribute service-oriented tasks to individuals within a specific geographical area' (Bérastégui 2021, p. 7). Here, the platform functions as mediator between customers' requests and a pool of workers immediately prepared to perform the task. Examples include food delivery, cleaning, Uber taxi service, or baby-sitting. The gig workers' job content varies according to the nature of tasks, and the same holds true for job qualification requirements. Although many workers are self-employed, it is sometimes difficult to clearly distinguish between self-employment and organization-dependent work, given the short-lived task assignments, and given a lack of companies' commitment to longer-term binding relationships with gig workers. Performing on-demand services carries the risk of job and income insecurity, or at least of high volatility. It deprives workers of the social security benefits and protection measures inherent in traditional employment contracts. Many such jobs are low-skilled, repetitive, monotonous, offering restricted autonomy and skill discretion, and resulting in poor pay. At the same time, given the independence of the working person, they may provide some individual freedom and flexibility in selecting tasks and organizing working time.
- **Crowd work:** This label is applied to a variety of virtual services that are based on micro-tasks. Work is performed online, without physical contact between customers and providers. In times of exponentially growing data collection and availability, crowd workers are typically committed to simple, highly repetitive tasks of data gathering, controlling, cleaning, or labelling on platforms. Often, transnational corporations outsource these jobs to a low-skilled workforce in developing countries. In principle, these jobs are threatened by digitization, as they are available to the extent only that technological progress of AI and machine learning has not yet been capable of replacing them. Again, main features of this type of gig work point to a highly precarious way of being employed.
- **Online freelancing:** Different from the two previous types, this category of gig work describes the provision of specialized skills in virtual

exchange. Frequent examples are accounting, translating, illustrating and computing texts. Human capital in the form of specific expertise, experience-based competencies, or individually developed skills improves the options of continued job demands. Still, the positive features of freelancing often do not outweigh its negative aspects related to instability, uncertainty, and the absence of long-term protection.

Despite the heterogeneity of tasks, the different types of gig work share a common feature as the performance of the economic activity largely occurs in social isolation. Apart from short-lived contacts with customers through on-demand services, tasks are accomplished in remote places, often at home, with exclusive access to computers and mobiles. The absence of several important aspects of social exchange in shared physical workplaces contributes to a poor quality of work. Importantly, social support from colleagues, advice and feedback from superiors and managers, including recognition and approval, are lacking. Equally so, jobs cannot be delegated, discussed, modified, or divided as usual in occupational settings offering teamwork. A disturbed work–life balance is a frequent consequence of physically and socially isolated work. There is no control of excessively long working hours, and unpredictable duty calls may interfere with time reserved for privacy and relaxation. An additional shared characteristic of gig work concerns a high amount of external control. Whenever a company or organization has assigned this work, digital surveillance of workers' performance is likely to occur. In many jobs, algorithms have been integrated into platform devices, enabling continuous monitoring and constant evaluation of performance. If people are on their way to accomplish on-demand services, global positioning systems (GPS) trace their movements, and several automatic rating systems are used to increase successive workload or to alter the amount of remuneration (Bérastégui 2021).

In summary, in an era of digitization, availability of big data, and continued innovation of ICT and AI, the proportion of people exposed to gig work is likely to grow at rapid pace. Most often, these jobs offer a low quality of work, are deprived of basic social security benefits, are performed in social isolation, impair a balanced work–life cycle, and share the main features of precariousness. It is premature to appraise their potential negative effects on health and well-being, but, as will be discussed later, major toxic effects, identified by the dominant, widely analysed models of a health-adverse psychosocial work environment, are expected to occur among people exposed to gig work as well. Analysing the burden of disease attributable to these new manifestations of nonstandard employment is an important task on the agenda of psychosocial occupational health research. It is important to mention that with an expansion of nonstandard employment, substantial parts of the workforce are now exposed to precariousness and its adverse effects on health and well-being, where a segmented labour market separates a disadvantaged population from a well-trained, privileged working population.

2.5 Tensions between economy and ecology

Economic growth is commonly defined as the total value of goods and services produced in a country during a year, the so-called Gross Domestic Product (GDP). GDP is determined by a variety of factors, with increased access to capital and labour as well as productivity gains being prominent. Although productivity gains due to technological advances are primary drivers, economic growth so far substantially depends on the exploitation of finite, non-renewable natural resources, in particular oil and coal. Fossil fuel burning is an essential element of energy production and of material transformation in industrial production. An oil-based energy culture affects large parts of everyday life in modern societies. In addition, it was recently estimated that some thirty-four billion tons of CO_2 are emitted into the air each year, and that exploitation of coal in earth and sea account for about half of all man-made CO_2 emission (Friedlingstein et al. 2020). At present, convincing scientific evidence points to a causal link between these emissions and global warming of the climate system, as indicated by ocean warming, rise of sea levels, and shrinking Arctic and Antarctic ice and glaciers in conjunction with increased concentrations of greenhouse gases in the atmosphere (Intergovernmental Panel on Climate Change 2014).

If not mitigated by far-reaching measures aiming at net-zero carbon emissions and their replacement by renewable energies, progressive global warming is expected to result in irreversible damage to living systems on earth, including threats to human health as well as societal and economic functioning. To name just some consequences of global warming on human health, substantial increases in the burden of disease are estimated due to altered exposure to heat and cold, increased exposure to UV radiation, air pollution, emerging infections, and decreased food security and water quality (Munro et al. 2020). Obviously, there is a fundamental tension between economic growth and environmental sustainability, with its direct effects on human well-being. Hopefully, continued growth at the expense of natural exploitation and destruction will no longer be allowed by national governments and international regulatory bodies. The main challenge will be to replace the exploitation of natural fossil resources by man-made capital (technological developments) and by establishing and promoting renewable, regenerative sources of energy (e.g. solar, water, wind energy). Moreover, efforts towards reducing energy consumption are essential.

Recent progress at global level along these lines became visible in 2015, when the United Nations achieved two important agreements. The first one consisted of the endorsement of the 2030 agenda on sustainable development goals by its member states. This agenda sets seventeen targets for sustainable global environmental, economic, and social development in the near future (United Nations 2015). Although the responsibility for implementation measures remains at national level, their progress is continuously monitored, and in many countries, strong political and social movements emerged to support and promote this process. The second achievement occurred in the same year, when the United Nations launched their agreement on climate change in Paris. For the first time, concrete climate protection goals were declared mandatory for all member states. Global warming should be restricted to a level below 2° Celsius, or even below 1.5° Celsius, an increase with reference to the earth's mean temperature before the start of its industrialization. To this end, a reduction of greenhouse gas emissions, in particular CO_2 and methane, was defined as the first priority. This aim should be reinforced by providing strong economic incentives towards compliance, most importantly by introducing a tax on carbon and by establishing international control mechanisms. A large majority of member states endorsed this agreement, and many countries are pioneering new protection measures. For instance, the European Union declared its aim to achieve net-zero carbon emissions by the year 2050. In the UK, decarbonization measures include national regulations for reducing fuel combustion in road transport (electrification of transport), power stations (replacing power generation), domestic heating, and carbon-intensive food products. These measures will also transform working and employment conditions, e.g. by extending working from home, reducing commuter traffic, expanding online communication, and reducing mean weekly working hours. A more radical shift towards a 'green economy' points to the growth of circular economy. It aims at reducing environmental resource and energy use through increased and smart efficiency in manufacturing, through extended recycling, as well as through restrictions on consumptive lifestyle behaviours (Munro et al. 2020).

At the policy level, several alternative strategies are available to implement the United Nations' sustainable development goals. A first strategy maintains that liberal market capitalism is capable of creating ecology-friendly technological innovations and of influencing consumer behaviour towards resource-saving habits. This strategy is favoured by influential economic organizations, interest groups, and corporations as well as by liberal and conservative political parties. A different approach, supported by many social-democratic governments, trade unions, and parts of the industry and service sector, posits that strong political institutions and regulations need to be developed and implemented in order to successfully govern sustainability measures. To this end, a broad spectrum of regulatory measures should be made available, including the extension of green taxes and the development of active policies of promoting climate-mitigating technologies. Even more distant from currently operating policies is a third strategy that favours a no-growth economy, taking potential negative consequences into account, such as reduced welfare and reduced employment. This strategy is supported by various bio-environmentalist movements and by organizations maintaining that the capitalist system is an obstacle against ecological and economic transformation (Hedenus et al. 2019).

At a fundamental level, these strategies illustrate the critical limitations of the concept of 'economic growth' that dominates national and international policies and decision-making agencies. With its unidimensional focus on material consumption, it disregards the vast negative side effects of externalized costs, the price of growth in terms of environmental damage and the burden on future generations. For instance, energy prices derived from nuclear power may be low and, thus, stimulate economic growth, but costs produced in the long run, such as ultimate decommissioning of dangerous materials, are not properly taken into account. A further critique of this unidimensional concept emphasizes the lack of including the many essential non-market goods produced in every society, such as child-care, housework, informal caring, or voluntary work. Restricting the evaluation of a society's economic output to the revenues derived from market exchange results in a fragmented, unbalanced view of the actual level of living conditions of a nation's population. Moreover, calculating a GDP value tells nothing about how wealth and income are distributed across the population. Income inequalities are one of the core concerns of global development policies. Finally, economic growth does not automatically increase human well-being. While a close link of economic progress with increased life expectancy remains undisputed, beneficial health effects largely depend on complementary developments of welfare policies and of public welfare in terms of educational progress and democratization of societies (Baum 2016). Moreover, there is no strong positive correlation between the level of socioeconomic progress and the increase of populations' well-being (Oswald 2010). For these reasons, several attempts were made to measure economic growth more adequately by broadening the range of indicators beyond GDP. The now famous Stiglitz–Sen–Fitoussi Commission delivered a report with some far-reaching recommendations. Accordingly, rather than focusing exclusively on productivity, economic progress should take income and consumption of households into account. Distribution of income and wealth should be a high priority, and objective indicators of quality of life should be complemented by subjective indicators, measuring human capabilities and developmental prospects, emotional prosperity, and well-being. Importantly, sustainability of economic growth in the face of environmental threats should be an overarching concern (Stiglitz et al. 2010). These considerations illustrate the basic tension between economic progress and ecological sustainability. They point to the urgency of unmet challenges and the need of searching new solutions. As far as modern working and employment conditions are concerned, these challenges will be addressed in later chapters of the book.

2.6 Summary

This chapter depicted far-reaching transformations of work and employment that need to be considered when dealing with the impact of occupational life on working people's health. Importantly, despite technological, economic, and social progress, several substantial threats remain in view of a globalized economy in conjunction with the growth of technological unemployment, nonstandard employment, and precarious work. Even at a more fundamental level, continuation of economic growth is no longer ensured, given the dangers of global warming and environmental degradation. Increased effort and investment in sustainable development is required.

2.7 Relevant questions

- Considering the potential impact of a growing digitization of work on people's health and well-being, what are the main positive and the main negative effects?

- The global trend of increased job insecurity and flexibility is often interpreted as undesirable. However, it may also promote workers' self-direction. What structural and personal measures are needed to strengthen this latter effect?
- What are the main obstacles against reconciling economic growth with ecological sustainability?

Recommended reading

❖   Arntz, M., Gregory, T., and Zierahn, U. (2019), *Digitalization and the future of work: Macroeconomic consequences*, IZA Discussion paper 12428. Bonn: Institute of Labor Economics (IZA).
❖   Kalleberg, A. L. (2018), *Precarious lives: job insecurity and well-being in rich democracies*. Cambridge: Policy Press.
❖   Munro, A., Boyce, T., and Marmot, M. G. (2020), *Sustainable health equity: achieving a net-zero UK*. London: Institute of Health Equity.

Useful websites

❖   International Labour Organization. Statistics.
      https://ilostat.ilo.org/
❖   World Bank: The World Development Report (WDR) 2019: the Changing Nature of Work.
      https://www.worldbank.org/en/publication/wdr2019
❖   Wikipedia: Occupational Safety and Health. https://en.wikipedia.org/wiki/Occupational_safety_and_health

References

Abrahamsson, K., and Larsson, A. (2021), 'How can Europe tackle the three employment challenges: the digital, the climate and the pandemic transition?', *Europ J Workpl Innov*, 6 (1), 8–18.

Arntz, M., Gregory, T., and Zierahn, U. (2016), *The risk of automation for jobs in OECD countries: a comparative analysis*, OECD Social, Employment and Migration Working Papers, No. 189. Paris: OECD Publishing.

Arntz, M., Gregory, T., and Zierahn, U. (2019), *Digitalization and the future of work: macroeconomic consequences*, IZA Discussion paper 12428. Bonn: Institute of Labor Economics (IZA).

Autor, D. H. (2015), 'Why are there still so many jobs? The history and future of workplace automation', *J Econ Perspect*, 29 (3), 3–30.

Backhaus, I., Hoven, H., Di Tecco, C., et al. (2022), 'Economic change and population health: lessons learnt from an umbrella review on the Great Recession', *BMJ Open*, 12 (4), e060710.

Baum, F. (2016), *The new public health* 4th ed. Oxford: Oxford University Press.

Bell, D. (1973), *The coming of post-industrial society*. New York: Basic Books.

Bérastégui, P. (2021), 'Exposure to psychosocial risk factors in the gig economy: a systematic review', *ETUI Research Paper - Report 2021.01*.

Bodin, T., Caglayan, C., Garde, A. H., et al. (2020), 'Precarious employment in occupational health—an OMEGA-NET working group position paper', *Scand J Work Environ Health*, 46 (3), 321–29.

Cockburn, W. (2021), 'OSH in the future: where next?', *Europ J Workplace Innov*, 6 (1), 84–97.

Eichhorst, W., and Portela de Souza, A. P. (2018), 'The future of work: Good jobs for all?'. In M. Webber and K. Bezanson (eds.), *Rethinking society for the 21st century: Report of the International Panel on Social Progress*, vol. 1. Cambridge: Cambridge University Press, 253–309.

Esping-Andersen, G. (1990), *The three worlds of welfare capitalism*. Oxford: Policy Press.

Frey, C. B., and Osborne, M. A. (2017), 'The future of employment: How susceptible are jobs to computerisation?', *Technological forecasting and social change*, 114, 254–80.

Friedlingstein, P., O'Sullivan, M., Jones, M. W., et al. (2020), 'Global carbon budget 2020', *Earth Syst Sci Data*, 12 (4), 3269–340.

German Federal Statistical Office (2022), 'Erwerbstätige im Inland nach Wirtschaftssektoren', https://www.destatis.de/DE/Themen/Wirtschaft/Konjunkturindikatoren/Lange-Reihen/Arbeitsmarkt/lrerw13a.html, accessed February 21, 2023.

Hedenus, F., Persson, M., and Sprei, F. (2019), *Sustainable development*. Lund: Studentlitteratur AB.

Hobsbawm, E. (1968), *Industry and empire*. London: Pelican.

Hyde, M., George, S., and Kumar, V. (2020), 'Trends in work and employment in rapidly developing countries'. In U. Bültmann and J. Siegrist (eds.), *Handbook of Disability, Work and Health*. Cham: Springer, 33–52.

Intergovernmental Panel on Climate Change (2014), *Climate change 2014: synthesis report*, Contribution of Working Groups I, II and III to the Fifth Assessment Report of the Intergovernmental Panel on Climate Change. Geneva: IPCC.

International Labour Organization (2013), *World of work report*. Geneva: ILO.

International Labour Organization (2018), *World employment and social trends*. Geneva: ILO.

Kalleberg, A. L. (2009), 'Precarious work, insecure workers: Employment relations in transition', *Am Soc Rev*, 74 (1), 1–22.

Kalleberg, A. L. (2018), *Precarious lives: job insecurity and well-being in rich democracies*. Cambridge: Policy Press.

Karasek, R. A., and Theorell, T. (1990), *Healthy work: stress, productivity and the reconstruction of working life*. New York: Basic Books.

Kreshpaj, B., Orellana, C., Burström, B., et al. (2020), 'What is precarious employment? A systematic review of definitions and operationalizations from quantitative and qualitative studies', *Scand J Work, Environ Health*, 46 (3), 235–47.

Labonté, R. (2015), 'Globalization and health', *International Encyclopedia of the Social & Behavioral Sciences* (2nd ed.), 198–205. doi:10.1016/B978-0-08-097086-8.14022-X

Marshall, T. H. (1965), 'The right to welfare', *The Sociological Review*, 13 (3), 261–72.

Marx, K. (1984), *Das Kapital. Buch III: Der Gesammtprocess der kapitalistischen Produktion*. Hamburg: Otto Meissner.

Munro, A., Boyce, T., and Marmot, M. G. (2020), *Sustainable health equity: achieving a net-zero UK*. London: Institute of Health Equity.

Oswald, A. J. (2010), 'IZA DP No. 5390: Emotional prosperity and the Stiglitz Commission', *Brit J Ind Relat*, 48 (4), 651–69.

Piketty, T. (2014), *Capital in the twenty-first century*. Cambridge, MA: Harvard University Press.

Piore, M. J., and Sabel, C. (1984), *The second industrial divide: possibilities for prosperity*. New York: Basic Books.

Rifkin, J. (1995), *The end of work: the decline of the global labor force and the dawn of the post-market era*: Putnam Publishing Group.

Stiglitz, J., Sen, A., and Fitoussi, P. (2010), *Mismeasuring our lives*. New York: The New Press.

Tomlinson, J., Baird, M., Berg, P., et al. (2018), 'Flexible careers across the life course: Advancing theory, research and practice', *Hum Relat*, 71 (1), 4–22.

United Nations (2015), 'Transforming our world: the 2030 Agenda for Sustainable Development', https://sdgs.un.org/2030agenda, accessed 27 Feb 2023.

Wood, A. J., Graham, M., Lehdonvirta, V., et al. (2019), 'Good gig, bad gig: autonomy and algorithmic control in the global gig economy', *Work, Employ Soc*, 33 (1), 56–75.

World Health Organization (2008), 'Closing the gap in a generation: health equity though action on the social determinants of health. Final report of the Commission on Social Determinants of Health', (Geneva: WHO).

PART II

ASSESSING PSYCHOSOCIAL WORK ENVIRONMENTS AND THEIR RELATIONSHIP WITH HEALTH

3
Theoretical concepts of psychosocial work

3.1 The role of theory in psychosocial occupational health

3.1.1 Basic notions

It is a major aim of scientific research to identify facts, to describe observations, and to analyse associations between different facts or observations in order to develop an explanation of how they interact. There are two main strategies of analysing associations between variables measuring observations or facts. With an exploratory approach, neither the selection of variables nor their interaction is predefined by the researcher. Using data mining techniques, findings result by chance and inform the researcher about further steps of analysis. Alternatively, the researcher selects distinct variables, based on an elaborated research hypothesis that proposes an explanation of the association between variables under study. The main task of research is then to search for ways of rejecting or confirming the hypothesis by structured data analysis. In practice, the two strategies are not always strictly separated. For instance, an unexpected association between variables may inspire the researcher to develop a new research hypothesis, or preliminary evidence for a research hypothesis may initiate exploratory analyses in new data sets. Yet, it is important that the way these two approaches were utilized is clearly described in scientific publications.

To develop a causal explanation between variables under study is a pre-eminent research interest in science. As explanations and predictions share the same logical structure, a causal explanation of associated facts enables their prediction in the future. If substantiated by empirical investigation, an interventive or preventive measure can be derived from an explanation or prediction. This sequence from explanation/prediction to prevention/

Psychosocial Occupational Health. Johannes Siegrist and Jian Li, Oxford University Press.
© Oxford University Press 2024. DOI: 10.1093/oso/9780192887924.003.0003

intervention documents the outstanding significance of scientific research for practice. In the basic sciences, the experimental method represents the classical approach to test a causal hypothesis. This method sets out to analyse changes of a dependent variable as a function of exposure to a systematic variation of an independent variable where, at the same time, potential confounding effects of additional interacting variables are controlled for. In many scientific disciplines, there are only limited opportunities for conducting experiments in order to test causal hypotheses. This certainly holds true for social and behavioural sciences, as well as for epidemiology and demography. In these disciplines, observational investigations represent the main methodological approach. Accordingly, conducting causal analysis within observational investigations presents an important challenge. To this end, study designs and statistical methods need to meet distinct requirements. In Chapter 5, these requirements are discussed in more detail. Notably, new statistical techniques are now available, developed in a counterfactual framework. Furthermore, to combine a hypothetical assumption about causality with steps of statistical analysis, a useful tool, the Directed Acyclic Graph (DAG), has been proposed to guide analytical decisions (Glymour and Kubzansky 2018) (see Chapter 5).

In order to explain the association between a variable A and a variable B, a causal hypothesis needs to refer to a general principle underlying this association. This can be illustrated by a simple example—the hypothesis 'If a person consumes three glasses of wine (A), then the reaction time in subsequent car driving (B) will be substantially reduced.' To explain the link between A and B, the general notion of a negative effect of a high level of alcohol in blood on the brain's capacity of attention regulation needs to be applied. This notion does not only provide a causal understanding, but it additionally allows for a generalization of the content of variable A (not only wine, but any kind of alcohol producing a certain level of concentration in blood). In many cases, a causal hypothesis is not an exclusive singular statement, but is part of a series of general statements. In our example, the effect of alcohol concentration in blood (A) on attention (B) also depends on the time interval (C) and on the role of modifying factors within the organism (D) (e.g. nutrition, hormones). Thus, additional general statements are needed to fully explain the causal link. A coherent set of general statements (hypotheses) is called a theory. The terms 'theory' and 'theoretical model' are often used interchangeably, but in the latter case, an attempt is made to visualize the structure and direction of relationships between the statements.

When talking about a general theory or general statements, we need to keep in mind again some basic methodological differences between the social and behavioural sciences and the basic sciences (see Box 3.1). In the latter case, in many areas of scientific inquiry, a high degree of certainty of a causal link underlying general statements has been documented. These statements are usually termed laws. Moreover, systematic experimental inquiry enables a stepwise extension of the scope of generalization, such that several laws with universal validity have been discovered and confirmed. In the social and behavioural sciences, achieving these two aims is much more difficult, given the variability, heterogeneity, and fluidity of the phenomena under study. Therefore, two basic restrictions are observed in these sciences. Firstly, given a lower degree of certainty of causal links, research hypotheses are expressed in terms of probability statements. Secondly, recognizing a principal limitation for the range of validity of general statements (bound to a certain time,

---

Box 3.1 Differences between basic and social and behavioural sciences

There are three fundamental differences in the ways causal hypotheses and theories are developed and tested between the basic sciences and the social and behavioural sciences:

- Concerning the methodology of scientific inquiry, the former mainly rely on experiments that enable a direct test of causality assumptions. Social and behavioural sciences have only limited access to experiments, as observational methods are their main approach.
- Concerning the quality of general statements, those derived from basic sciences often contain a high degree of certainty, qualifying them as laws, whereas general hypotheses derived from the social and behavioural sciences are expressed in terms of probability statements.
- Concerning the validity of theories, their range of generalization can be universal in the basic sciences, while in social and behavioural sciences, middle-range theories prevail, given their focus on a specific time, place, population, or context, preventing universal generalization.

a certain space, a certain context, etc.), theories in these disciplines cannot claim universal validity for their general statements. Rather, the validity of their hypotheses is restricted to a middle range. The notion of 'middle-range theories' was introduced by sociologist Robert K. Merton in recognition of the differences mentioned between basic and social sciences (Merton 1968).

To summarize, developing and testing causal hypotheses is a core aim of scientific inquiry. To offer an explanation, causal hypotheses need to refer to a general principle underlying the association between phenomena or observations. Full explanation of a causal link often requires a set of several interconnected hypotheses, called a theory or a theoretical model.

A substantial body of research evidence in the field of psychosocial occupational health is derived from the social and behavioural sciences. In view of the methodological limitations mentioned, we want to know how the scientific quality of this evidence can be judged. What are the criteria that allow for an evaluation of the scientific significance of research hypotheses and theories, or theoretical models, developed in this field?

3.1.2 Application to research on psychosocial occupational health

The following sections of this chapter will present a variety of causal hypotheses and theoretical models that were developed over the past few decades of international research on psychosocial occupational health. How can their scientific significance be evaluated? Starting with the simple case of a causal hypothesis linking a psychosocial occupational exposure to a health outcome, we find at least six criteria that enable evaluation of the scientific significance of evidence for this type of hypothesis. These criteria were first elaborated and published in mainstream epidemiology by Austin Bradford Hill, and they are generally referred to as the Hill criteria of causality in epidemiologic research (Hill 1965):

- **Consistency of results** on the association: The higher the number of independent confirmations, the higher the validity of the hypothesis.
- **Strength of the association** observed in investigations, expressed as relative risk of incident disease as a function of exposure: the higher the relative risk, the higher the validity of the hypothesis.
- **Temporal sequence**: A prospective study design is required to ensure that the exposure precedes the incident disease. The validity of causal hypotheses can only be examined with this study design.

- **Dose–effect relation:** With a higher amount of exposure (duration, intensity), a higher risk of incident disease is expected. Confirmation of this relation supports the validity of the hypothesis.
- **Biological plausibility:** If the statistical association is supported by additional scientific evidence on pathways linking exposure with disease development (e.g. psychobiological stress mechanisms), the validity of a causal hypothesis is strengthened.
- **Risk reduction through intervention:** If measures of reducing the amount of exposure result in a subsequent reduction of the risk of incident disease (e.g. by intervention studies), the validity of a causal hypothesis is strengthened.

In Chapters 6 and 7 (and, in part, in Chapter 10), selected research findings relating psychosocial work environments to elevated disease risks are discussed with regard to these criteria, allowing readers to judge their scientific significance. However, these research findings concern theoretical models rather than single causal hypotheses. To evaluate the scientific significance of a theoretical model is more challenging than to evaluate a single causal hypothesis. In this case, a set of interrelated general statements representing a theoretical construct needs to be tested. Obviously, it is particularly difficult to achieve a high degree of consistency across these interrelated statements, even more so, if a model is analysed in populations with different sociocultural or socioeconomic backgrounds. Therefore, evaluating the scientific quality of a theoretical model includes an assessment of the six quality criteria mentioned and a judgment on the consistency of findings related to the different hypotheses supporting a theoretical construct.

In the main part of this chapter, theoretical models of psychosocial work environments with relevance to health are introduced. Based on explicit selection criteria, four such models are described in more detail by elaborating their research hypotheses, while other concepts are only briefly characterized. Differences and similarities between the four models are discussed, and some recent theoretical developments are highlighted (Section 3.2). In the final part, one of the main quality criteria of causal evidence is addressed, that is the availability of convincing scientific information on pathways linking occupational exposures to the development of disease among working people. Stress-physiologic processes and health-adverse behaviours are the two main pathways (Section 3.3).

Before extending our arguments in these two sections, a note of caution is justified. All statements on the role of research hypotheses and theories in science in general, and in the social and behavioural sciences in particular, including the field of psychosocial occupational health, refer to the dominant scientific paradigm of nomological, quantitative analytical research. In this paradigm, scientific statements are based on empirical data subjected to interpersonal control. These data are collected by standardized measurement approaches, where variables represent observable facts as well as unobserved phenomena that are identified by latent constructs. Beyond providing a valid description of selected aspects of reality, this paradigm aims at developing causal explanations for associations between phenomena of interest by subjecting single research hypotheses—or a set of hypotheses representing a theory—to empirical confirmation or rejection. Independent replication of hypothesis testing and extension of findings promote a stepwise process of inductive generalization that may ultimately result in some nomological statements with strong explanatory power.

Although dominant in empirical research in the main disciplines that analyse associations of working conditions with health (see Chapter 1), the nomological paradigm has been supplemented by alternative ways of conducting scientific enquiry, specifically within social and behavioural sciences, where they are applied under the umbrella of 'qualitative methodology'. Importantly, rather than predefining constructs and measurements, scientists accord primacy to the subjective views of people and their interpretations of social reality, collecting their open statements as the basis of a process of analytical reconstruction. These approaches reflect the significance of subjective representations of the social reality, thus complementing and enriching a researcher-based process of data collection. The analysis of data obtained through qualitative methods is characterized by intimate links between data interpretation and theoretical reasoning. In this frame, it is quite difficult to meet the criteria of intersubjective reproduction of results, of empirical confirmation or rejection of research hypotheses, and of generalizing statements through systematic empirical testing. Basic principles of qualitative methods are briefly described in Chapter 4, where the promise of applying a mixed-methods approach, that is, a combination of quantitative and qualitative methods, is mentioned.

3.2 Main theoretical models and new developments

Theoretical models analysing psychosocial work environments with relevance to health aim to explain these links by selectively focusing on a restricted set of elements within the complexity and diversity of work environments. The selection of these elements and the description of their relations represent a genuine scientific effort to gain new insights into phenomena that so far remain poorly understood. These elements and their associations are delineated at a level of generalization that allows for their identification in a wide range of different occupations and contexts. Given their selective approach, these theoretical models explore limited aspects of the complexity of the world of work. Yet, by proposing innovative ways to view aspects of relationships between the elements under study, they may produce new knowledge.

During several decades of research, many theoretical constructs were proposed and examined, originating mainly from the disciplines of psychology and sociology. In this book, no attempt is made to provide an exhaustive or representative review of these theoretical developments. In line with our main teaching objectives, we restrict the description of theoretical models to those that meet the following selection criteria:

- repeated and independent empirical examination by epidemiological investigations of employed populations;
- application of a prospective study design that allows for testing causal hypotheses;
- inclusion of clinical or otherwise validated data on distinct mental and physical disorders;
- availability of information on pathways linking psychosocial exposures with the development of incident disease.

When applying these criteria, four theoretical models have attracted a substantial amount of international research interest in recent times, thus contributing to the development of a stock of evidence-based knowledge. These models are described in the next section. Readers should keep in mind that this choice reflects current, state-of-the-art knowledge (see also Kivimäki et al. 2018). Priorities may change as a result of future research activities. To illustrate the rich and fertile dimension of this field of research, some additional promising theoretical concepts are listed here (for review, see also Cooper and Quick 2017; Cunningham and Black 2021; Theorell 2020), before the four selected models are described in more detail:

- **Person-environment fit** (Edwards et al. 1998): Originating from classical work conducted in the 1980s at the University of Michigan, person-environment (P-E) fit theory assumes that stress arises from misfit between the working person and the environment. Misfit can be due to discrepancies between objective characteristics (e.g. demands vs abilities) or to discrepancies between subjective perceptions of these characteristics (e.g. perceived insufficiency preventing desired goals). The theory predicts that stress responses are particularly strong in this latter case.

- **Vitamin model** (Warr 1987): Distinct from approaches focused entirely on harmful effects, this model delineates twelve principal characteristics of work environments with positive effects on mental health and happiness. In analogy to vitamins, these effects reach an optimum at a certain level, with no further benefit beyond that level. In addition, person-centred characteristics, both longer-term and shorter-term, impact mental health, mainly by inducing situation-based mental processes. This model, thus, offers a broad framework open to more detailed specifications (Warr 2017).

- **Conservation of resources** (Hobfoll 1989): This concept focuses on persons' coping options in stressful situations (within and beyond the world of work). Options are defined as resources (objects, conditions, person characteristics) whose conservation by relevant investments is considered essential for health and well-being. Importantly, loss and threat of loss of resources is the main cause of stressful experience, where 'resource loss is disproportionately more salient than resource gain' (Hobfoll et al. 2016, p. 69).

- **Stressor-detachment model** (Sonnentag and Fritz 2015): Starting from an earlier 'effort-recovery' concept, this model elaborates the negative effects of strain reactions that often persist after tackling severe work demands and prevent recovery. Ways of restoring resources through recovery include psychological detachment from work, experiences of mastery and control, and psychophysiological relaxation.

- **Stress as offence to self** (Semmer 2020): This model considers a broad spectrum of experienced interpersonal devaluation at work (e.g. disrespect, abuse, unfair treatment) as a main source of stress. In these cases, the self of a person, that is, his or her social identity, is threatened, causing negative affect, anger, and intention to retaliate. Costs of devaluation include negative stress-related health effects as well as increased levels of social conflicts at work.

- **Psychosocial safety climate** (Dollard et al. 2019): This notion emphasizes the organizational climate perceived by employees where investments in psychological safety and health are weighted against productivity imperatives. Management commitment and support, transparent communication, and organizational participation are means of strengthening this climate, with documented positive effects on employees' well-being.

- **Workplace social capital** (Kouvonen et al. 2006): Applying the two components of social capital—structural aspects of social interactions, and cognitive aspects of norms and attitudes—to the work context is the aim of this concept. Measured by eight items, this approach demonstrates some construct validity in terms of limited overlap with prevailing theoretical models.

One major gap in our analysis relates to the concept of work-life balance (or work-family conflict; or work- life interference). Given its importance and given an extensive literature on its role as an additional determinant—or as a protective factor—in work-health associations, this topic deserves an own comprehensive analysis, as documented by several excellent publications (e.g. Berkman et al. 2014; Brough et al. 2020). In the context of a book focusing on the psychosocial work environment and its direct effects on health, the integration of this knowledge complicates the analysis as it is difficult to disentangle the health effects due to extra-work factors vs factors attributable to work, or to estimate their joint contribution. Moreover, at the theoretical level, research on work-life balance so far heavily relies on the main theoretical concepts discussed in this chapter, leaving the development of genuine theoretical approaches to capture the interference between two different domains of everyday life to future research.

3.2.1 Four main theoretical models

3.2.1.1 Demand-control

The Demand-Control (DC) model is one of the most widely applied and best-known models of psychosocial stress at work. It was first proposed by American sociologist Robert Karasek (1979), with close-links to psychobiological stress theory, as applied to cardiovascular disease (Karasek and Theorell 1990), and with an extension to include social support at work as a third dimension (Johnson and Hall 1988). Its scientific roots are grounded in sociological alienation theory, where low control among workers was studied in relation to their well-being and personal development (Kornhauser 1965), and in occupational health research on high workloads (Frankenhaeuser and Gardell 1976). Karasek's original idea of combining the two dimensions of psychological demands and decision latitude (or control) to explain elevated health risks associated with job task characteristics was supported by survey data. Soon, it became apparent that the control dimension was composed of two different aspects: the worker's influence on performing the work (decision authority) and his or her ability to use their own resources (skill discretion). Jobs defined by high psychological demands and low decision latitude were proposed to generate stress and to reduce health and well-being ('high strain'), whereas demanding jobs with a high level of control and autonomy ('active') were thought to buffer stress and to strengthen the experience of mastery and active learning (Karasek and Theorell 1990). Accordingly, four quadrants can be defined in a two-dimensional scheme: active jobs, low strain jobs, passive jobs, and high-strain jobs (Fig. 3.1). A close linkage of these sociological components with psychobiological stress theory is considered a particular strength of this model. Specifically, jobs defined by a combination of high demand and low control ('high strain' or 'job strain') were shown to simultaneously activate two stress axes within the organism, the sympathetic-adreno-medullary axis and the hypothalamic-pituitary-adrenocortical axis, and this synergistic activation contributes to the pathology of stress-related disorders, such as ischaemic heart disease (Henry and Stephens 1977; see 3.3.2).

Karasek's concept (defined as Job Strain or Demand-Control (DC) model) meets the criteria for a theoretical model, as it contains a set of interrelated research hypotheses. It claims that distinct features of job task profiles matter for health. Moreover, different combinations of these features can have positive or negative effects on workers' health and well-being (e.g. 'active' vs 'high strain' conditions). Importantly, the combined effect of high demand and low control is expected to exert higher risks for health than each single component of the model. Finally, social support at work mitigates the effect of work stress on health, whereas lack of support in combination with high strain (iso-strain) results in the strongest negative health effects (Johnson and Hall 1988). It is important to mention that this model is often labelled 'Demand-Control-Support (DCS) Model', in view of the third dimension included. Yet, in stress theory, its basis is the differential association of demand with control. Moreover, many epidemiologic studies contain data only on these two dimensions. For these reasons, in this book, we use the definition 'Demand-Control (DC) model', and we mention social support explicitly in cases where research evidence refers to results with particular significance of this component.

As the components of this model are mainly measured by the psychometrically validated scales of the Job Content Questionnaire (see Chapter 4), the individual research hypotheses as well as the set of hypotheses representing the theoretical model can be confirmed or rejected. In fact, rich empirical evidence supporting the validity of the model is currently available. A substantial part of main findings of this model will be documented and discussed in Chapters 6 and 7, with a focus on the explanation and prediction of stress-related disorders.

In summary, the DC model has been investigated more thoroughly than any other similar concept in occupational health research, and, based on strong evidence, it has exerted considerable impact on practical measures of worksite health promotion in several countries (see Chapters 10 and 11). Its scientific significance mainly relies on the core stress-theoretical notion of control/autonomy in human agency (Steptoe and Poole 2016). Therefore, its range of generalization has been extended beyond paid work, including household work (Chandola et al. 2004) and educational work (Gädin and Hammarström 2000). The proposer of this model, Robert Karasek, recently extended the original concept into a multilevel framework termed 'associationalist demand-control theory' (Karasek 2020) but sufficient empirical support is not available so far.

3.2.1.2 Effort-reward imbalance

The Effort-Reward Imbalance (ERI) model represents a complementary approach towards analysing a health-adverse psychosocial environment. It focuses on the employment contract as the core element of employment relations, emphasizing the role of social reciprocity in costly transactions for health and well-being (Siegrist 1996). Rooted in sociological and social psychological theories of exchange and equity (Adams 1965; Gouldner 1960) and referring to sociological role theory (Merton 1968), the model assumes that failed reciprocity, experienced in terms of 'high cost-low gain' conditions, threatens the working person's self-esteem, causing negative emotions and psychobiological stress responses. Importantly, three basic types of reward are transmitted: salary or wage (financial reward), career promotion or job security (status-related reward), and recognition or appreciation (socio-emotional reward). In addition to these extrinsic factors, the model contains an intrinsic motivational factor, the working person's inability to withdraw from work obligations and excessive striving ('overcommitment'). This risky pattern of coping may be due to an underlying need for approval and esteem at work, but it can also be reinforced by

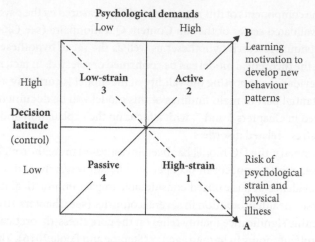

Figure 3.1 The demand-control model (Karasek 1979).

Source: Reproduced with permission from Berkman, L. F., Kawachi, I., and Theorell, T. (2014), 'Working conditions and health'. In L. F. Berkman, I. Kawachi, and M. M. Glymour (eds.), *Social epidemiology*. Oxford: Oxford University Press, 153–81. [Figure 5.1, p. 159]; license no.: 79235.

group pressure at work. Contrary to expectancy-value theory, the model posits that 'high cost-low gain' conditions are often maintained by those who have no alternative choice in the labour market, those working in highly competitive jobs, and those who are overcommitted to their work, thus being widely prevalent in the current economy. The ERI model has a strong transdisciplinary link to neuroscience-based stress theory, as sustained experience of reward deficiency at work activates distinct brain reward circuits, including such regions as the nucleus accumbens, anterior cingulate cortex, and insula (Schultz 2006). This threat or loss of significant social reward is associated with sustained activation of the stress axes (see Section 3.2.1.1), and it may additionally stimulate addictive behaviour. In the long run, allostatic load is triggered within several regulatory systems of the body, thus precipitating the development of stress-related disorders (McEwen 1998).

A series of interrelated hypotheses define the theoretical model. Firstly, negative health effects of violated reciprocity in costly exchanges are restricted to conditions where costs are high and gain is low. Secondly, prevalence of this imbalance is high among less skilled workers (due to lack of alternative job choice), and among those exposed to heavy competition and job insecurity. Thirdly, there is a dose-response relationship between the extent of this imbalance and the level of reduced health. Moreover, although the combination of high effort and low reward is expected to produce relatively stronger effects on health, each model component exerts negative effects on health as well. This also holds true for the three sub-components of 'reward' that are of comparable importance. Finally, over-commitment moderates the effect of effort-reward imbalance on health, with a higher level increasing the risk (Fig. 3.2).

Similar to the demand-control model, the ERI model is measured by psychometrically validated scales of a standardized Likert-scaled questionnaire (see Chapter 4). The model with its research hypotheses has been tested in a number of cohort studies, largely supporting its validity. Chapters 6 and 7 give an overview of the main findings, and their strengths and limitations are discussed. Although not as widely applied as the demand-control model, the ERI model has received continued interest in international research, including occupational research in rapidly developing countries. Its scientific significance mainly relies on the emphasis on reward/recognition in costly social exchange, a notion that links labour market conditions and daily individual work experience with the brain's reward system and its effects on health and well-being. In terms of generalization, the model has been successfully applied to unpaid work, such as caring, volunteering, household and family work, and educational work, and to unbalanced 'costs' in close social relationships (Siegrist and Wahrendorf 2016). These extensions underline the relevance of the universal norm of social reciprocity for social functioning and individual well-being.

3.2.1.3 Organizational justice

The third concept selected for this contribution, Organizational Justice (OJ), has a long tradition in research on social and organizational psychology, where three basic notions of justice are distinguished: distributive, procedural, and interactional (or relational) justice (Bies and Moag 1986; Greenberg and Cohen 1982). The first notion points to the fairness of distribution of resources and rewards between members of a group, whereas the second notion stresses fair decision-making procedures and equal application of rules in organizational behaviour. The third notion concerns respectful and trusting behaviour between colleagues, and specifically between leaders or managers and employees within the organization, thus avoiding prejudice, bullying, and discrimination. For decades, research on organizational justice was devoted to the study of its effects

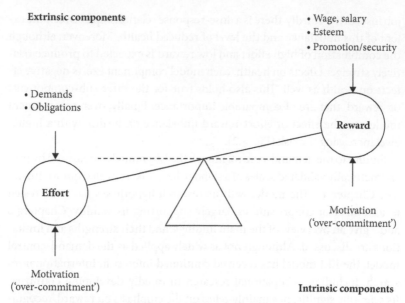

Extrinsic components

- Wage, salary
- Esteem
- Promotion/security

- Demands
- Obligations

Reward

Effort

Motivation
('over-commitment')

Motivation
('over-commitment')

Intrinsic components

Figure 3.2 The effort-reward imbalance model.

Source: Adapted with permission from Siegrist, J. and Wahrendorf, M. (2016),
'A theoretical model in the context of economic globalization'. In J. Siegrist and
M. Wahrendorf (eds.), *Work stress and health in a globalized economy*. Cham: Springer,
3–19. [Figure 1.1, p. 11]; license no.: 5493640227794.

on working people's behaviour within their companies and businesses. Analyses revealed that perceived injustice within organizations increased the likelihood of dissatisfaction, absenteeism, turnover intention, and attitudes of disengagement or even revenge (Greenberg and Colquitt 2005). Therefore, these findings were of direct practical interest for improving leadership behaviour, management styles, teamwork collaboration, and work motivation. In 2002, Finnish psychologist Marko Elovainio and his team applied this model to the explanation of stress-related ill health and disease, documenting associations with mental health and sickness absence (Elovainio et al. 2002; Elovainio and Virtanen 2020). In fact, this is the reason why the concept is often labelled 'Organizational Injustice'. The model contains a series of research hypotheses with direct relevance for health. Most importantly, all three notions of perceived injustice in an organization have a direct impact on health, as unjust acts violate binding norms of organizational behaviour and evoke stress reactions. Moreover, perceived organizational injustice adversely affects health and well-being even in the absence of personally experienced offence. This latter effect may be due to a worsened organizational climate reducing trust, security, and fairness. In addition to these direct effects, perceived organizational injustice exerts an indirect effect on health by reinforcing health-adverse behaviours, such as cigarette smoking and risky alcohol use. In line with main stream research on organizational justice the OJ model, as applied to health, assumes independent effects of each one of the three core components, distributive, procedural, and interactional justice (Elovainio and Virtanen 2020). This assumption has been visualized in Figure 3.3.

In epidemiological investigations, the OJ model so far was mainly measured by a set of standardized questionnaire items developed in 1991 (Moorman 1991). However, a detailed, psychometrically validated measurement approach was developed by Colquitt and Rodell (2015) where the three dimensions were supplemented by a fourth dimension termed 'informational justice' (see also Eib et al. 2022). The empirical evidence testing the model's hypotheses is impressive and covers both direct and indirect effects. It supports the validity of this model, as documented, among others, in two reviews (Elovainio and Virtanen 2020; Ndjaboué et al. 2012). The focus of the former review is on direct effects (especially cardiovascular health and stress-physiological parameters) and on health-adverse behaviour, whereas the latter publication reviews effects on mental health (see also Chapter 6). However, it should be mentioned that empirical support for the main hypothesis is stronger for procedural and relational injustice than for distributive injustice. With its emphasis on perceived organizational injustice and unfairness, the model adds a relevant feature to the dimensions of work-related stress, and it offers an option of generalizing this notion beyond paid work (Elovainio and Virtanen 2020).

3.2.1.4 Job demands-resources

The Job Demands-Resources (JD-R) model is considered the dominant theoretical approach to organizational psychology, with a substantial extension to occupational health research. It has been developed in two steps, first as a construct explaining impaired health (mainly burnout) as a negative outcome and work motivation as a positive outcome (Demerouti et al. 2001). Later, it was extended to the more complex Job Demands-Resources Theory, 'a heuristic and flexible model' (Bakker and Demerouti 2017, p. 278). In this brief summary, it is not possible to give elaborated comprehensive account of the many interrelated research hypotheses supporting the model (see Bakker and Demerouti 2017). Yet, essential propositions

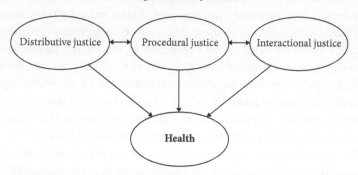

Figure 3.3 The model of organizational justice. Visualization of the model's basic assumption.

Source: Data from Marko Elovainio (Elovainio et al. 2002; Elovainio and Virtanen 2020) (see text).

are as follows: (1) All job characteristics can be classified as either demands or resources; (2) High demands and low resources reduce workers' health, while high demands and high resources strengthen work motivation; (3) Two types of resources operate in these processes, job-related and person-related resources; (4) There are bi-directional processes between demands/resources (predictors) and health or motivation (outcomes), such that reversed causal effects can occur; (5) Job demands are not always externally determined, but can be influenced proactively by workers ('job crafting'), with positive effects on health and motivation.

As a general framework, the JD-R model builds on distinct psychological theories of coping with demands and of strengthening resilience and recovery, in order to explain the observed associations. Such approaches include conservation of resources, social, cognitive, and self-determination theories (Schaufeli and Taris 2014). The model has also been influenced by the demand-control model mentioned above. With its emphasis on direct and indirect effects of job resources on personal and organizational outcomes, the JD-R model adds an important dimension to the field of occupational health research, and it links this field with research on job design and human resource management (Bakker and Demerouti 2017) (see Fig. 3.4).

Abundant empirical support was documented for the model's central hypotheses of direct positive effects of job resources on work engagement and of job demands on reduced well-being, while job resources also protect against reduced well-being. Fewer studies tested moderation and mediation effects, including personal resources. A meta-analytic review of seventy-four longitudinal studies found substantial support for the central hypotheses (Lesener et al. 2019). In Chapter 6, more information on health outcomes is provided, although most studies so far use self-reported rather than objectively documented health information. Despite the wide acceptance of this model, the authors also point to a number of unresolved conceptual and methodological problems, not least a clear conceptual distinction between demands and resources, more information on underlying mechanisms, and the need for a multilevel approach (Bakker and Demerouti 2017). In conclusion, this impressive amount of innovative work offers a stimulating framework, deserving special attention in future research in this field.

3.2.2 New developments

The theoretical models described so far reflect major developments during the past few decades. Two questions arise: What can we conclude as potential next steps from these developments? And how well can these models address new phenomena of work and employment that became manifest in recent times? When dealing with the first question, one has to remember that the four models emerged from different scientific backgrounds. Although originating from a shared body of knowledge and reasoning, they propose different theoretical priorities within their selective scope, focusing on 'control/autonomy in human agency', 'reward/recognition in social exchange', 'justice/fairness in interpersonal relationships', and 'balance between demands and resources'. A closer inspection reveals some minor overlap between some of their components (e.g. 'demand'/'effort'), but comparative tests of the models documented their independent contribution towards explaining workers' health risks. One future step might consist in combining these models in order to increase their explanatory power (see Chapter 6). While the analysis of co-manifestation of different stress dimensions is scientifically instructive, further extension seems problematic. With this extension, an integration of the different stress-dimensions at a higher level of theoretical generalization is proposed. For instance, in the frame of data analysis of the European Working Conditions Survey, it was proposed to classify all work stress dimensions into two broad categories of 'demands' and 'resources' (Eurofound 2019). This proposition was later modified into a 'job quality framework' containing seven distinct dimensions (Eurofound 2021). In a similar way, OECD proposed a concept with six dimensions of physical and social environments: job tasks; organizational characteristics; working-time arrangements; job prospects, and intrinsic job aspects (OECD 2017). These overarching frameworks are operationalized by combining scales or their proxies from established models, in line with an earlier influential measurement approach, the Copenhagen Psychosocial Questionnaire (Kristensen et al. 2005). Yet, the interpretation of results seems problematic from a theoretical perspective. As discussed above, any theoretical explanation requires a level of generalization that reduces the complexity of scientific inquiry. It is essentially the function of a theoretical model to reduce this complexity by proposing a selective heuristic focus of analysis. A strong theory is characterized by parsimony, that is, by a restricted number of elements (or statements or mathematical formulae) that explain a large number of phenomena under study. Each one of the four theoretical models represents such an attempt towards parsimony. By merging them all together, as proposed by these recent claims, one loses their distinct explanatory contribution. Apart from these attempts towards overarching concepts, there are some remarkable theoretical propositions linking expanded work-related models with work-redesign practices and policies, such as an extended demand-control-support model of worker well-being (Lovejoy et al. 2021), or a framework that analyses worker well-being along three dimensions of diversity, inclusion, and equity (Wilcox and Koontz 2022).

With the second question, we ask how well the models can capture newly emerging phenomena in the world of work. The rise in nonstandard employment, as described in Chapter 2, is one such phenomenon. In essence, all main models are rooted in the notion of a rather stable job that is maintained over a longer period of one's occupational trajectory. In methodological terms, long-term exposure to the same circumstances is an essential prerequisite of estimating incident disease risks. Some longitudinal studies examined the duration of exposure to adverse psychosocial work environments. In fact, a large majority of workers continued their job over several years without substantial change. For instance, in a Swedish cohort study, work stress, as measured by effort-reward imbalance, remained unchanged over four measurement waves covering seven years in almost ninety per cent of participants (Leineweber et al. 2020). Nevertheless, mobility and discontinuity of employment need to be addressed in conceptual terms as well. With the recent development of life-course studies in occupational epidemiology, new evidence on the impact of the dynamics of working life became available.

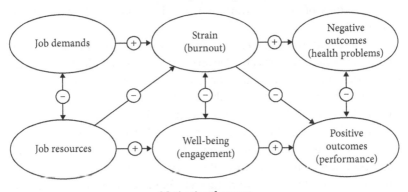

Figure 3.4 The revised job demands-resources (JD-R) model.
Source: Reproduced with permission from Schaufeli, W. B. and Taris, T. W. (2014), 'A critical review of the job demands-resources model: implications for improving work and health'. In G. F. Bauer and O. Hämmig (eds.), *Bridging occupational, organizational and public health*. Cham: Springer, 43–68. [Figure 4.1, p. 46]; license no.: 5493640813808.

By assessing employment histories retrospectively or prospectively, information on exposure duration and number and duration of interruptions and job changes can be obtained. As input to a stress-theoretical framework, this information serves to identify different types of critical occupational trajectories. For example, based on retrospectively collected data on work histories of a large cohort of employees in France from age 25 to age 45, three types of critical occupational trajectories were identified:

- precarious careers (e.g. temporary contracts, repeated job changes);
- discontinuous careers (e.g. involuntary interruptions; temporary unemployment);
- careers with cumulative disadvantage (e.g. being 'locked' in a hazardous, low skill job).

Employees exposed to these critical careers exhibited elevated risks of poor health functioning after age 45 (Wahrendorf et al. 2019). On similar grounds, a cohort study in the United States revealed that precarious and unstable job conditions during late midlife worsened functional limitations after age 65 and contributed to higher mortality risk (Donnelly 2022). Therefore, adapting established work stress models to the new reality of discontinued, disruptive, and mobile work careers may result in new conceptualizations of stressful work and its effects on health (Wahrendorf et al. 2023).

New attempts towards defining and measuring precarious work, including self-employed jobs and delivery services through digital platforms (gig work), are currently under way (see e.g. Bodin et al. 2020; Kreshpaj et al. 2020). In this context, the analysis of distance work and its association with health and well-being deserves attention. Telework, work from home, and other forms of distance work, flexible work arrangements with part-time physical attendance, and extended virtual meetings are becoming more common. Starting in 2020, the COVID-19 pandemic forced large parts of the workforce into working from home as a preventive measure against infection. It is likely that this sudden, radical shift of work environment accelerates the diffusion and extension of distance work, at least in several employment sectors, such as office and administrative support, communication, information, and service occupations and professions whose work is amenable to online exchange. Established notions and categories of analysis, such as supervision and leadership, control, feedback, teamwork, work climate, and social support call for revision. Emerging challenges of extensive social isolation, of struggling with technical problems, of aligning and coordinating work and private obligations, and of coping with an omnipresent virtual reality deserve the attention of scientists (Kniffin et al. 2021).

It seems premature to deal with a further line of new developments at work, the impact of digitization on work organization, job performance, and workers' health (Cockburn 2021). Large-scale automation is penetrating industrial production. Cyberphysical systems and interconnected, automated data exchange of supply chains enhance production efficacy, enabling factories to reduce their personnel. Job tasks, not only in industrial production, but also in a variety of service occupations, are often defined by on-screen control monitoring, an activity with risks of attention deficit and monotony, but also with the stress of coping with interruptions and technical failures. Working with digital wearable technology can aggravate one's workload in settings susceptible to technostress, especially if options of task definition and job discretion are restricted. Human-robot interaction is a further source of potential strain, depending on the intimacy, speed, and variety of tasks to be exchanged. It is often argued that automation and digitization contribute to a reduction of physical and mental workload among employees. However, several reports indicate that this benefit is lost due to increased work intensity and work pressure (Diebig et al. 2020). The growth of nonstandard employment with its discontinuity and fragmentation of occupational trajectories, including a rise of precarious work, the expansion of distance work, and specifically telework, as well as the dynamic increase of digitization and automation, are powerful recent developments of the modern world of work. To prevent their adverse effects on workers' health and to promote decent, sustainable work, research needs to analyse its core features with innovative conceptual and methodological approaches. Available theoretical frameworks and models can fertilize these developments.

Having discussed the main theoretical models, we now ask how the explanations offered by them are substantiated by two powerful underlying pathways, psychobiological processes and health-adverse behaviours.

3.3 Stress-theoretical and behavioural pathways

3.3.1 Basic notions

In scientific literature, the term 'stress' is used in different ways. We therefore clarify the terminology and its underlying conceptualization in the context of this book. Importantly, in a biopsychosocial frame of health and disease, stress basically refers to a bodily reaction and a subjective human experience in the presence of a challenge. As a reaction to an extrinsic demand, the organism responds by providing the energy needed to cope with the situation. To adapt to environmental demands and challenges with physiological reactions, the organism uses two interrelated regulatory systems termed 'catabolism' and 'anabolism'. The former system mobilizes energy for action, whereas the latter system restores a state of equilibrium by promoting regeneration and relaxation. These systems are activated by the autonomic nervous system and associated neuroendocrine patterns of response, where the sympathetic nervous system triggers catabolic reactions and the parasympathetic nervous system triggers anabolic reactions. Accordingly, stress at the physiologic level is a catabolic response. To adapt to the demands of everyday life, the organism recurrently activates its catabolic reactions as a sign of vitality and survival. Therefore, stress responses are part of a normal and healthy life experience.

At the same time, stress is a subjective experience; we evaluate core features of a demand or challenge, and we judge our capacity to respond to it. If the result of this evaluation is positive, the experience is favourably appraised, meaning that we can master the challenge. This positive response is often termed 'eustress' (in the Greek language, 'eu' means 'good'). Conversely, a difficult challenge with uncertain success of coping, or even a demand that exceeds the capacity to respond is negatively appraised, termed 'distress'. Emotional as well as physiological responses differ according to this evaluation. In addition to the quality and intensity of demand, its duration matters most. Even a positive challenge that is easily mastered can harm the organism if continued over a long time. Chronic activation of the catabolic system overtaxes the physiologic responses in the long run, precipitating a state of exhaustion in the absence of anabolic restoration. However, in a majority of cases, the duration of positively evaluated challenges can be controlled by the person, as part of the capacity for coping. This is less likely in the case of negatively evaluated challenges, as options to control them through personal coping are often restricted. In order to further clarify the distinctions between positively and negatively appraised challenges and the persons' emotional and physiologic responses, several definitions are proposed here, before the stress process is described in more detail (see Box 3.2).

As indicated in Box 3.2, we propose to restrict the term 'stressor' to a challenge that taxes or exceeds a person's coping capacity. Such a challenge is experienced as a threat, due to its risk of uncontrollability and unpredictability. Accordingly, the term 'stress reaction' is used exclusively to indicate the emotional and physiologic reaction to a stressor (Koolhaas et al. 2011). Given the connectivity between affective and physiological stress reactions, these latter are termed 'psychobiological stress responses' (Steptoe 2006) (see Chapter 7). Threatening experiences evoke negative emotions of fear, anxiety, anger or helplessness, and the brain activates 'catabolic' stress axes, mobilizing the body's energy for survival responses of 'fight or flight'. The psychobiologic stress response is described in more detail in the next section, where the body's complex interplay of stress- and anti-stress reactions is further explored. Here, we emphasize that stressors can originate from the natural environment (e.g. as a disaster) as well as from the social environment. It is generally believed that chronic stressors originating from the social environment have a major impact on the development of stress-related disorders among humans (Weiner 1992). This may be due to the long duration and perseverance of many socio-environmental exposures to large population groups, to their frequent occurrence, and to their significance for people's material

Box 3.2 **Stressor and stress response: Definitions**

- An environmental challenge is negatively evaluated if it taxes or exceeds the person's coping capacity. This challenge is termed a 'stressor'.
- Uncontrollability of the event and unpredictability of the outcome of coping efforts are core features of a stressor, evoking experiences of threat.
- The physiological and emotional reaction to a stressor is termed 'stress response'.
- A stress response is characterized by negative emotions of fear, anxiety, anger, or helplessness as a reaction to threat.
- Simultaneously, the brain activates distinct 'stress axes' mobilizing the body's energy for alarm reactions of 'fight or flight'. In view of its close connection with emotions, this reaction is termed 'psychobiological response'.
- Sustained chronic stress responses induce functional and structural changes in distinct organ systems and subsequent health risks.
- Chronic stressors arising from the social environment in general, and the work environment in particular, act as major determinants of elevated health risks mediated by sustained stress responses.

and psychosocial preferences in life. As this holds true for stressors originating from the wider social environment, it is equally relevant for stressors evolving from the work environment.

Stress research with relevance to human health and disease has a history of more than a hundred years. It is impossible to summarize here its major developments (see e.g. Fink 2016; Weiner 1992). However, it may be instructive to briefly mention what we consider the most significant advances within this field, thus justifying the selective approach that guides our further analysis of the topic. Undoubtedly, two pioneers stand out in the history of stress research—Walter B. Cannon (1871–1945) and Hans Selye (1907–1982). Cannon's ground-breaking discovery concerned the fight or flight response of the organism to an external threat. He successfully delineated a direct link from the sympathetic nervous system to the adrenal medulla, which induces release of catecholamines into the bloodstream. This catabolic response prepares the organism for active coping by increasing heart rate and blood flow, breathing and oxygen delivery to muscles and brain, and metabolic processes (glucose, free fatty acids). As an old evolutionary pattern of surviving life-threatening dangers, this sympathetic-adreno-medullary (SAM) axis is the principal bodily response to all types of challenging situations, and its intensity is particularly enhanced in the face of stressors (Cannon 1929). With his main discovery, Selye identified recurrent activation of the hypothalamic-pituitary-adrenocortical (HPA) axis as a stereotyped response to a variety of noxious stimuli. Again, this bodily response was shown to promote adaptation to challenging situations, thus acting as another old evolutionary pattern of surviving life-threatening dangers (Selye 1936). Importantly, glucocorticoids (mainly cortisol) are released into the bloodstream from the adrenal cortex, unfolding a wide spectrum of physiological reactions, including elevated glucose levels and reduced functioning of the immune system. Based on his animal experiments, Selye maintained that the stress response was a general adaptation system that was indifferent to various properties of noxious stimuli. This assumption was later rejected by the seminal work of James Mason (1968) who demonstrated that psychobiological stress responses differed according to the quality and severity of a stressor. More specifically, whether the HPA axis or the SAM axis is the main response, and whether or not they are simultaneously activated, largely depends on the degree of controllability of a stressor. Supported by innovative animal research conducted by James P. Henry, there was evidence for a primary activation of the HPA axis under conditions of loss of control, whereas both axes are aroused if active coping with a taxing stressor occurs (Henry and Stephens 1977). The prominent role of cognitive appraisal and coping efforts in the modulation of psychobiological stress responses was elucidated in the highly influential work of psychologist Richard S. Lazarus (Lazarus and Folkman 1984). Despite a decisive role of cognitive appraisal in the stress process, sensory input of an environmental stressor may eventually bypass a person's awareness, thus directly targeting the brain circuits that process affect and affect-induced neuroendocrine activation. Joseph LeDoux and his team contributed significantly to this new knowledge (LeDoux and Daw 2018). This latter pathway is particularly relevant if habituation occurs in the presence of a chronic stressor. More recently, concepts were developed that reveal the mechanisms of long-term outcomes of sustained stress responses, most importantly Bruce McEwen's paradigm shifting analysis of 'allostatic load' (McEwen 1998).

Many more stress researchers with innovative findings deserve to be mentioned here, but with our specific interest in the associations of chronic work stressors with health risks, as triggered by sustained stress responses, insights from the scientists mentioned are particularly valuable. Accordingly, we will now proceed to describe the dynamics of psychobiological stress responses in more detail.

3.3.2 Dynamics of psychobiological stress responses

Analysing a complex matter that requires a textbook unto itself is not feasible within the constraints of a few pages. Therefore, in an attempt to shed some light on basic processes, we selectively focus on the following aspects. Firstly, the pathway from sensory input of stressful experience to the brain's limbic structures and the stress axes activated by them is described. Secondly, the endocrine, cardiovascular, immune- and inflammation-related responses of this activation are described. Very briefly, we also point to some newly discovered molecular mechanisms. Finally, the dynamics of psychobiological stress responses with longer-term outcomes of functional and structural lesions triggering distinct physical and mental disorders are highlighted.

3.3.2.1 Role of the brain's limbic structures

Stressful socio-environmental stimuli are processed by structures in the prefrontal cortex as entry points of the brain's salience network, where the results of cognitive appraisal and affective evaluation are projected downward via limbic structures, including the anterior cingulum and insula. To actuate the stress response, the amygdalae, in conjunction with the hippocampus, stimulate the hypothalamus through efferent neurons (Osborne et al. 2020). More specifically, prelimbic and infralimbic regions of the ventral medial prefrontal cortex are particularly sensitive to the processing of the experience of control and its loss (Steptoe and Poole 2016). At the same time, the nucleus accumbens, anterior cingulum, and insula, as parts of the brain's reward circuit—process the experience of reward and its frustration or denial, and of emotional pain associated with loss (Schultz 2006). Notably, insular activation is modulated by the magnitude of loss following effort (Hernandez Lallement et al. 2014), and the experience of disadvantageous inequity in social exchange is associated with heightened arousal of different parts of the limbic circuit (Tricomi et al. 2010).

As mentioned, stress-related neural activity reflecting fear, anxiety, anger, frustration, and helplessness is projected to the amygdalae, causing an increase in metabolic activity and stimulation of efferent signalling to the hypothalamus. The hypothalamus plays a central role within the stress process, transducing activity from the central nervous system to distinct peripheral systems of the organism. As one main pathway of this transduction, heightened arousal of the sympathetic nervous system triggers the SAM axis, with release of catecholamines into the bloodstream. A second main pathway involves the synthesis of CRF (corticotropin-releasing factor) with subsequent release of ACTH (adrenocorticotropic hormone) from the anterior pituitary, further stimulating the HPA axis to secrete glucocorticoids from the adrenal cortex (Chrousos and Gold 1992). These two axes act partly independent of each other, partly in conjunction, depending on the quality of the stressor and the coping requirements. Yet, restricting the analysis to these two stress axes neglects the complexity of regulatory systems within the organism, where additional stress- and anti-stress axes operate, such as the hypothalamic-pituitary gonadal axis and the hypothalamic-pituitary growth hormone axis. These latter systems provide regenerative, anabolic responses, thus 'counterbalancing' noxious effects of continued SAM- and HPA-activation (Theorell 2016) (see Chapter 7). Protective effects mitigating the stress response were also documented for distinct hypothalamic hormones and neurotransmitters, in particular oxytocin (Meyer-Lindenberg et al. 2011). Taken together, the brain's regulatory network and subsequent structures enables compensatory, balancing effects between the different stress- and anti-stress axes, protecting the organism against a rapid 'breakdown' process (see Fig. 3.5).

3.3.2.2 Endocrine, cardiovascular, immune, and inflammation-related responses

Activation of the SAM axis initiates an instant energy-promoting process through neuronal noradrenergic-mediated firing and through the release of adrenalin from the adrenal medulla into the systemic circulation. A cascade of cardiovascular and metabolic responses supports this process, which has been described on many occasions. Circulating catecholamines increase heart rate, cardiac output, and blood pressure, oxygen supply and breathing—they promote vasoconstriction of vessels and stimulate metabolism via glycogenolysis and lipolysis, changing insulin sensitivity. Moreover, noradrenergic activation impairs parasympathetic control, thus reinforcing a sympathetically dominated imbalance of the autonomic

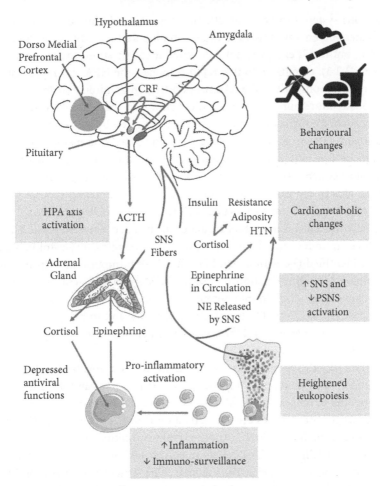

Figure 3.5 Overview of psychobiological pathways and effects. ACTH, adrenocorticotropic hormone; CRF, corticotropin-releasing factor; HPA, hypothalamic pituitary adrenocortical axis; HTN, hypertension; NE, norepinephrine; PSNS, parasympathetic nervous system; SNS, sympathetic nervous system.

Source: Reproduced with permission from Osborne, M. T., Shin, L. M., Mehta, N. N., et al. (2020), 'Disentangling the links between psychosocial stress and cardiovascular disease', *Circ Cardiovasc*, 13 (8), e010931. [Figure 3, p. 5]; license no.: 5497040748078.

nervous system (Thayer et al. 2012). As mentioned, this sudden increase of catabolic energy serves the organism's life-saving activities of fight or flight, but if this energy is not consumed it causes strain to the organism (see 3.3.2.3). Compared to this rapid response, the HPA axis represents a delayed response where the release of cortisol from adrenal cortex into the bloodstream requires several minutes. However, the physiological effects of cortisol on the organism are far-reaching, given its substantial control function. Glucocorticoids enhance circulating levels of energy substrates (glucose, free fatty acids), and they exert regulatory effects on the cardio-vascular system. At the same time, if released over a longer time period, these effects decrease immunosurveillance by suppressing natural killer cells and proinflammatory cytokines. An immune-neuro-endocrine net-work with feedback loops that regulates the balance between humoral and cellular immunity and the modulating role of inflammatory cytokines has been identified (Besedovsky and Del Rey 2007). Importantly, chronically dampened immune function and continued low-grade systemic inflamma-tion have several important consequences for health. Among others, they increase the susceptibility to infectious diseases and to malignancy, they impair wound healing, and they promote atherosclerotic developments in arteries.

More recently, several basic molecular mechanisms involved in the stress response were identified. They include oxidative stress and the enhanced expression of nuclear factor kB (NF-kB) as transmitters of stress-induced sympathetic arousal into cellular activation (Bierhaus et al. 2003; Ghaemi Kerahrodi and Michal 2020). Another pathway linking psychosocial stress with elevated disease risk via cellular mechanisms concerns the telomere ef-fect (Blackburn and Epel 2017). Telomeres are structural elements of DNA located at the non-coding ends of chromosomes. Their length is reduced at each cell division. An important protective effect is produced by the enzyme telomerase that adds base pairs to the ends of chromosomes to prevent cel-lular death. Innovative research demonstrates that chronic psychosocial stress results in accelerated shortening of telomere length, and that acceler-ated shortening of telomere length increases the risk of developing a variety of non-communicable diseases. In agreement with the above-mentioned evidence, short telomere length was shown to be promoted by high levels of oxidative stress and pro-inflammatory cytokines (Blackburn and Epel 2017). In addition, ground-breaking epigenetic mechanisms of activating the genetic code were identified. DNA methylation acts as a major pro-cess of gene transcription, and by this process extrinsic stimuli from the material and psychosocial environment can affect transcription factors in specific promoter genes. Altered levels of methylation in inflammation- and immune-function-related genes are of special interest in this context. Environmental stimuli can include sustained psychosocial stress, as demonstrated in pioneering experimental animal research with altered DNA-methylation of the promotor glucocorticoid receptor gene that regulates the stress hormone system (Weaver et al. 2004). In humans, an influential study documented associations of chronic social adversity with epigenetic modifications of inflammatory genes (Stringhini et al. 2015). In Chapter 7, several recent discoveries with relevance to occupational stress research are listed. They illustrate an innovative line of scientific inquiry.

3.3.2.3 Long-term effects of sustained psychobiological stress responses

So far, we can summarize findings showing that chronic psychosocial stress is a relevant predictor of impaired health if defined as a response to continued, long-lasting demands that tax or exceed the persons' coping resources, occurring in an unpredictable manner and with a low probability of control. To explain how stressful experience 'gets under the skin', we pointed to some research in neuroscience, where the processing of threatening information by the brain's salience network was analysed. In this network, distinct limbic circuits operate, with a central role of the amygdalae. The SAM and HPA stress axes transmit stress responses to peripheral systems within the body, affecting cardiovascular functioning, metabolic regulation, inflammatory activity, and immune competence. In a more recent stage of stress research, the cellular and subcellular processes underlying these psychobiological stress responses were explored, demonstrating a crucial role for oxidative stress and redox-sensitive transcription factors, such as nuclear factor kB (NF-kB). An important discovery concerns the telomere effect, where noxious conditions such as chronic psychosocial stress contribute to a shortening of telomere length in the DNA, thus precipitating cellular death. Finally, it became evident that stressful stimuli arising from the material and psychosocial environment can influence gene transcription, thus enhancing or suppressing the function of distinct promoter genes through DNA methylation.

Is there a unifying concept that integrates these different levels of analysis and their temporal sequence? Does such a concept convincingly explain the long-term effects of sustained psychobiological stress responses? An answer to these questions was proposed by Bruce McEwen with the concept of allostatic load (McEwen 1998). Unlike homeostasis, an essential state of the organism's functioning, allostasis describes a further fundamental physiological principle of 'maintaining stability through change'. As the organism has to adapt to environmental challenges, the boundaries of control may change. Distinct physiological mediators regulate this maintenance of balance under conditions of adaptive change, including stress hormones, pro- and anti-inflammatory cytokines, and the parasympathetic nervous system (primary mediators) (McEwen 2016). However, when occurring chronically and sustained over months and years, these adaptive regulations become exhausted. For instance, they lose the propensity to respond (e.g. by down-regulation of receptors), or they fail to recover from activity, triggering subtle dysfunctions within each regulatory system (secondary outcomes). Different dysfunctions reinforce each other, contributing to a physiological burden that manifests itself in abnormal levels of metabolic, cardiovascular, and immune parameters, triggering tissue damage and structural lesions of organs and vessels. Ultimately, allostatic load (or overload) results in incident disease manifestation (tertiary outcomes).

The question of whether an integrative pathophysiological process links chronic psychosocial stress with several physical and mental disease manifestations via this process of allostatic load is currently still open. One hypothesis maintains that systemic chronic inflammation with its breakdown of immune tolerance represents one such integral pathway, increasing the susceptibility of cardiovascular disease, cancer, type 2 diabetes, and neurodegenerative disorders (Furman et al. 2019). Another hypothesis proposes a neuro-immune-arterial axis with a determining effect of sustained amygdalar activation on the development of cardiovascular events (Osborne et al. 2020; Tawakol et al. 2017) and of diabetes (Osborne et al. 2019). In an attempt to reconcile the two hypotheses, a further approach supports a leading role of stress-induced limbic structure activation and its effects on systemic chronic inflammation. Yet, two distinct categories of disorders resulting from allostatic load are proposed. The first category includes atherosclerotic disorders, in particular ischaemic heart disease and stroke, hypertension, obesity, metabolic syndrome, and type 2 diabetes, whereas the second category includes major depression and anxiety disorders, where stress-induced inflammation seems to play an important role (Ghaemi Kerahrodi and Michal 2020). While suggestive, these hypotheses deserve further exploration, but they point to a prominent role of chronic psychosocial stress in the development of major non-communicable diseases in modern societies (see also Chapter 7).

3.3.3 The role of coping

From an evolutionary perspective, threat-induced physiological stress responses serve the aim of enhancing survival through rapid fight or flight reactions. These rapid reactions are triggered by downward signals from the amygdalae, targeting the periaqueductal gray, an area in the brain that coordinates sensory and motor circuits, and the brain stem, causing those immediate movements that are required for defensive action (Koutsikou et al. 2015). This evolutionary stable mechanism of survival was modified rather substantially by pre-historic and historic developments in human societies. For a long time, stress-induced fight or flight reactions were a dominant pattern among humans, where physical power and violence against enemies was used to tackle stressful threats. However, in modern societies, a far-reaching attempt has been made to minimize the exertion of direct physical power and violence in interpersonal exchanges. To this end, the monopoly of physical power was accorded to two societal institutions—the police and the military—thus gradually replacing aggression through physical action in social relationships by legally binding procedures of negotiation and conflict resolution. This process of preventing the exertion of physical power in social exchange is considered a main accomplishment of the civilizing process of societal life (Elias 2000).

Modern working life, as well as other domains of social life, does not allow people to face extrinsic stressors with 'fight or flight' responses. Often, these are 'no exit' situations where escaping from the challenge is not possible. In these instances, people cannot deplete their augmented energy level induced by physiological arousal. Rather, prolonged autonomic nervous system activation and negative emotions persist, unless coping efforts other than those resulting in a depletion of energy are available. In modern economies, in the vast majority of cases, jobs do not require the expenditure of continued physical effort at work. Here, psycho-mental and socio-emotional efforts are recurrently required, while enhanced autonomic activity persists. Sedentary jobs exposed to work pressure or work intensification, piecework, and other forms of machine-paced work, and the many different service jobs with clients are examples where stressful autonomic arousal persists. Or take the case of interpersonal conflicts at work. How can people who experience workplace bullying and harassment, mistreatment, humiliation, disrespect, and discrimination from superiors, colleagues, subordinates, or clients respond to these stressful events? Options of defence by overt behaviour, such as a spontaneous aggressive act expressing anger or fear, are prohibited. In all these instances, ways of coping other than fight or flight are required.

The central role of coping in dealing with work-related stressors was empha-sized in the conceptual framework depicted in Figure 1.1 (see Chapter 1). When facing a stressor, two instantaneous cognitive appraisals occur, one evaluating the severity and intensity of the challenge (its potential threat to the working person), and one evaluating the person's available means of meeting this chal-lenge. 'Coping' is defined as the person's response to the evaluation of this challenge, including mobilizing thoughts, emotions, motivations, and actions to solve the problem. As described in Figure 1.1, the effectiveness of this ac-tivity largely depends on the person's coping capabilities. As mentioned, the direct pathway from sensory input to appraisal, coping activity, and psycho-biological stress response is of crucial concern in stress research, whereas the analysis of the coping process was traditionally a domain of psychological sci-ence. For a long time, an influential theory, proposed by Lazarus and Folkman (1984), distinguished between two different ways of coping—problem-based and emotion-based coping. The former is directed to addressing the situation, whereas the latter aims to reduce the stressor's adverse effects on personal health and well-being. However, as emotion-based coping was mainly de-scribed in terms of avoidance and escape, this dichotomy may be less useful in our context of dealing with stressors at work. The main dimensions of problem-solving coping at work concern the person's competences and skills in meeting the challenge, the availability of material and social resources, and eventually the option of modifying the challenge (e.g. by redefining the task, changing the division of work). Importantly, competences and skills of coping at work include psychological capabilities, such as perseverance, self-efficacy, and op-timism. In addition, mood control through the exertion of relaxation, and cognitive reappraisal (e.g. threat reduction through comparison with worse events) provide means of strengthening active coping at work. In the concep-tual framework of Figure 1.1, a second pathway was included. Extrinsic and in-trinsic constraints often limit successful coping efforts on the job. Under these circumstances, an indirect pathway is likely to be mobilized. Here, people tend to reduce their emotional strain by the consumption of stress-relieving sub-stances. This consumption may offer an instantaneous relief, but as it does not target the sources of stressful experience, its chronic use is likely, with risks of inducing or reinforcing addictive health-damaging behaviours (e.g. smoking, alcohol or drug consumption, unhealthy food). The consumption of these sub-stances is used as an alternative to problem-solving strategies at work, resulting from the experience that active coping may not be successful, or may be too costly and time-consuming. Drug use, in particular, can reduce tension imme-diately, by evoking relaxation and a rewarding experience. If applied repeatedly, there is an increased risk of transition from casual use to addiction. The close link between chronic stress and the consumption of stress-relieving substances points to shared pathways in the brain limbic structures that govern reward responses (mesolimbic dopaminergic systems) (Roche et al. 2017). At the level of epidemiological investigations, a couple of longitudinal studies demonstrate elevated risks of health-adverse behaviours, including use of addictive substances, among employed populations exposed to stressful psychosocial work environments. Some of these findings are documented in Chapter 6.

In view of the critical role of coping within the pathways linking exposure to work stressors with workers' health, we need to clarify how the main work stress models discussed in this chapter deal with the concept of coping. When reviewing the demand-control model and the organizational justice model, it appears that coping efforts or coping capabilities are not part of their explanatory frameworks. These models can be labelled black-box models as personal characteristics are excluded from the analysis. This exclusion can be justified by the argument that demonstrating a direct association between exposure and health outcome is the primary task of scientific analysis in this field. However, including information on coping can enrich the models' explanatory contribution. Thus, the effort-reward imbalance model and the job demands-resources model explicitly include personal characteristics in their concepts, in line with basic propositions of stress research. In the former model, 'over-commitment' has been introduced as a motivational pattern of coping with work demands, and its role was specified in two hypotheses. The first states that scoring high on this intrinsic characteristic is an independent risk factor for reduced health, whereas the second maintains that scoring high on over-commitment modifies the effect of effort-reward imbalance on health. In the job demands-resources model, the role of coping is emphasized by the introduction of the category of 'personal resources' into a frame that initially only considered characteristics of the work environment. According to a review of this model, personal resources act in various ways as coping characteristics: they may exert a direct effect on health; they may moderate or mediate the relation between job features and health; and they may influence the perception of job characteristics (Schaufeli and Taris 2014). By proposing several personal resources (e.g. self-efficacy, optimism, self-esteem), this model adds complexity to the analysis. This short commentary on differences between the four theoretical models with respect to the inclusion or exclusion of personal coping factors reveals an urgent need to extend the theoretical discussion between sociologically and psychologically oriented researchers in this field.

To summarize, the way working people address the challenges in their job has a decisive impact on psychobiological stress responses and their consequences for health. Given a prominent role for psycho-mental and socio-emotional demands in the modern world of work, coping efforts usually cannot result in a depletion of physical energy. Rather, autonomic arousal persists, requiring problem-solving strategies that mobilize workers' thoughts, emotions, motivations, and actions. Successful coping is largely contingent on the working persons' competences and skills and on the availability of material and social resources. Conversely, unsuccessful coping attempts increase susceptibility to consumption of stress-relieving substances that offer instantaneous relaxation and reward, while augmenting the risk of addiction in the longer run. In view of a critical role of these direct and indirect ways of coping with work-related stressors, a final paragraph briefly discussed whether and how the main work stress models presented in this chapter deal with this topic. Two models exclude the concept of coping from their analysis, whereas two other models enrich their explanatory framework by integrating distinct personal coping characteristics in the analysis.

3.4 Summary

This chapter laid the conceptual ground for subsequent parts of the book. By elaborating core terms and mechanisms of the stress process, by comparing four main models of psychosocial work environments with relevance to health, and by discussing the role of coping with demands and threats at work, this chapter offers essential knowledge enabling students and professionals to advance their understanding and their analytical skills in dealing with the complexities of modern work and their impact on workers' health.

3.5 Relevant questions

- Why is it important to introduce theoretical models in research on psychosocial work environments and their effects on health?
- Some, but not all theoretical models mentioned include information on coping with the burden of work. What are the main arguments in favour of including this information?

- In view of far-reaching, recent changes in the nature of work and employment relationships, which relevant aspects have not received adequate attention in the models discussed in this chapter?

Recommended reading

❖ Berkman, L. F., Kawachi, I., and Theorell, T. (2014), 'Working conditions and health'. In L. F. Berkman, I. Kawachi, and M. M. Glymour (eds.), *Social epidemiology*. Oxford: Oxford University Press, 153–81.

❖ Fink, G. (ed.), (2016), *Stress: concepts, cognition, emotion, and behavior*. London: Academic Press.

❖ Kivimäki, M., Batty, G. D., Kawachi, I., et al. (2018), *The Routledge international handbook of psychosocial epidemiology*. Abingdon, New York, NY: Routledge/ Taylor & Francis Group.

Useful websites

❖ International Labour Organization (ILO): Psychosocial risks and work-related stress. https://www.ilo.org/safework/areasofwork/workplace-health-promotion-and-well-being/WCMS_108557/lang--en/index.htm

❖ European Foundation for the Improvement of Living and Working Conditions (Eurofound): Work-related stress. https://www.eurofound.europa.eu/publi cations/report/2010/work-related-stress

❖ American Psychological Association (APA): Coping with stress at work. https://www.apa.org/topics/healthy-workplaces/work-stress

❖ Job Content Questionnaire (JCQ) center. https://www.jcqcenter.com/

❖ Effort-Reward Imbalance (ERI) website. https://www.uniklinik-duesseldorf. de/patienten-besucher/klinikeninstitutezentren/institut-fuer-medizinische-soziologie/das-institut/forschung/the-eri-model-stress-and-health

❖ Job Demands-Resources (JD-R). https://de.wikipedia.org/wiki/Job-Dema nds-Resources-Modell

References

Adams, J. S. (1965), 'Inequity in social exchange'. In B. Leonard (ed.), *Advances in experimental social psychology*, vol. 2. New York: Academic, 267–99.

Bakker, A. B., and Demerouti, E. (2017), 'Job demands-resources theory: taking stock and looking forward', *J Occup Health Psychol*, 22 (3), 273–85.

Berkman, L. F., Kawachi, I., and Theorell, T. (2014), 'Working conditions and health'. In L. F. Berkman, I. Kawachi, and M. M. Glymour (eds.), *Social epidemiology*. Oxford: Oxford University Press, 153–81.

Besedovsky, H. O., and Del Rey, A. (2007), 'Physiology of psychoneuroimmunology: a personal view', *Brain Behav Immun*, 21 (1), 34–44.

Bierhaus, A., Wolf, J., Andrassy, M., et al. (2003), 'A mechanism converting psychosocial stress into mononuclear cell activation', *Proc Natl Acad Sci USA*, 100 (4), 1920–5.

Bies, R. J., and Moag, J. S. (1986), 'Interactional justice: communication criteria for fairness'. In B. Sheppard (ed.), *Research on negotiation in organizational behavior* vol. 1. Greenwich, CT: JAI Press, 43–55.

Blackburn, E., and Epel, E. (2017), *The telomere effect: a revolutionary approach to living younger, healthier, longer*. New York, NY: Grand Central Publishing.

Bodin, T., Caglayan, C., Garde, A. H., et al. (2020), 'Precarious employment in occupational health - an OMEGA-NET working group position paper', *Scand J Work Environ Health*, 46 (3), 321–29.

Brough, P., Timms, C., Chan, X. W., et al. (2020), 'Work-life balance: definitions, causes, and consequences'. In T. Theorell (ed.), *Handbook of socioeconomic determinants of occupational health: from macro-level to micro-level evidence*. Cham: Springer, 473–87.

Cannon, W. B. (1929), *Bodily changes in pain, hunger, fear, and rage* 2 edn. New York, NY: D. Appleton.

Chandola, T., Kuper, H., Singh-Manoux, A., et al. (2004), 'The effect of control at home on CHD events in the Whitehall II study: gender differences in psychosocial domestic pathways to social inequalities in CHD', *So Sci Med*, 58 (8), 1501–09.

Chrousos, G. P., and Gold, P. W. (1992), 'The concepts of stress and stress system disorders: overview of physical and behavioral homeostasis', *JAMA*, 267 (9), 1244–52.

Cockburn, W. (2021), 'OSH in the future: where next?', *Europ J Workplace Innov*, 6 (1), 84–97.

Colquitt, J. A., and Rodell, J. B. (2015), 'Measuring justice and fairness'. In R. Cropanzano and M. L. Ambrose (eds.), *The Oxford handbook of justice in the workplace*. New York: Oxford University Press, 187–202.

Cooper, C. L., and Quick, J. C. (eds.) (2017), *The handbook of stress and health*. Chichester: Wiley Blackwell.

Cunningham, C. J. L., and Black, K. J. (2021), *Essentials of occupational health psychology*. New York, NY: Routledge.

Demerouti, E., Bakker, A. B., Nachreiner, F., et al. (2001), 'The job demands-resources model of burnout', *J Appl Psychol*, 86 (3), 499–512.

Diebig, M., Müller, A., and Angerer, P. (2020), 'Impact of the digitalization in the industry sector on work, employment, and health'. In T. Theorell (ed.), *Handbook of socioeconomic determinants of occupational health: from macro-level to micro-level evidence*. Cham: Springer, 305–19.

Dollard, M. F., Dormann, C., and Idris, M. A. (2019), *Psychosocial safety climate: a new work stress theory*. Cham: Springer.

Donnelly, R. (2022), 'Precarious work in midlife: long-term implications for the health and mortality of women and men', *J Health Soc Behav*, 63 (1), 142–58.

Edwards, J. R., Caplan, R. D., and Van Harrison, R. (1998), 'Person-environment fit theory'. In C. L. Cooper (ed.), *Theories of organizational stress*. Oxford: Oxford University Press, 28–67.

Eib, C., Leineweber, C., and Bernhard-Oettel, C. (2022), 'Fairness at work'. In P. Brough, E. Gardiner, and K. Daniels (eds.), *Handbook on management and employment practices*. Cham: Springer Nature International Publications, 285–310.

Elias, N. (2000), *The civilizing process (revised edition)*. Oxford: Blackwell.

Elovainio, M., and Virtanen, M. (2020), 'Organizational justice and health'. In T. Theorell (ed.), *Handbook of socioeconomic determinants of occupational health: from macro-level to micro-level evidence*. Cham: Springer, 383–96.

Elovainio, M., Kivimäki, M., and Vahtera, J. (2002), 'Organizational justice: evidence of a new psychosocial predictor of health', *Am J Public Health*, 92 (1), 105–8.

Eurofound (2019), 'Working conditions and workers' health', (Luxembourg: Publications Office of the European Union).

Eurofound (2021), 'Working conditions and sustainable work: an analysis using the job quality framework. ', (Luxembourg: Publications Office of the European Union).

Fink, G. (ed.), (2016), *Stress: concepts, cognition, emotion, and behavior*. London: Academic Press.

Frankenhaeuser, M., and Gardell, B. (1976), 'Underload and overload in working life: outline of a multidisciplinary approach', *J Human Stress*, 2 (3), 35–46.

Furman, D., Campisi, J., Verdin, E., et al. (2019), 'Chronic inflammation in the etiology of disease across the life span', *Nat Med*, 25 (12), 1822–32.

Gädin, K. G., and Hammarström, A. (2000), 'School-related health: a cross-sectional study among young boys and girls', *Int J Health Serv*, 30 (4), 797–820.

Ghaemi Kerahrodi, J., and Michal, M. (2020), 'The fear-defense system, emotions, and oxidative stress', *Redox Biol*, 37, 101588.

Glymour, M. M., and Kubzansky, L. D. (2018), 'Causal inference in psychosocial epidemiology'. In M. Kivimäki, G. D. Batty, A. Steptoe, and I. Kawachi (eds.), *The Routledge international handbook of psychosocial epidemiology*. Abingdon, New York, NY: Routledge/Taylor & Francis Group, 21–45.

Gouldner, A. W. (1960), 'The norm of reciprocity: a preliminary statement', *Am Soc Rev*, 25 (2), 161–78.

Greenberg, J., and Colquitt, J. A. (2005), *Handbook of organizational justice*. New York, NY, London: LEA/Taylor & Francis Group.

Greenberg, J., and Cohen, J. R. (eds.) (1982), *Equity and justice in social behaviour*. New York: Academic.

Henry, J. P., and Stephens, P. A. (1977), *Stress, health, and the social environment*. New York: Springer.

Hernandez Lallement, J., Kuss, K., Trautner, P., et al. (2014), 'Effort increases sensitivity to reward and loss magnitude in the human brain', *Soc Cogn Affect Neurosci*, 9 (3), 342–9.

Hill, A. B. (1965), 'The environment and disease: association or causation?', *Proc R Soc Med*, 58, 295–300.

Hobfoll, S. E. (1989), 'Conservation of resources. A new attempt at conceptualizing stress', *Am Psychol*, 44 (3), 513–24.

Hobfoll, S. E., Tirone, V., Holmgreen, L., et al. (2016), 'Conservation of resources theory applied to major stress'. In G. Fink (ed.), *Stress: concepts, cognition, emotion, and behavior* London: Academic Press, 65–71.

Johnson, J. V., and Hall, E. M. (1988), 'Job strain, work place social support, and cardiovascular disease: a cross-sectional study of a random sample of the Swedish working population', *Am J Public Health*, 78 (10), 1336–42.

Karasek, R. A. (1979), 'Job demands, job decision latitude, and mental strain: implications for job redesign', *Adm Sci Q*, 24 (2), 285–308.

Karasek, R. A. (2020), 'The associationalist demand-control (ADC) theory'. In T. Theorell (ed.), *Handbook of socioeconomic determinants of occupational health: from macro-level to micro-level evidence*. Cham: Springer, 573–610.

Karasek, R. A., and Theorell, T. (1990), *Healthy work: stress, productivity and the reconstruction of working life*. New York: Basic Books.

Kivimäki, M., Batty, G. D., Kawachi, I., et al. (2018), *The Routledge international handbook of psychosocial epidemiology*. Abingdon, New York, NY: Routledge/ Taylor & Francis Group.

Kniffin, K. M., Narayanan, J., Anseel, F., et al. (2021), 'COVID-19 and the workplace: implications, issues, and insights for future research and action', *Am Psychol*, 76 (1), 63–77.

Koolhaas, J. M., Bartolomucci, A., Buwalda, B., et al. (2011), 'Stress revisited: a critical evaluation of the stress concept', *Neurosci Biobehav Rev*, 35 (5), 1291–301.

Kornhauser, A. (1965), *The mental health of the industrial worker: a Detroit study*. New York, NY: John Wiley & Sons.

Koutsikou, S., Watson, T. C., Crook, J. J., et al. (2015), 'The periaqueductal gray orchestrates sensory and motor circuits at multiple levels of the neuraxis', *J Neurosci*, 35 (42), 14132–47.

Kouvonen, A., Kivimäki, M., Vahtera, J., et al. (2006), 'Psychometric evaluation of a short measure of social capital at work', *BMC Public Health*, 6, 251.

Kreshpaj, B., Orellana, C., Burström, B., et al. (2020), 'What is precarious employment? A systematic review of definitions and operationalizations from quantitative and qualitative studies', *Scand J Work, Environ Health*, 46 (3), 235–47.

Kristensen, T. S., Hannerz, H., Hogh, A., et al. (2005), 'The Copenhagen Psychosocial Questionnaire, a tool for the assessment and improvement of the psychosocial work environment', *Scand J Work Environ Health*, 31 (6), 438–49.

Lazarus, R. S., and Folkman, S. (1984), *Stress, appraisal and coping*. New York, NY: Springer.

LeDoux, J., and Daw, N. D. (2018), 'Surviving threats: neural circuit and computational implications of a new taxonomy of defensive behaviour', *Nat Rev Neurosci*, 19 (5), 269–82.

Leineweber, C., Eib, C., Bernhard-Oettel, C., et al. (2020), 'Trajectories of effort-reward imbalance in Swedish workers: differences in demographic and work-related factors and associations with health', *Work Stress*, 34 (3), 238–58.

Lesener, T., Gusy, B., and Wolter, C. (2019), 'The job demands-resources model: a meta-analytic review of longitudinal studies', *Work Stress*, 33 (1), 76–103.

Lovejoy, M., Kelly, E. L., Kubzansky, L. D., et al. (2021), 'Work redesign for the 21st century: promising strategies for enhancing worker well-being', *Am J Public Health*, 111 (10), 1787–95.

Mason, J. W. (1968), 'A review of psychoendocrine research on the pituitary-adrenal cortical system', *Psychosom Med*, 30 (5), 576–607.

McEwen, B. S. (1998), 'Protective and damaging effects of stress mediators', *N Engl J Med*, 338 (3), 171–9.

McEwen, B. S. (2016), 'Central role of the brain in stress and adaptation: allostasis, biological embedding, and cumulative change'. In G. Fink (ed.), *Handbook of stress*, vol. 1: Stress: Concepts, Cognition, Emotion, and Behavior. San Diego, CA: Academic Press/Elsevier, 39–55.

Merton, R. K. (1968), *Social theory and social structure*. New York, NY: The Free Press.

Meyer-Lindenberg, A., Domes, G., Kirsch, P., et al. (2011), 'Oxytocin and vasopressin in the human brain: social neuropeptides for translational medicine', *Nat Rev Neurosci*, 12 (9), 524–38.

Moorman, R. H. (1991), 'Relationship between organizational justice and organizational citizenship behaviors: do fairness perceptions influence employee citizenship?', *J Applied Psychol*, 76 (6), 845–55.

Ndjaboué, R., Brisson, C., and Vezina, M. (2012), 'Organisational justice and mental health: a systematic review of prospective studies', *Occup Environ Med*, 69 (10), 694–700.

OECD (2017), *OECD guidelines on measuring the quality of the working environment*. Paris: OECD.

Osborne, M. T., Shin, L. M., Mehta, N. N., et al. (2020), 'Disentangling the links between psychosocial stress and cardiovascular disease', *Circ Cardiovasc*, 13 (8), e010931.

Osborne, M. T., Ishai, A., Hammad, B., et al. (2019), 'Amygdalar activity predicts future incident diabetes independently of adiposity', *Psychoneuroendocrinology*, 100, 32–40.

Roche, A., Kostadinov, V., and Fischer, J. (2017), 'Stress and addiction'. In C. L. Cooper and J. C. Quick (eds.), *The handbook of stress and health: a guide to research and practice*. Chichester: Wiley Blackwell, 252–79.

Schaufeli, W. B., and Taris, T. W. (2014), 'A critical review of the job demands-resources model: implications for improving work and health'. In G. F. Bauer and O. Hämmig (eds.), *Bridging occupational, organizational and public health*. Cham: Springer, 43–68.

Schultz, W. (2006), 'Behavioral theories and the neurophysiology of reward', *Annu Rev Psychol*, 57, 87–115.

Selye, H. (1936), 'A syndrome produced by diverse nocuous agents', *J Neuropsychiatry Clin Neurosci*, 138, 32.

Semmer, N. K. (2020), 'Conflict and offense to self'. In T. Theorell (ed.), *Handbook of socioeconomic determinants of occupational health: from macro-level to micro-level evidence*. Cham: Springer, 1–31.

Siegrist, J. (1996), 'Adverse health effects of high-effort/low-reward conditions', *J Occup Health Psychol*, 1 (1), 27–41.

Siegrist, J., and Wahrendorf, M. (2016), 'A theoretical model in the context of economic globalization'. In J. Siegrist and M. Wahrendorf (eds.), *Work stress and health in a globalized economy*. Cham: Springer, 3–19.

Sonnentag, S., and Fritz, C. (2015), 'Recovery from job stress: the stressor-detachment model as an integrative framework', *J Organ Behav*, 36 (S1), S72–S103.

Steptoe, A. (2006), 'Psychobiological processes linking socio-economic position with health'. In J. Siegrist and M. Marmot (eds.), *Social inequalities in health: new evidence and policy implications*. Oxford: Oxford University Press, 101–26.

Steptoe, A., and Poole, L. (2016), 'Control and stress'. In G. Fink (ed.), *Handbook of stress, vol. 1: Stress: Concepts, Cognition, Emotion, and Behavior*. San Diego, CA: Academic/Elsevier, 73–80.

Stringhini, S., Polidoro, S., Sacerdote, C., et al. (2015), 'Life-course socioeconomic status and DNA methylation of genes regulating inflammation', *Int J Epidemiol*, 44 (4), 1320–30.

Tawakol, A., Ishai, A., Takx, R. A. P., et al. (2017), 'Relation between resting amygdalar activity and cardiovascular events: a longitudinal and cohort study', *Lancet*, 389 (10071), 834–45.

Thayer, J. F., Ahs, F., Fredrikson, M., et al. (2012), 'A meta-analysis of heart rate variability and neuroimaging studies: implications for heart rate variability as a marker of stress and health', *Neurosci Biobehav Rev*, 36 (2), 747–56.

Theorell, T. (2016), 'Reward, flow and control at work'. In J. Siegrist and M. Wahrendorf (eds.), *Work stress and health in a globalized economy*. Cham: Springer, 315–32.

Theorell, T. (ed.), (2020), *Handbook of socioeconomic determinants of occupational health: from macro-level to micro-level evidence*. Cham: Springer.

Tricomi, E., Rangel, A., Camerer, C. F., et al. (2010), 'Neural evidence for inequality-averse social preferences', *Nature*, 463 (7284), 1089–91.

Wahrendorf, M., Hoven, H., Goldberg, M., et al. (2019), 'Adverse employment histories and health functioning: the CONSTANCES study', *Int J Epidemiol*, 48 (2), 402–14.

Wahrendorf, M., Chandola, T., and Descatha, A. (eds.) (2023), *Handbook of life course occupational health*. Cham: Springer.

Warr, P. B. (1987), *Work, unemployment, and mental health*. Oxford: Oxford Univresity Press.

Warr, P. B. (2017), 'Happiness and mental health'. In C. L. Cooper and J. C. Quick (eds.), *The handbook of stress and health*. Chichester: Wiley Blackwell, 57–74.

Weaver, I. C., Cervoni, N., Champagne, F. A., et al. (2004), 'Epigenetic programming by maternal behavior', *Nat Neurosci*, 7 (8), 847–54.

Weiner, H. (1992), *Perturbing the organism: the biology of stressful experience*. Chicago, ILL: University of Chicago press.

Wilcox, A., and Koontz, A. (2022), 'Workplace well-being: shifting from an individual to an organizational framework', *Sociology Compass*, 16 (10), e13035.

4
Measurement, methods, data collection, and study designs

4.1 Measuring psychosocial work environments

4.1.1 Basic notions

Scientific statements are based on data representing empirical facts. They are open to independent confirmation or rejection. This principle is termed 'intersubjectivity'. To this end, the terms or elements of a scientific statement need to be operationalized as variables. A variable represents a unit of observation that is expressed in discrete or continuous form. In the former case, its characteristics are classified into two or more distinct categories. If classified exclusively into two categories, a variable is termed 'binary' or 'dichotomous'. If expressed as a continuous variable, the unit is indicated along a spectrum of quantitative differences (e.g. time as measured in seconds). Importantly, 'measurement' is the systematic attribution of numbers to the characteristics of a variable. This attribution can be performed at different scale levels. A scale defines the quality of the relationship between the characteristics of a variable and the numbers attributed to them. The following scale levels are distinguished:

- **Nominal scale**: Numbers indicate distinct, mutually exclusive categories of a variable, without specifying their relationships. Data analysis is restricted to the frequency of categories. Examples of nominal scale data are blood group and employment status.
- **Ordinal scale**: Numbers indicate differences between categories of a variable along an order, without assuming equal distance between the categories. Data analysis does not allow monotonous transformation, such as addition, subtraction, or arithmetic mean. Examples of ordinal scale data are school marks, educational degrees, or any characteristic

Psychosocial Occupational Health. Johannes Siegrist and Jian Li, Oxford University Press.
© Oxford University Press 2024. DOI: 10.1093/oso/9780192887924.003.0004

with differences in intensity or quality that lack a measure of equal distance.

- **Metric scale:** Numbers indicate differences between categories of a variable along an order by defining an equal distance between them. Full numbers represent equal distance between categories, based on a calibrated metric. If a metric scale includes a natural 'zero' point (e.g. zero degree temperature), it is termed 'ratio scale'. In all other cases, the term interval scale is used. Data analysis is open to all basic statistical procedures (mean, median, etc.) Examples of metric scale data are seconds or minutes (time), metres (space), or Euros (money).

In basic sciences, metric scales represent the standard of measurement. However, in the social and behavioural sciences, many phenomena under study lack a calibrated metric (see 4.1.2.1.2). Moreover, the range of variables representing observable facts that can be quantified along the scales mentioned is limited. Many properties or features of interest are not accessible to direct observation. Rather, they indicate latent phenomena that are measured indirectly, by distinct indicators describing an underlying latent construct. 'Intelligence' is an example of a latent psychological construct. Its indicators are usually assessed by a standardized test measuring core cognitive abilities. 'Social class' is an example of a latent sociological construct. Its conventional measurement applies one or several indicators of people's socioeconomic standing in the hierarchy of differences in income, education, and occupational position. When applying more than one indicator to this measurement, an index needs to be constructed. If measured by more than one indicator, a latent construct is assessed by an index, a test, or a psychometric scale (see 4.1.2.1).

Whatever the scale level of scientific data, they need to meet the substantial quality criteria of reliability and validity. Reliability indicates the degree of accuracy of a measurement. For instance, high reliability is achieved if the results of a series of repeated measurements are highly consistent. Equally so, reliability is high if the results of a measurement obtained from different researchers are highly consistent. A special case of reliability concerns the quality of psychometric scales, where a high degree of internal consistency between scale items is given. This criterion is measured by Cronbach's Alpha, which indicates the strength of correlations between items of a scale (intra-correlation). Reliability is a precondition but not a proof of validity. The notion of validity refers to the degree to which the measurement of a phenomenon truly represents this phenomenon. To this end, the aspects of content, construct, and criterion validity are distinguished. Content validity requires an external judgment about the adequacy of a respective measurement. Often, expert judgments are used to assess content validity. As mentioned, latent constructs are often used in social and behavioural sciences. One way of examining the accuracy of operationalizing a construct is defined by the convergent validity. In this case, the same construct is measured by different methods (e.g. survey and experiment), and coherent results of both measurements indicate high convergent validity. At the same time, the validity of differences between similar, but not identical constructs needs to be examined as well. To this end, procedures of discriminant validity are applied. Criterion validity describes a further relevant aspect as it requires a high amount of agreement of a measurement with an independent but closely associated criterion. For instance, the theory of psychosocial stress at work assumes that significantly elevated disease risks result from this exposure. If this holds true for separate measurements of work stress, these assessments are considered valid in terms of criterion validity. Finally, in view of the fact that many phenomena change over time, a further criterion of validity relates to the ability of a measurement to indicate such changes over time. A successful empirical test of this assumption confirms high sensitivity to change.

The content of this part of the chapter is divided into three sections. Firstly, the measurement of psychosocial work environments is described in terms of self-reported (subjective) assessment. Here, the main part is devoted to quantitative methods, and the rest to qualitative methods. Secondly, independent (objective) measures are presented, with a focus on observational ratings and job exposure matrices. A final section deals with core methodological questions.

4.1.2 Self-reported (subjective) measures

In line with a biopsychosocial framework of analysis, and as explained in the conceptual model depicted in Figure 1.1, psychosocial work environments are composed of a variety of dimensions. Some of these dimensions are easily observable and can be objectively assessed as facts, by answering factual questions. The size of a company, its economic standing, the composition of and fluctuation in its workforce, wage and salary differences, or the division of work tasks are examples. Other dimensions are less easily observable, such as competition between employees, conflicts between managers and subordinates, work pressure, job insecurity, unfair treatment, or lack of social support. As these latter dimensions matter for workers' affective and psychobiological responses, the researcher has to rely on the working persons' experiences and appraisal of these dimensions. In fact, in line with substantial evidence from basic stress research, the working person's interpretation of his or her working situation exerts a crucial impact on the quality and intensity of affective and psychobiological responses to the stressor at work (see Chapter 3). Therefore, the collection of self-reported information on the perceived and appraised work environment represents a methodological approach of outstanding significance. At the same time, using self-reported information as scientific data provides a methodological challenge that needs to be critically discussed.

We describe the two main methodological traditions of assessing self-reported, subjective information on psychosocial work environments from working people, the quantitative and the qualitative tradition. The main difference between these two traditions concerns the role of the two participants, the researcher and the responding person, in defining the research content. According to the quantitative methodology, the research content—the questions to be asked and the way they are answered, the content and sequence of statements offered for response—is predefined by the scientist. It represents the operationalization of concepts and hypotheses derived from the state of art in this field. To this end, a high degree of standardization of the data collection process is required to ensure comparability and reliability of information. Ideally, each category of answer is given a numerical value, such that a system of empirical relations can be transformed into a system of numerical relations. It is this latter system that defines the essence of results derived from quantitative analysis. In the qualitative methodology, the researcher communicates with his or her respondent in a much more open way. Prepared by a set of research questions and interests, the researcher leaves much more room for the respondent's views, thoughts, and feelings in answering questions. The aim is to deepen the understanding of the topic under study and to seek new insights by carefully analysing the content of the dialogue that is usually tape-recorded and analysed ex post by the researcher. Despite these differences, the two approaches are often combined. For instance, a pre-test is conducted with a qualitative approach to explore the feasibility of a standardized assessment. As an alternative, the findings of a quantitative study fail to offer substantial new insights, therefore requiring a supplementary qualitative inquiry.

4.1.2.1 Quantitative methods

4.1.2.1.1 Standardized questionnaires

Answering standardized questionnaires represents the essential method of data collection used in quantitative social and behavioural science research, as applied to occupational health. This method is available in two forms, either as an oral interview conducted between the researcher and the responding person, or as a survey. In this latter case, data are collected in written form by self-administration of the responding person. Interviews are realized as face-to-face communication or as telephone interviews. Surveys using self-completion questionnaires are sent to study participants by mail, or they are distributed to them at a convenient place, such as the worksite or a screening centre. To date, internet-based surveys using a software procedure are applied more and more frequently (Bethlehem and Biffignandi 2011). Online-based surveys are increasingly administered via mobile phones and tablets, thus requiring technical and layout adaptation.

Each method of data collection has specific strengths and weaknesses that are discussed in detail by a rich methodological research literature (Dillman et al. 2014). Notably, the choice of a method is contingent on the research topic and on the opportunities and constraints of conducting an empirical research project. For instance, in occupational health research, epidemiologic studies that require a large number of participants are often applied. In these cases, face-to-face interviews may be too costly in terms of time and costs. As another example, disclosing sensitive information, for instance on bullying and harassment at work, may be more difficult in a face-to-face interview than in the anonymous context of providing written self-completion answers. On the other hand, if a research question requires an active role of the participants by providing feedback and expression of own opinions, a direct communication by interview is indicated. To date, the computer-assisted telephone interview (CATI) offers an ideal method to this end as responses can be recorded immediately by the interviewer, and queries can be clarified by further conversation. Computer-assisted devices are equally used as in face-to-face (personal) interviews (CAPI) and in video-guided interviews (CAVI).

It is the quality of a standardized questionnaire that matters most in this area of research (see Box 4.1). This type of questionnaire is composed by a series of questions or statements that require answers in pre-defined categories. If the response to a statement requires a judgment beyond 'yes' or 'no', by quantifying the degree of acceptance or rejection or the intensity of an experience to be evaluated, then this statement is termed an 'item'. In

Box 4.1 **Quality criteria of questionnaires**

Among the many quality criteria to be observed in designing a questionnaire, the following ones may need particular consideration:

- Bias-free questions/statements: Use neutral terms, avoid value judgments in statements, avoid preference of a distinct answer category;
- Unambiguous meaning of terms: Use simple questions/statements with terms that are well understood in the general population; avoid specialized technical terms;
- Distinction of different types of questions/statements: Use factual questions if the content can be objectively described; use attitudinal or evaluative questions if the content refers to subjective appraisals or judgements;
- Visualisation of questions/statements: Use a vignette illustrating a typical content or providing a reference to a standard if a complex topic needs to be answered;
- Splitting relevant questions/statements into parts: Instead of asking a global question, specify number, duration, cause and consequence of the event in subsequent questions;
- Exhaustive and disjunctive answer categories: Avoid questions/statements requiring two answers; provide an exhaustive list of answer categories that are mutually exclusive;
- Time frame of content: If past events are explored, use a time frame that provides reliable recollection (fair reliability was documented for events that occurred two to three years ago; extraordinary life events are remembered over longer periods of time);
- Sequence of questions: Carefully consider the impact of content on subsequent questions/statements. Assessing self-rated health after a series of questions on adverse working and living conditions may provoke more negative answers;
- Length of questionnaire: To reduce attrition inform and motivate participant. Questionnaires should not exceed ten pages. Attrition accumulates with time used.

this case, specific response formats are available to quantify the information. Such sets of items are mainly used to measure latent constructs. If they meet distinct criteria of statistical proof, they are termed psychometrically validated scales (see below).

As can be seen from this non-exhaustive enumeration of quality aspects the design of a questionnaire is a difficult task requiring careful, dedicated teamwork. It is mandatory to pre-test a questionnaire before its application in a study. Useful guidelines of designing and pre-testing a questionnaire are available for readers requiring more in-depth information (e.g. Beatty et al. 2019; Presser et al. 2004; Willis 2004).

4.1.2.1.2 Psychometric scales

The term 'scale' is not only used to define the different levels of measurement, it also describes a specific method of answering questions or evaluating statements. In this context, a scale is defined as a set of items measuring a construct, answered by an identical form of rating. Ratings are given as judgments on a scale with equal-distanced numbers, where numbers indicate the degree of agreement or disagreement, the frequency or intensity of a condition. Thus, items are answered at the level of an interval scale (see below). The Likert scale is the most widely established rating procedure. Answers are rated, e.g. on a 5-point scale with 5 = fully agree, 4 = agree, 3 = neither agree nor disagree, 2 = disagree, 1 = fully disagree. Another version points to the frequency: 1 = rarely or never, 2 = sometimes, eventually; 3 = often, 4 = very frequently, permanent. In comparative studies 5-point scales have been shown to be the best balance between individual ability to differentiate and precision of measurement. However, this preference depends on socio-cultural contexts. For instance, in an Eastern Asian culture influenced by a religious 'doctrine of the mean' (Confucius), a 4-point scale avoiding 'neither agree nor disagree' may work better (Lee et al. 2002). Similar to the Likert scale, the Visual Analogue Scale offers a line drawn from 0 to 10, where respondents have to indicate the frequency or intensity of the condition. To achieve a summary measure of the set of items measuring a construct, these ratings are summarized to a sum score. This score reflects the severity, frequency, or intensity of the underlying phenomenon. Latent constructs that are measured by scales are composed by different components. Accordingly, scores are calculated for the single components or additionally for the total construct.

Of notice, sets of items are scales to the extent only that they meet distinct psychometric properties (see below). In the social and behavioural sciences, many latent constructs are operationalized by scales. This also holds true for occupational health research, where two types of latent constructs are most often studied. Firstly, many health-related outcomes are measured by scales. Examples are depression (e.g. CES-D scale; Radloff 1977), anxiety (e.g. HADS; Zigmond and Snaith 1983), health functioning (e.g. SF-36; Ware et al. 1994), or burnout (e.g. BAT; Schaufeli et al. 2020). The second type of latent constructs assessed by scales relates to self-reported exposures. In fact, the theoretical models of psychosocial work environments with relevance to health (described in Chapter 3) are measured by psychometrically validated scales (see Box 4.2). Accordingly, scores of these scales indicate summary estimates of the manifestation of single components of a latent construct. Eventually, a score can also indicate the overall manifestation of this construct. For instance, depression as measured by the CES-D scale is composed by a component indicating mental symptoms and a component indicating somatic symptoms. Separate scores for these two components are calculated. In addition, a total score measuring depression is computed (on a range from 0 to 80 points). This sum score can be graded into categories of absence, presence, and severity of depressive symptoms, and it can also be used for clinical decision making, based on a clinically validated cut-off value (>22 points; Radloff 1977). In a similar way, analyses of latent constructs of stressful psychosocial work environments apply scores for single components of these constructs. Based on these scores, summary measures are proposed to operationalize the theoretical construct. For instance, in the demand-control (DC) model (Karasek and Theorell 1990), a combination of scores of the scale 'demand' and the scale 'control' serves to define the risk condition 'job strain' (see Box 4.2). Concerning the measurement of the four theoretical models described in Box 4.2, several versions, including proxy measures, were applied in a variety of studies (see also chapters 3 and 6). Often, such measures were added to pre-existing batteries of questionnaires used in surveys and cohort studies. An excellent collection of survey questions representing scales, sub-scales, or proxies of these models, with particular reference to European data, was prepared and published by an expert team of OECD (OECD 2017).

The measurement of latent constructs in the social and behavioural sciences gave rise—and continues to give rise—to a series of debates and methodological controversies with far-reaching implications. As occupational health researchers, we are not in a position to give an account of these controversies that are the subject of highly specialized experts in psychology and statistics. One of the fundamental problems concerns the

---

Box 4.2 Scales of theoretical models measuring psychosocial wok environments

---

- Demand-control (DC model) (Karasek et al. 1998): Job Content Questionnaire (JCQ) as standard assessment: Psychological demand 5 items; Decision latitude (skill discretion 6 items; decision authority 3 items); Social support (8 items) (4-point Likert agree-disagree). Confirmatory factor analysis (CFA); convergent and criterion validity; standard scores (e.g. Chungkham et al. 2013). As option of a summary measure: 'job strain' from quadrant split half above (demand) or below (latitude) median (Figure 3.1);
- Effort-reward imbalance (ERI model) (Siegrist et al. 2004): Original version: Effort 5 items (without physical effort); Reward 11 items (3 subscales); Over-commitment 6 items. CFA, factorial and criterion validity (CV) with self-rated health. Short version (Leineweber et al. 2010): Effort 3 items; Reward 7 items; Over-commitment 6 items; (4-point Likert agree-disagree); 2nd order CFA; CV with depressive symptoms. As option of a summary measure: Effort-reward ratio;
- Organizational justice (OJ model) (Elovainio et al. 2002): Original version: 2 scales Procedural justice (7 items); Relational justice (6 items) (5-point Likert agree-disagree; derived from Moorman 1991). CV with a number of health indicators. For a further comprehensive measurement, using four dimensions of OJ see Colquitt and Rodell (2015);
- Job demands-resources (JD-R model) (Demerouti et al. 2001): Original version: Demands (D) 5 items; Resources (R) 6 items (4-point Likert-scale agree-disagree; partly based on previous sources); CFA with 2 latent factors (D; R); CV: exhaustion and disengagement (differential prediction of burnout components). Multiple replications (e.g. Lesener et al. 2019).

measurement model underlying the construction of a psychometric scale. Here, two distinct approaches are discussed, a reflexive and a formative model. The former model assumes that answers of an item directly reflect aspects of the latent construct, whereas the formative model allows a modifying effect of answers to an item on the latent construct (Bollen and Lennox 1991). As the classical psychological test theory relies on the reflexive approach, and as this also holds true for scales measuring the main theoretical models of psychosocial work environments, our short description of scale construction follows this classical approach (Cooper 2019). Nevertheless, an important more recent development, the item response theory (IRT) deserves attention (Embretson and Reise 2000). This approach 'represents mathematical functions which relate person and item parameters to the probability of the responses on a discrete outcome, such as a correct response to an item' (Tsutsumi et al. 2008, p. 110), thus improving measurement accuracy and reducing measurement error. This new approach is also useful in dealing with the problem of equal distance between rating categories. In fact, the transformation of ordinal-scaled data to interval scaled data requires a methodological justification, given the absence of a calibrated scale. While such justification can be provided ex post by examining the degree of violation of this assumption in a given data set, applying non-linear main component analysis (Maydeu-Olivares 2005), IRT offers a direct test by "calibrating the scores to a logit scale and then comparing the distances in raw-score units between successive scores on the equal-interval logit scale' (Tsutsumi et al. 2008, p. 116). IRT has eventually been applied to scales measuring psychosocial work stress models. The study of Akizumi Tsutsumi and colleagues (2008) is an instructive example, comparing an early measurement approach to effort-reward imbalance (ERI) at work, based on classical test theory, with item response theory. Findings demonstrated an improved measurement accuracy of scale items and a somewhat improved correlation with depressive symptoms, used as an indicator of criterion validity. This comparison was useful to the authors of the original ERI scales (Siegrist et al. 2004), as it motivated them to develop strictly unidimensional scales (see e.g. Leineweber et al. 2010).

According to classical test theory, scales measuring a latent construct must meet core psychometric quality criteria:

- Components of the construct are represented by unidimensional scales;
- Scales demonstrate a high degree of internal consistency (Cronbach's alpha > 0.70), test-retest reliability, and/or split-half reliability;
- The theoretical construct is adequately represented by the factorial structure of the scales, as documented by confirmatory factor analysis with adequate fit indices;

- Content, construct, and criterion validity of the scales or their summary measure are demonstrated by independent replications;
- If scales are applied over time, the changes of their score are valid (sensitivity to change);
- If applied across different samples or different times, the equivalence of factor loadings and factorial structure of the construct is confirmed (factorial validity).

To conclude, psychometrically validated scales measuring latent constructs of self-reported exposures, and in particular theoretical models of stressful work environments, play a crucial role in psychosocial occupational health research. As a large proportion of empirical results is based on this measurement approach (see Chapters 6 and 7), its accuracy is of outstanding importance. Although further improvements at the methodological level are required, the current state of scales implemented in this field of research provides a robust evidence base (for a comprehensive textbook, see Finch and French 2018).

4.1.2.1.3 Ecological momentary assessment

The methods of quantitative data collection described so far share a common methodological problem: they ask participants to respond to a predefined instrument by answering questions at a certain time point (the date of an interview or the deadline for completing a questionnaire). This approach assumes that in answering the questions or statements, participants usually refer to their current (or a typical) working situation. Sometimes, the time frame is specified in the text (e.g. 'summarizing your experience over the past twelve months'). However, it remains unknown whether answers provided by the participants share a common time frame of reported experiences. In addition, we do not know to what extent contextual influences at the time of answering the questions interfere with the appraisal of working conditions. These sources of bias remain uncontrolled. Therefore, a supplementary methodological approach termed 'ecological momentary assessment' (EMA) was developed (Shiffman et al. 2008). It defines a standardized time frame to which the participant's appraisal of working conditions refers. This can be an instantaneous assessment in a real life setting during a working day or at the end of a working day. Furthermore, it enables participants to conduct repeated assessments of their work experience (e.g. over a week), thus providing detailed information on the stability of assessments and their change over time. With the use of advanced technology (e.g. smartphones), brief inventories of stressful work environments and participants' responses can be filled in. This methodological innovation has also been applied to main models of psychosocial work environments.

In a real-time study with digital-assistant-based EMA, Derek W. Johnston and his team collected short work stress measures every 90 minutes over three shifts in a group of 254 nurses (Johnston et al. 2013). Features of the DC and ERI models were monitored in combination with scales measuring positive and negative affect. Fixed effects derived from multilevel linear modelling showed an increase of negative affect with increasing demand/effort and decreasing control at work. In addition, control moderated the effect of demand/effort. Reward was associated with increased positive affect, and it moderated the effect of demand/effort as predicted (Johnston et al. 2013; see also Chapter 5).

To summarize, quantitative methods of collecting self-reported data on working conditions with relevance to health offer a wide spectrum of standardized approaches (questionnaires as applied by interviews or surveys, psychometric scales, EMA). Their choice depends on the study aim and the research opportunities. Up to now, they represent the mainstream method of psychosocial occupational health research, in particular of epidemiological investigations. Their strengths and limitations need to be carefully considered (see below).

4.1.2.2 Qualitative methods

The principal difference between quantitative and qualitative methodology concerns the sequence between the two steps of defining scientific statements and collecting data. As mentioned, in the former case, scientific statements or hypotheses are predefined by the researcher, and the process of data collection serves to examine their validity by confirmation or rejection. In qualitative research, the two steps are intertwined. While the researcher starts data collection with a prepared mind, defining core questions and core topics of interest, the dialogue is much more open, and the counterpart's views and experiences are valued as potential contributions to the researcher's progress of scientific understanding. Therefore, the ideal qualitative interview is a face-to-face communication based on mutual trust and openness, guided by the researcher's empathy. The communication should aim at providing rich and dense information without narrowing the content by formal prescriptions. To this end, qualitative interviews are usually recorded, and their content analysis performed by the researcher after data collection provides essential scientific insights.

Interpretation of content is the common link between different types of qualitative research. For instance, this method can be applied in the analysis of written documents (e.g. diaries, protocols) and in the analysis of communication recorded during sessions of focus groups. A focus group is defined as an open-ended interview by an expert or coordinator with a small homogeneous group of participants that aims at exploring different views on a common topic and at gaining insights by contrasting opinions and reflections. The outcomes of these groups are particularly helpful at two stages of the research process, first in the exploratory phase of developing a research plan, and second, following termination of data analysis when results are to be translated into practice.

The crucial step of data analysis in qualitative research deserves closer consideration as it deviates remarkably from quantitative procedures. Extensive reviews of this topic are available for more information (Corbin and Strauss 2015; Denzin and Lincoln 2011; Schreier 2012). Here, we briefly refer to the following essential aspects:

- To provide a systematic interpretation of a written text the researcher needs to develop a categorical framework. Categories are delineated at a level of generalization that allows for their application to a broad range of statements contained in the text. This application is termed 'coding';
- Coding is expected to be performed according to some defined principles. Ideally, the coding process is performed by two independent researchers in order to assess the reliability of this procedure;
- Reducing the complexity of content by coding its essential elements and by comparing the categories of coding and their relations across a variety of texts enables the researcher to obtain new insights that stimulate theoretical reasoning;
- To this end, it is important to generate a certain heterogeneity of content by including subgroups into the sample that differ in their views and attitudes on the topic under study;
- As a result, qualitative methods, if compared to quantitative methods, offer a more comprehensive understanding of the phenomena under study, based on the researcher's reconstruction and interpretation of actors' perspectives;
- Important quality criteria of quantitative research, in particular replication, reliability, validity, and generalizability of findings, are not easily met by qualitative methodology.

To our knowledge, there are not many qualitative studies of psychosocial work environments with relevance to health. A narrative approach to understanding nursing work serves as example (McGillis Hall and Kiesners 2005). In this study, eight nurses were extensively interviewed to detail their work experience, with the researchers' interest in elucidating the experience of ERI at work. One of the findings emphasized the relevance of esteem received from patients for satisfying care, and the nurses' feelings of frustration and guilt due to a high workload preventing the delivery of high-quality care. Obviously, the few standard questions of the original ERI questionnaire would fail to capture these detailed observations obtained from a qualitative method. On the other hand, it remains unknown how robust and generalizable these few observations are. When deciding about the choice of applying a method, researchers need to be aware of these strengths and weaknesses.

4.1.3 Independent (objective) measures

4.1.3.1 Observation

Independent assessment of work environments can be realized in different forms. An original, rarely used, and controversial approach is represented by participant observation. In this case, the researcher, as observer, takes an active role as collaborator in a work setting he or she is observing. For ethical reasons, this role has to be declared to the other persons (overt observation). Due to the researcher's active involvement, observations are selective, non-systematic, and biased by this role, and their independent replication is not possible. Data collection is restricted to some field notes or reports after work shifts. For these reasons, the scientific quality of this method is limited, and its application may be restricted to rare and exceptional circumstances. Differing from this approach, systematic non-participant observation has been developed as an important alternative method of assessing material and psychosocial work environments, based on objective rather than subjective judgments. Here, the researcher is introduced to the field with an unambiguous role, and the research aims are openly disclosed. The observation process is highly standardized, based on a prepared set of categories to be monitored. Systematic observation can be performed simultaneously by two or more observers, thus providing information on the reliability of measurement. Moreover, by training observers to correctly categorize observations, data quality can be improved. Although this method is costly and time-consuming, it has been—and continues to be—successfully applied in occupational health research. Three examples support this conclusion.

Firstly, an observational instrument based on Action Regulation Theory is of special interest in this context (Hacker 1994). Focusing on the mental structure of work tasks it assesses requirements for skill utilization and hindrances (work barriers) to identify stressful experiences at work. The instrument consists of a combination of a protocol-guided on-site observation by trained experts and interview questions. In an updated version, it was applied, among others, in a study of hypertension among bus drivers in San Francisco (Greiner et al. 2004). Of interest, externally assessed observational data on task features were compared with the bus drivers' self-reported appraisal of stressful work. The findings indicated a significant association between observed work barriers and hypertension, whereas self-reported data were unrelated to hypertension. In a second landmark study, the British Whitehall II study of civil servants, the degree of job control was assessed by two complementary methods, a standardized measurement of the relevant scale of the Job Content Questionnaire, and an independent rating of each individual job by skilled personnel managers (Bosma et al. 1997). Although the correlation between the two assessments was moderate, both measures were successful in predicting significantly increased relative risks of incident ischaemic heart disease events, with estimates of similar magnitude. The wording of the question to be rated by observers was, 'How often does the job permit complete discretion and independence in determining how, and when, the work is to be done?' (Bosma et al. 1997, p. 564). However, the paper presenting the results did not describe how exactly the observer rating was accomplished. As a third example, a German study of employees from the health and finance sector was conducted to compare observer ratings of job tasks' demand and control with self-reported data (Rau et al. 2010). The sample was divided into a group with documented past or present depression and a disease-free group, and the hypothesis was tested whether the two work stress components of the DC model were significantly different between these two groups. Ten rating scales based on Action Regulation Theory were applied, and trained job analysists rated each single workplace. The main finding indicated that observer-based demands, but not control, significantly predicted disease status. Moreover, this effect was partly mediated by self-rated job demands.

The three study findings support the notion that independent ratings of stressful work provide relevant information in addition to self-reported data. Nevertheless, some methodological limitations should be considered. Even among well-trained job experts, these ratings may not be free from observer bias (person characteristics; job preference; selective attention). Another limitation concerns the inability to identify the meaning of an observed task for the working person. For instance, a small decision latitude in handling a task may be judged as 'low degree of control' by the observer and considered as a stressful experience in the frame of the DC model. However, the worker may appraise low control as a relief, given the absence of pressure due to responsibility, accountability, or risk of a personal mistake. Moreover, observation is restricted in terms of time and space, thus reducing the external validity of observational evidence. Despite these limitations, the method offers innovative insights, and its application is particularly promising if combined with quantitative methods. This latter procedure approach is used rather frequently in some areas of social and behavioural science research, known as 'mixed methods' approach.

4.1.3.2 Job exposure matrix

As a powerful alternative to self-reported data, job exposure matrices (JEMs) are used as approximate estimates of individual extent of exposure, and these data are linked with available health information to assess the exposure's potential health risk. Material and psychosocial work exposures with relevance to health are mainly derived from representative surveys. For instance, in a Norwegian study, expert-based items specifying physical work hazards (mechanical workload) and scales measuring stressful psychosocial work environments (DC model) were assessed by survey data from two panels, where item values for each one of eight mechanical and five psychosocial indicators were dichotomized (Hanvold et al. 2019). Individual occupations were classified according to the International Standard Classification of Occupations (ISCO-88) using 353 job titles. Mean scores of exposure indicators were computed for each job title, and individual exposure data were compared with job exposure data, using different measures of agreement (e.g. kappa, specificity, sensitivity). Moreover, criterion validity was analysed by associations with self-reported data on low back pain. Results demonstrated moderate to fair agreement between individual and job title-based exposure estimates, with somewhat better agreement for the mechanical compared to the psychosocial indicators. Applying mean values of individual exposures from surveys to job titles as a basis for large-scale estimates of exposures provides an attractive and efficient epidemiological approach. It offers a standardized exposure assessment between studies, and it enables the translation of retrospectively assessed job histories into specific exposures (Peters 2020). In addition, refined methodological analyses based on a linear multilevel (random intercept) model were developed where different levels of job classification can be distinguished and where adjustment for individual data (e.g. age, gender) effects provides more robust estimates than those based on mean levels (Kroll 2011).

The relevance of JEMs as applied to psychosocial occupational health is illustrated by two recent investigations. In France, Isabelle Niedhammer and her team developed a JEM that was based on all three scales of the DC model and additional summary measures with data derived from two large-scale surveys (Niedhammer et al. 2018). In addition to occupational position, company size, and economic sector were included to define job categories although the first indicator remained most important. A sophisticated classification method (Classification and Responses Tree) was applied to identify homogeneous occupational groups for psychosocial work variables, providing a hierarchical JEM classification, separately for working women and men. Correlation coefficients and additional association measures revealed moderate or fair agreement between individual scores and JEM scores, where the performance varied between the different dimensions of exposure. Highest agreement was observed for 'decision latitude'. In a subsequent publication, this team applied the JEM measuring job strain to a nationally representative prospective cohort of about 1.4 million employees with data on job title histories from 1976 to 2002, and this data set was linked to the national mortality database, where mortality from cardiovascular disease (and additionally from ischaemic heart disease and stroke) was used as independent and valid outcome criterion (Niedhammer et al. 2020). Table 4.1 demonstrates a subset of results from this comprehensive study. Here, the hazard ratios of cardiovascular mortality risk are given for the three main dimensions of the job strain model (adjusted for each other), and additionally for two summary measures (job strain; iso-strain (high strain)). The sample includes participants who died before retirement, thus estimating cumulative exposure over their job histories. As can be seen, most estimates are statistically significant with moderately elevated mortality risks. The findings of cardiovascular mortality were replicated for the two subcategories, but consistency was lower among women than among men (Niedhammer et al. 2020).

Table 4.1 Associations between cumulative exposure and cardiovascular mortality (CM) on-the-job among men and women.

	Men (N = 789 547) HR (95% CI) CM N= 2988	Women (N = 697 785) HR (95% CI) CM N= 474
High psychological demands[a]	1.11 (1.00; 1.23)	0.99 (0.79; 1.25)
Low decision latitude[a]	1.41 (1.28; 1.55)	1.31 (1.00; 1.70)
Low social support[a]	1.07 (0.97; 1.17)	1.50 (1.16; 1.93)
Job strain	1.33 (1.18; 1.50)	1.26 (1.02; 1.56)
Iso-strain	1.34 (1.18; 1.52)	1.30 (1.05; 1.61)

CI, confidence interval; CM, cardiovascular mortality; HR, hazard ratio. Adjusted for calendar time, biomechanical, physical, chemical, and biological exposures and age was used as the time scale.

[a]The three dimensions were adjusted for each other.

Source: Adapted with permission from Niedhammer, I., Milner, A., Geoffroy-Perez, B., et al. (2020), 'Psychosocial work exposures of the job strain model and cardiovascular mortality in France: results from the STRESSJEM prospective study', *Scand J Work Environ Health,* 46 (5), 542–51. [table 2, p. 546]. (Creative Commons Attribution 4.0 International License, https:// creativecommons.org/licenses/by/4.0/).

This investigation is not the first one testing the job strain model in terms of a JEM with prospectively assessed health outcomes, but it documents the robustness and validity of this method. Along these lines, a further study combined three JEMs, one based on the DC model, one based on the ERI model, and a third one based on the construct of emotional demands. This investigation analysed associations of psychosocial work characteristics with blood pressure among 63,800 employees from the Netherlands (Faruque et al. 2022). JEMs that had been derived from a representative Danish cohort with questionnaire data where job title scores according to ISCO-88 classification were applied to the sample. Findings revealed positive associations of job strain with systolic and diastolic blood pressure and of ERI with diastolic blood pressure, but negative associations of emotional demands with systolic blood pressure and prevalence of hypertension. Prevalence of hypertension was also significantly higher among those with high job strain, but not among those with high imbalance. Combining the exposures did not substantially improve the findings (Faruque et al. 2022).

These examples illustrate the strengths and limitations of the job exposure approach. The most significant limitation concerns the lack of information on inter-individual variability within each job title category. This problem is particularly pertinent in crude job classification systems. On the other hand, higher-level job classifications require a large sample size to obtain reliable exposure measures. Moreover, JEM estimates are less precise and less predictive than individual-level data, and they disregard a core aspect in a stress-theoretical perspective, the quality of individual experience of exposure. For these reasons, the methodological strength of avoiding reporting bias inherent in self-reported data needs to be carefully weighed against these weaknesses.

4.1.4 Methodological discussion

How valid is the measurement of psychosocial work environments? As is the case with all latent constructs, the test of their validity relies on approximate procedures, construct, and criterion validity as already described. Triangulation is a frequently used approach to ensure data validity as the same topic is assessed by two different methods. For instance, observational ratings are compared with self-reported data on work environments, as mentioned. We have already pointed to a mixed methods approach where results of a quantitative study are compared with those of a qualitative investigation. Importantly, the validity of self-reported data on work and employment is threatened by the presence of a reporting bias, that is, a systematic source of error that may invalidate the information. Recall bias (or recording bias) is one such source. Respondents may not be able to accurately record their recent experience. Distorting the perception of previous experience in retrospect represents a mechanism of cognitive adaption that can result in an under- or overestimation of lived experience. Recall bias is a major methodological challenge in longitudinal studies dealing with the previous life course. Interestingly, this challenge was examined in research on occupational histories, with the results satisfying agreement of self-reported information with administrative record data, even if events dating far back were reported (Baumgarten et al. 1983; Wahrendorf et al. 2019). As another systematic source of error, reporting bias can be due to specific psychological characteristics of the responding individual. For instance, 'neuroticism' as a personality trait characterized by emotional lability, irritability, and negative mood is expected to distort perceptions of psychosocial work environments by over-emphasizing their negative aspects. To control for this source of bias, studies often include a measure of a particular personality trait or psychological coping pattern as a confounding factor in their design. This is also the case in several investigations mentioned in Chapter 6. In general, the strength of associations of psychosocial predictors with health outcomes was reduced after statistically controlling for personality traits, but it remained significant in most cases. A responding person's prevalent disease or disability represents another source of error in data on psychosocial work environments. This is most obvious in cases of depression. Emotional, perceptual, and cognitive features associated with this disorder are likely to systematically bias reported information (de Lange et al. 2005; see Chapter 8). Again, adjusting for this potential confounding effect in cohort studies is a measure to strengthen the validity of findings. Another source of reporting bias concerns 'response set', a tendency to apply the same answer category to items irrespective of their content (e.g. as a way of abbreviating the task).

To summarize, control of reporting bias is a major methodological challenge in research on occupational psychosocial health. Different approaches are available to this extent. They include the method of aggregating the measures of individual employees to those of a group of employees within a relatively homogeneous work unit. With this procedure, individual reporting bias is minimized (Juvani et al. 2014). Threats to the internal validity of data on psychosocial work environments are not restricted to employed people participating in research. They are also present, perhaps to a lesser extent, among interviewers and observers, as indicated by low inter-rater reliability of observational scales or, among interviewers, by the identification of unnoticed person preferences or suggestive ways of asking questions. Clearly, bias control must be part of any rigorous scientific work. As far as it concerns the study population (selection bias) or the test of hypotheses (confounding), additional approaches will be described (see below and Chapter 5).

4.2 Data collection and study designs

4.2.1 Basic notions

Scientists in search of data collection and data analysis have different choices in how to proceed. For a long time, the collection of new data by available methods and study designs has been—and often continues to be—the master approach. While costly and time consuming, this strategy enables a high degree of autonomy in defining and testing research questions and in acquiring innovative knowledge (primary data). With the micro-electronic revolution and the availability of internet-processed data sets, new options of accessing data collected by other research teams for scientific analysis were developed (secondary data). One way of using secondary data concerns registry data. They offer systematically and repetitively collected information on target populations, either with regard to specific diseases (disease registries) or with regard to administrative aims of local, regional, or national populations (e.g. health insurance data) (Blewett et al. 2018). Several institutions and organizations collect administrative data on their members for management purposes, such as health insurance or pension funds. In all these cases, one needs to carefully study the aims, restrictions, and quality aspects of available data. For instance, administrative health data may not be based on standardized diagnostic criteria. They may be restricted to selective populations, or they may contain single rather than continued information. Often, the scientific value of administrative data depends on the opportunity of their linkage with primary data sets, and this opportunity may be restricted, e.g. due to legal regulations. A further, increasingly used way of accessing secondary data relates to public/scientific files of research data. In many countries, funding for large research projects, such as epidemiological cohort studies or surveys, involves the obligation of researchers to provide access to data for external users, with regulations of entitlement and extent of data access. A large number of scientific analyses in the field of psychosocial occupational health rely on secondary data analysis. To mention just two frequent sources in Europe, the European Working Conditions survey (EWCS; Eurofound 2019) and the Survey of Health, Aging and Retirement in Europe (SHARE; Börsch-Supan et al. 2011). Finally, 'big data' are available for secondary data analysis through social media, through institutions collecting transfer data (e.g. consumer transactions), or through sensor-based data (e.g. GPS) (Khoury and Ioannidis 2014). With this broad access to large datasets new challenges of analysing this information became obvious, and new techniques of data inspection and analysis were developed, in line with accelerated operation speed and capacity of computers.

The collection of primary data continues to be an indispensable option in research on work and health. Most frequently used strategies are the internet-based survey, the telephone interview, the questionnaire sent out by mail or administered at a specific location, and the face-to-face interview. This latter method offers a variety of approaches, reaching from a highly structured short communication to an extensive, open-ended narrative encounter registered for subsequent analysis and interpretation within a qualitative framework. Other methods of primary data collection include systematic and participatory observation, group discussions (e.g. focus groups), experiments, and interventions (see below, study designs). All these methods focus on verbal and/or visual information. If feasible, they can be combined with methods collecting biological information (e.g. obtained from medical screening, from the collection of biological samples, or from online-registered data transfer).

4.2.2 Study samples

It is an ultimate aim of scientific research to produce generalizable knowledge. Yet, any empirical study suffers from limitations that threaten its external validity. One such limitation concerns the study population. Defining a study population that enables the researcher to draw some valid conclusions from the results is therefore an important aim, specifically if primary data are to be collected. As access to a total population (of a country or region, an occupational category, an enterprise or organization etc.) is usually not feasible, selection criteria have to be defined to establish a study sample. How can we ensure that the findings of a restricted study sample are representative of the larger population? Recruiting a random sample of a distinct size out of the total population is one such approach. However, this method disregards the variation of major phenomena of interest according to core characteristics of subgroups in the population (e.g. age, gender, socioeconomic position). Such subgroups are termed 'strata'. It is therefore unknown to what extent findings derived from a random sample are representative for these subgroups. To this end, proportionate stratified random sampling is the method of choice. Here, the target sample is composed of relevant strata whose size is proportionate to the respective characteristic in the population at large. For instance, a study of full-time employees must consider the unequal proportion of women and men working full-time. To be representative, the sample composition needs to reflect these unequal proportions of the two strata. Based on probabilistic assumptions, this method avoids systematic selection bias, thus meeting high quality criteria. In practice, the procedure of proportionate random sampling may be time-consuming. Therefore, a somewhat easier approach is often chosen, the quota sampling method. This method takes into account the basic principle of stratification, but selection of subjects into a stratum is not done at random. For instance, interviewers are free to recruit participants within a stratum according to their preference, up to the pre-determined stratum size. This is done at the risk of producing some bias due to an unbalanced representation of subgroups.

Whatever the method of recruiting a study sample, a major question relates to the sample size. As a general principle, a large sample size increases the precision of estimates of randomly distributed characteristics, but it is the trade-off between sample size and precision of estimates that matters most. To determine the size of a sample required to obtain a solid answer of a research question several aspects are important: What is the study design, and how many measurement waves are planned? How many variables are included in the analysis, and how complex are the hypotheses to be tested? To estimate the minimum size of a sample required to ensure the detection of statistically significant differences or associations between variables of interest, online tools of statistical power analysis are available for calculation.

Once the sampling method has been fixed and the sample size, including stratification, has been determined, researchers need to choose how participants are recruited (e.g. by mail, phone, internet). If we consider the process from an initially fixed sample size to the number of those people who finally participated in the research project, three important sources of sample loss need to be considered as they can result in a systematic bias of study outcomes:

- Sample loss due to non-accessibility: Specific subgroups of the sample may not be reached as they do not use the media advertising the study, or do not use a telephone, or do not have a permanent address. Usually, people living in socioeconomically deprived circumstances are at elevated risk of non-accessibility.
- Sample loss due to non-response: the proportion of people who refuse to participate with or without justification varies from study to study, but it is generally rather high. Applying several strategies of motivating people was shown to substantially augment final participation rates (Dillman et al. 2014). To estimate the bias due to this loss, comparisons of available characteristics of the two samples are required.
- Sample loss during follow-up (attrition): Whenever participants are expected to continue their commitment beyond a first wave, their

probability of continuation decreases. This attrition of the sample size is particularly critical in longitudinal studies involving several measurement waves over a longer period of time. Again, it is crucial to compare the initial sample with the final study population to account for systematic dropouts, and thus for potentially biased findings.

Hence, the analysis of changes in sample size from beginning to end of a research programme is a relevant scientific task. In case of longitudinal studies in occupational epidemiology, a further potential source of systematic bias needs to be considered, the 'healthy worker effect'. It defines an increased probability of loss-to-follow-up of participants who are exposed to particularly demanding or unfavourable jobs, irrespective of whether or not resulting in absenteeism, job change, or job loss. As a result, the association of stressful occupational exposure with incident disease risk may be weakened, thus underestimating the severity of risk. To analyse the potential bias due to non-response, several statistical approaches are available. For instance, in the French CONSTANCES study, a large longitudinal investigation of occupational and environmental determinants of health (Goldberg et al. 2017), characteristics of non-response were determined by analysing data from a large random sample of invited, but non-responding individuals whose basic sociodemographic data were retrieved in the official database. This enabled the identification of variables discriminating between the two samples and a subsequent correction for non-response by applying a re-weighting technique (Santin et al. 2014). In conclusion, to generalize research findings, the composition of study samples has to be determined in accordance with established selection procedures. Moreover, control of systematic bias due to sample loss is an important scientific task.

4.2.3 Study designs

As indicated in Figure 1.1 (Chapter 1), most studies dealing with occupational psychosocial health are interested in the analysis of associations between occupational and socio-environmental characteristics and health, studying bi-directional pathways including the effects of interventions. Here, individual-level data are of primary interest, while ecological data collected at aggregate level are relevant by providing supplementary contextual information. There are four main types of study designs available for collection of primary data: cross-sectional studies, cohort studies, case-control studies, and experimental studies.

4.2.3.1 Cross-sectional studies

This study design is characterized by the fact that a single measurement wave is realized and that all variables, whether measuring independent (predictive) or dependent (criterion) features, are simultaneously assessed. Prevalence data are the main outcome of this type of studies. Information such as prevalence of risk factors and diseases, of health care utilization, is highly relevant for aims of health planning and surveillance, specifically if prevalence data are collected in standardized form covering representative population samples. Cross-sectional studies are also used to analyse associations of exposures with health risks. Likewise, relationships between distinct health conditions and resulting behavioural or social consequences are investigated. These studies are useful for exploratory reasons, but they cannot provide evidence on causality, given the lack of a temporal dimension between exposure and health outcome, or between health status and behavioural or social consequences. At the level of statistical analysis, hypotheses linking an exposure with an elevated health risk are tested in terms of odds ratios or regression coefficients, adjusting for relevant confounders in multivariable logistic or linear regression models (see Chapter 5).

4.2.3.2 Cohort studies

The prospective observational cohort study represents the gold standard of research in occupational epidemiology as it allows researchers to document distinct occupational or socio-environmental exposures as determinants of elevated health risks in the framework of probabilistic causal inference. To this end, two population groups are included in the study, a group defined by exposure to the determinant of interest (e.g. a stressful psychosocial work environment), and a group without this exposure. Importantly, at study entry, all participants must be free from the disease that is suspected to result from this exposure. Subsequently, both groups are followed over several years, with repetitive health examinations that document the incidence of the disease of interest. Comparing the relative risk of cumulative disease incidence between the exposed vs unexposed group over the observation period is the main aim of this study design. In practice, this design is often enriched by inclusion of additional determinants entering the analysis as confounding, mediating, or moderating factors; by repetitive assessment of exposure; and by measuring biological (e.g. cardiovascular, metabolic, immune) markers of the pathway underlying the association between exposure and disease. Appropriate statistical models are available to quantify the relative risk of disease incidence in the exposed vs the unexposed group and to assess the statistical significance of this difference. In Chapter 5, these models are described in more detail, and subsequent chapters offer a series of illustrations selected from recent epidemiological research (esp. Chapter 6).

The longitudinal nature of cohort studies is considered a major strength as the temporal sequence between the experience of an exposure and the development of a disease is a principal prerequisite of analysis. Although most investigations have a prospective design, retrospective cohort studies are also conducted. In this case, the working population with manifest disease has already been identified, and exposure data are collected in retrospect, either by primary or secondary data. Despite their strengths cohort studies are not free from limitations. Loss-to-follow-up is a major threat to the generalization of research findings. Moreover, several uncontrolled influences can have an impact on the association under study, including health-care interventions or behavioural changes. The fact of being part of a scientific investigation can exert an intended or unintended effect ('Hawthorne effect'). As diseases under study are often determined by a set of different exposures, it may be difficult to capture all relevant determinants within a single study design. In addition, the statistical analysis of multiple exposures, their accumulation, and interaction is considered a challenging scientific task. In conclusion, carefully conducted cohort studies, representing the gold standard in this field of research, produce new scientific knowledge with high quality. In fact, a range of relevant discoveries in occupational epidemiology evolved from this study design.

4.2.3.3 Case–control studies

As cohort studies are time consuming and expensive, case–control studies represent a less difficult, but also less conclusive approach. In this study design, differences of exposure are explored between a group of individuals with the disease under study and a control group of individuals without this disease. Importantly, the control group needs to be matched according to important confounding factors (e.g. age, gender, socioeconomic status). By definition, the exposure assessment occurs in retrospect. The aim of case–control studies consists in identifying a distinct exposure as a potential risk factor of a specific disease. For instance, long working hours are assumed to increase the risk of acute myocardial infarction. In a Japanese study, 195 men surviving their acute myocardial infarction were compared to 331 healthy men matched by age and occupational position. Retrospectively assessed working hours were compared between the two groups, where critical exposure was defined as working eleven hours or more per day. The adjusted odds ratio of this risk factor in the disease group was 2.44 (95% confidence interval 1.26; 4.73) compared to 1.00 in the healthy group (Sokejima and Kagamimori 1998). Obviously, findings derived from this design need to be replicated by prospective evidence, as they are not free from several risks of bias. In fact, this finding was confirmed by a large meta-analysis based on cross-national prospective data (World Health Organization and International Labour Organization 2021). Selection bias may occur in the choice of both case and control groups. The probability of reporting bias, including recall bias, is particularly high in the disease group as the retrospective assessment of exposure can be distorted by cognitive and affective responses resulting from processes of coping with the disease.

4.2.3.4 Experiments

The uncertainties of causal explanations even in most sophisticated designs of observational studies are overcome by experiments. They represent the classical approach in basic science. In social and behavioural sciences, their application is often less feasible, and the main problem of experimental results is given by their restricted external validity. Experimental studies are based on three principles. Firstly, at least two groups of participants are distinguished, with one group (intervention group) exposed to a treatment condition and the other (control) group unexposed to this condition. Secondly, individuals are randomly assigned to these two groups to avoid selection effects. Thirdly, the treatment condition is systematically varied by the leader of the experiment, such that its independent effects on an outcome can be analysed in comparison with the control group. If these principles are less strictly followed, for instance by avoiding randomization, these investigations are termed quasi-experiments. In clinical research, the randomized controlled trial is considered the gold standard of evaluating treatment effects of therapeutic interventions. As an important precondition, randomization is done in blind or even double-blind ways, such that participants (and physicians, including study leaders) are not aware of whether participants received the intervention or a placebo. In the field of psychosocial occupational health, experimental designs are not often applied. Ethical and logistic reasons prevent or reduce opportunities of randomizing workers into an intervention and control group. Intervention studies in real work settings are important, and their potential beneficial effects are exemplified below (see Chapter 10) despite the many methodological and procedural challenges.

4.3 Summary

Basic methodological knowledge is an indispensable precondition of critical appraisal of the scientific state of art. In this chapter, we provided some essential aspects of this knowledge, while being aware that each topic deserves additional in-depth elaboration. The focus of this part of the book was on quantitative methods. This was done in line with a major part of current empirical evidence on psychosocial occupational health. Future research developments may broaden the spectrum of analysis. As an important practical message, we maintain that scientific research is a privileged, precious activity that merits the application of highest standards of quality. Thus, the standards of data collection, sample composition, and study design mentioned deserve attention from all readers.

4.4 Relevant questions

- What are the main reasons of assessing theoretical models of psychosocial work environments primarily by psychometric scales?
- Which types of bias in the process of data collection can you distinguish? Why is it important to aim at controlling their impact?
- Qualitative methods were rarely applied in this field of research. What are the reasons for this shortage? And what are the most promising aspects you are expecting from a stronger implementation of qualitative methods in this research?

Recommended reading

❖ Cooper, C. (2019) *Psychological testing. Theory and practice.* Abingdon: Routledge/Taylor & Francis.

❖ Finch, W. H. and French, B. F. (2018) *Educational and psychological measurement.* New York, NY: Routledge.

❖ OECD (2017) *OECD Guidelines on measuring the quality of the working environment.* Paris: OECD.

❖ Schreier, M. (2012) *Qualitative content analysis in practice.* London: Sage Publications.

Useful websites

❖ World Health Organization: Health research methodology: a guide for training in research methods. https://iris.who.int/handle/10665/206929

❖   U.S. Centers for Disease Control and Prevention (CDC): Principles of Epidemiology in Public Health Practice Course. https://stacks.cdc.gov/view/cdc/6914

❖   American Psychological Association: Testing, assessment, and measurement. https://www.apa.org/topics/testing-assessment-measurement

References

Baumgarten, M., Siemiatycki, J., and Gibbs, G. W. (1983), 'Validity of work histories obtained by interview for epidemiologic purposes', *Am J Epidemiol*, 118 (4), 583–91.

Beatty, P. C., Collins, D., Kaye, L., et al. (2019), *Advances in questionnaire design, development, evaluation and testing*: John Wiley & Sons.

Bethlehem, J., and Biffignandi, S. (2011), *Handbook of web surveys*. Chichester: Wiley.

Blewett, L. A., Call, K. T., Turner, J., et al. (2018), 'Data resources for conducting health services and policy research', *Annu Rev Public Health*, 39, 437–52.

Bollen, K., and Lennox, R. (1991), 'Conventional wisdom on measurement: a structural equation perspective', *Psychol Bull*, 110 (2), 305.

Börsch-Supan, A., Brandt, M., Hank, K., et al. (2011), *The individual and the welfare state: life histories in Europe*. Heidelberg: Springer.

Bosma, H., Marmot, M. G., Hemingway, H., et al. (1997), 'Low job control and risk of coronary heart disease in Whitehall II (prospective cohort) study', *BMJ*, 314 (7080), 558–65.

Chungkham, H. S., Ingre, M., Karasek, R. A., et al. (2013), 'Factor structure and longitudinal measurement invariance of the demand control support model: an evidence from the Swedish Longitudinal Occupational Survey of Health (SLOSH)', *PLoS One*, 8 (8), e70541.

Colquitt, J. A., and Rodell, J. B. (2015), 'Measuring justice and fairness'. In R. Cropanzano and M. L. Ambrose (eds.), *The Oxford handbook of justice in the workplace*. New York: Oxford University Press, 187–202.

Cooper, C. (2019), *Psychological testing: theory and practice*. Abingdon: Routledge/Taylor & Francis.

Corbin, J., and Strauss, A. (2015), *Basics of qualitative research: techniques and procedures for developing grounded theory* 4 edn. Thousand Oaks, CA: Sage Publications.

de Lange, A. H., Taris, T. W., Kompier, M. A., et al. (2005), 'Different mechanisms to explain the reversed effects of mental health on work characteristics', *Scand J Work Environ Health*, 31 (1), 3–14.

Demerouti, E., Bakker, A. B., Nachreiner, F., et al. (2001), 'The job demands-resources model of burnout', *J Appl Psychol*, 86 (3), 499–512.

Denzin, N. K., and Lincoln, Y. S. (2011), *Handbook of qualitative research*. Thousand Oaks, CA: Sage Publications.

Dillman, D. A., Smyth, J. D., and Christian, L. M. (2014), *Internet, phone, mail, and mixed-mode surveys: the tailored design method*. Hoboken, NJ: John Wiley & Sons.

Elovainio, M., Kivimäki, M., and Vahtera, J. (2002), 'Organizational justice: evidence of a new psychosocial predictor of health', *Am J Public Health*, 92 (1), 105–8.

Embretson, S. E., and Reise, S. P. (2000), *Item response theory for psychologists*. Mahwah, NJ: Psychology Press.

Eurofound (2019), 'Working conditions and workers' health', (Luxembourg: Publications Office of the European Union).

Faruque, M. O., Framke, E., Sorensen, J. K., et al. (2022), 'Psychosocial work factors and blood pressure among 63,800 employees from The Netherlands in the Lifelines Cohort Study', *J Epidemiol Community Health*, 76 (1), 60–66.

Finch, W. H., and French, B. F. (2018), *Educational and psychological measurement*. New York, NY: Routledge.

Goldberg, M., Carton, M., Descatha, A., et al. (2017), 'CONSTANCES: a general prospective population-based cohort for occupational and environmental epidemiology: cohort profile', *Occup Environ Med*, 74 (1), 66–71.

Greiner, B. A., Krause, N., Ragland, D., et al. (2004), 'Occupational stressors and hypertension: a multi-method study using observer-based job analysis and self-reports in urban transit operators', *So Sci Med*, 59 (5), 1081–94.

Hacker, W. (1994), 'Action regulation theory and occupational psychology: review of German empirical research since 1987', *German J Psychol*. 18, 91–120.

Hanvold, T. N., Sterud, T., Kristensen, P., et al. (2019), 'Mechanical and psychosocial work exposures: the construction and evaluation of a gender-specific job exposure matrix (JEM)', *Scand J Work Environ Health*, 45 (3), 239–47.

Johnston, D. W., Jones, M. C., Charles, K., et al. (2013), 'Stress in nurses: stress-related affect and its determinants examined over the nursing day', *Ann Behav Med*, 45 (3), 348–56.

Juvani, A., Oksanen, T., Salo, P., et al. (2014), 'Effort-reward imbalance as a risk factor for disability pension: the Finnish Public Sector Study', *Scand J Work Environ Health*, 40 (3), 266–77.

Karasek, R. A., and Theorell, T. (1990), *Healthy work: stress, productivity and the reconstruction of working life*. New York: Basic Books.

Karasek, R. A., Brisson, C., Kawakami, N., et al. (1998), 'The Job Content Questionnaire (JCQ): an instrument for internationally comparative assessments of psychosocial job characteristics', *J Occup Health Psychol*, 3 (4), 322–55.

Khoury, M. J., and Ioannidis, J. P. (2014), 'Big data meets public health', *Science*, 346 (6213), 1054–5.

Kroll, L. E. (2011), 'Construction and validation of a general index for job demands in occupations based on ISCO-88 and KldB-92', *MDA - Methoden, Daten, Analysen (Methods, Data, Analyses)*, 5 (1), 63–90.

Lee, J. W., Jones, P. S., Mineyama, Y., et al. (2002), 'Cultural differences in responses to a Likert scale', *Res Nurs Health*, 25 (4), 295–306.

Leineweber, C., Wege, N., Westerlund, H., et al. (2010), 'How valid is a short measure of effort-reward imbalance at work? A replication study from Sweden', *Occup Environ Med*, 67 (8), 526–31.

Lesener, T., Gusy, B., and Wolter, C. (2019), 'The job demands-resources model: a meta-analytic review of longitudinal studies', *Work Stress*, 33 (1), 76–103.

Maydeu-Olivares, A. (2005), 'Linear item response theory, nonlinear item response theory, and factor analysis: a unified framework'. In A. Maydeu-Olivares and J. J. McArdle (eds.), *Contemporary psychometrics: a festschrift for Roderick P. McDonald* Hillsdale, NJ: Lawrence Erlbaum Associates Publishers, 73–100.

McGillis Hall, L., and Kiesners, D. (2005), 'A narrative approach to understanding the nursing work environment in Canada', *Soc Sci Med*, 61 (12), 2482–91.

Moorman, R. H. (1991), 'Relationship between organizational justice and organizational citizenship behaviors: do fairness perceptions influence employee citizenship?', *J Applied Psychol*, 76 (6), 845–55.

Niedhammer, I., Milner, A., LaMontagne, A. D., et al. (2018), 'Study of the validity of a job-exposure matrix for the job strain model factors: an update and a study of changes over time', *Int Arch Occup Environ Health*, 91 (5), 523–36.

Niedhammer, I., Milner, A., Geoffroy-Perez, B., et al. (2020), 'Psychosocial work exposures of the job strain model and cardiovascular mortality in France: results from the STRESSJEM prospective study', *Scand J Work Environ Health*, 46 (5), 542–51.

OECD (2017), *OECD guidelines on measuring the quality of the working environment*. Paris: OECD.

Peters, S. E. (2020), 'Although a valuable method in occupational epidemiology, job-exposure matrices are no magic fix', *Scand J Work Environ Health*, 46 (3), 231–34.

Presser, S., Couper, M. P., Lessler, J. T., et al. (2004), 'Methods for testing and evaluating survey questions'. In S. Presser, J. M. Rothgeb, M. P. Couper, et al. (eds.), *Methods for testing and evaluating survey questionnaires*: John Wiley & Sons, 1–22.

Radloff, L. S. (1977), 'The CES-D scale: a self-report depression scale for research in the general population', *Appl Psychol Meas*, 1 (3), 385–401.

Rau, R., Morling, K., and Rösler, U. (2010), 'Is there a relationship between major depression and both objectively assessed and perceived demands and control?', *Work & Stress*, 24 (1), 88–106.

Santin, G., Geoffroy, B., Benezet, L., et al. (2014), 'In an occupational health surveillance study, auxiliary data from administrative health and occupational databases effectively corrected for nonresponse', *J Clin Epidemiol*, 67 (6), 722–30.

Schaufeli, W. B., Desart, S., and De Witte, H. (2020), 'Burnout Assessment Tool (BAT) - Development, validity, and reliability', *Int J Environ Res Public Health*, 17 (24), 9495.

Schreier, M. (2012), *Qualitative content analysis in practice*. London: Sage Publications.

Shiffman, S., Stone, A. A., and Hufford, M. R. (2008), 'Ecological momentary assessment', *Annu Rev Clin Psychol*, 4, 1–32.

Siegrist, J., Starke, D., Chandola, T., et al. (2004), 'The measurement of effort-reward imbalance at work: European comparisons', *Soc Sci Med*, 58 (8), 1483–99.

Sokejima, S., and Kagamimori, S. (1998), 'Working hours as a risk factor for acute myocardial infarction in Japan: case-control study', *BMJ*, 317 (7161), 775–80.

Tsutsumi, A., Iwata, N., Wakita, T., et al. (2008), 'Improving the measurement accuracy of the effort-reward imbalance scales', *Int J Behav Med*, 15 (2), 109–19.

Wahrendorf, M., Marr, A., Antoni, M., et al. (2019), 'Agreement of self-reported and administrative data on employment histories in a German cohort study: a sequence analysis', *Eur J Popul*, 35 (2), 329–46.

Ware, J., Kosinski, M., and Keller, S. (1994), *SF-36 physical and mental health summary scales* 5th ed., *A user's manual*. Boston, MA: Health Assessment Lab.

Willis, G. B. (2004), *Cognitive interviewing: a tool for improving questionnaire design*. SAGE Publications.

World Health Organization, and International Labour Organization (2021), 'WHO/ILO joint estimate of the work-related burden of disease and injury. 2000-2016', (Geneva: WHO, ILO).

Zigmond, A. S., and Snaith, R. P. (1983), 'The Hospital Anxiety and Depression Scale', *Acta Psychiatr Scand*, 67 (6), 361–70.

5

Data analysis and statistical modelling

5.1 Regression analysis, structural equation, and multilevel modelling

In Chapter 4, different types of data collection and measurement requirements were discussed. This chapter deals with data analysis, a core step of scientific work. It informs readers about some of the main approaches to quantitative data analysis. Despite its importance, we do not address the topic of qualitative data analysis. Readers can find excellent textbooks on this matter, with a main focus on social science research (e.g. Denzin and Lincoln 2011; Schreier 2012). Moreover, we do not provide information on descriptive statistics as detailed analyses are provided in standard textbooks (e.g. Celentano and Szklo 2018; Checkoway et al. 2004). In short, descriptive information on variables assessed by continuous or discrete data is given as mean and standard deviation (SD) in case of normal distribution of values, and as median in case of skewed distribution of values. If variables are assessed as categorical data (binary, nominal, ordinal), their absolute and relative frequencies are given. For outcomes of interest, prevalence and incidence of events are given. As a standard requirement of scientific publications in epidemiological research, a table informs readers about basic descriptive data of the study, either as numerical or as graphical summaries. A website with information on how to calculate descriptive statistics and producing graphs with reference to the program R is indicated at the end of this chapter. This first part of the chapter is devoted to a short introduction to basic approaches of statistical modelling.

5.1.1 Regression analysis

Analytical statistics deal with relationships between two (bivariate) or more (multivariate) variables, with an attempt to identify their associations. Such

Psychosocial Occupational Health. Johannes Siegrist and Jian Li, Oxford University Press.
© Oxford University Press 2024. DOI: 10.1093/oso/9780192887924.003.0005

associations may be analysed in order to test a research hypothesis or to instruct further inquiry in search of an explanation of observed associations. As a crucial assumption, the analysis between two or more variables is defined as relationship between a dependent variable and one or more independent variables. The respective statistical approach, termed regression analysis, estimates parameters from the data that summarize the relationship between the independent variables and the dependent variable, using established mathematical formulae. The most widely used types of regression analysis are linear regression, logistic regression, Poisson regression, and Cox regression.

If the relationship between an independent variable and a dependent variable is supposed to be linear (which can be illustrated by a scatter plot), linear regression is the preferable choice. The dependent variable must be continuous, while independent variables can be measured as continuous/discrete or categorical. The simplest linear regression consists of one independent variable X and one dependent variable Y. In this model, the mean value of the dependent variable, denoted by $E(Y)$, is linearly related with the independent variable X. This can be expressed as $E(Y) = a + b \times X$. In this equation, the regression coefficients a and b define the intercept of the line and the slope respectively. This latter coefficient provides a measure of the contribution of the independent variable X towards explaining the dependent variable Y. If an independent variable is measured as continuous information (such as age), the slope of the regression coefficient represents a change in the dependent variable (e.g. systolic blood pressure in mmHg) per unit of change in the independent variable (e.g. age in years). To test the statistical significance of this linear regression, the 95 per cent confidence intervals (CI) for the regression coefficient are calculated. To this end, values must not include zero (0) to indicate a significant association at the 0.05 level. In an analogous way, regression coefficients are calculated for associations with categorical data of the independent variable.

In epidemiological research, this simple form of analysis is rarely used as research questions often require a more complex approach. In multivariable linear regression effects of multiple independent variables on a dependent variable are estimated, expressed by the equation $E(Y) = a + b_1 \times X_1 + b_2 \times X_2 + \ldots + b_n \times X_n$. Each coefficient b_i reflects the effect of the corresponding individual independent variable X_i, taking account of the potential impact of remaining independent variables by X_i. In other words, multivariable regression analysis enables multiple independent variables to be entered into the same equation, with adjustment of their regression coefficients for possible confounding effects between variables.

Many epidemiological investigations require a stepwise linear regression analysis, given the interrelationships between independent variables and their associations with the dependent variable. In this procedure a stepwise definition of successive regression models occurs, where independent variables are added that may contribute to the explanation, and where variables are removed when not contributing, based on a test of statistical significance. A final model is expected to represent the relevant explanatory contribution, adjusted for included confounders. It informs readers about the proportion of variance explained in Y by the resulting combination of independent variables (i.e. R^2). The same procedure is applied in case of other regression models, such as logistic regression or Cox proportional hazards regression. Below, in the context of Cox proportional hazards regression, the topic of confounder control will be illustrated by an example.

Applying logistic regression is indicated if the dependent variable is defined as a binary (dichotomous) outcome. In this case, independent variables can be assessed at nominal, ordinal, or interval scale. The logistic regression transforms the probability (range 0–1) of an event occurring into its odds, reflecting the ratio of two probabilities (i.e. the probability of an event to occur or not to occur). The regression coefficients represent the odds ratio (OR) in the logarithmic scale. The results of this analysis are presented in the original OR scale.

In case–control studies, the OR represents the odds that a disease will occur given a particular exposure, compared to the odds of the disease occurring in the absence of that exposure. In prospective studies, the relative risk (RR) is used to estimate the effect of a risk factor on disease onset. It is defined as the ratio of incident disease events in an exposed vs an unexposed group. When comparing ORs with RRs, the former measure is likely to overestimate a relative risk, particularly in cases of a high prevalence/incidence of the disease under study. In Chapter 6, examples of RRs derived from logistic regression analyses in prospective investigations are given, where exposure is defined in terms of constructs of adverse psychosocial working conditions. In some instances with a rare disease as outcome, ORs are used as approximate estimates.

This statistical approach can be extended to polytomous logistic regression and ordinal logistic regression. In the former, the dependent variable is defined by more than two discrete (non-ordinal) categories, where the mathematical model is based on a generalized logit. In contrast, ordinal logistic regression includes an ordinal dependent variable with more than two categories (e.g. health status: good; moderate; bad). For more information on this approach, see Bender and Grouven (1997). Furthermore, regression analysis is applied if outcomes are defined in countable quantities, such as days of hospitalization or days of sickness absence. The distribution of such data is often skewed, with many values being relatively low and few being high. To this end, Poisson regression analysis is applied (Hayat and Higgins 2014). Like linear regression and logistic regression, multiple independent variables (either continuous or categorical) are included, and a linear relationship is assumed between the independent variable(s) and the natural logarithm (ln) of the expected value of the dependent variable. The slope regression coefficient in Poisson regression is interpreted as estimate of the ratio of two event rates (or incidence rates), expressed as RR. The RR represents the estimated risk of outcome of interest.

As an example of a Poisson regression analysis with a count variable, a Danish cohort study used the number of sickness absence days as a count outcome variable and explored whether job burnout increased this risk (Borritz et al. 2006). In this study, the RR = 1.21 (1.11; 1.32) was observed after adjustment for relevant confounders. This means that an increment of one standard deviation of the job burnout score (assessed at baseline) predicted a 21 per cent increase in the number of sickness absence days at follow-up (Borritz et al. 2006). A modified Poisson regression analysis containing a robust error variance was developed for calculation of relative risks of dichotomous outcomes (e.g. a specific disease event) in prospective epidemiological investigations (Zou 2004). This approach has been widely applied in research on psychosocial occupational health outcomes (e.g. Matthews et al. 2021; Wege et al. 2018).

Finally, Cox proportional hazards regression represents a fourth type of regression models, when the dependent variable represents the time an event takes to happen during the follow-up period. This method simultaneously investigates the effect of several predicting variables on the time-to-event outcome. In this model, the risk of suffering an event at some exact time point is called the hazard, and the hazard ratio (HR) associated with a predictor is given by the exponent of its coefficient. The HR is defined as the ratio of the number of observed to expected events occurring in two comparable groups (an exposed vs an unexposed group) within a defined time period.

As an often used practical application of time-to-event dependent variable analysis survival rates are plotted in a curve called Kaplan–Meier curve. On the X-axis of this curve participants' survival time is given, and on the Y-axis survival probability is indicated, ranging from 0 to 1. When comparing survival time of participants from different groups, a log-rank

Table 5.1 Overview of basic regression analyses

Regression model	Dependent variable	Independent variables	Effect estimate
Linear regression	Continuous variable	Continuous and/ or categorical variables	Beta coefficient
Logistic regression	Dichotomous variable		Odds ratio
Poisson regression	Count variable or rare event		Relative risk
Cox regression	Time to first event		Hazard ratio

test is applied using available data during the whole follow-up period. With this method, censored data are analysed as well. Specifically, right-censoring data indicating loss of participants during follow-up are included in the plot (Hosmer et al. 2008). Many cohort studies apply Cox regression models when estimating survival from or risk of incident events during a defined follow-up time. Participants are followed until time of first onset of an event. The HR indicates the increased probability of event manifestation among exposed vs unexposed people within this period. For instance, in a Canadian cohort study among 967 workers who returned to work after recovering from their first acute myocardial infarction, 205 recurrent coronary events occurred during a mean observation period of 5.9 years. The adjusted HR of a recurrent event was 1.67 (1.10; 2.53) among those working ≥ 55 hours/week compared to those working 35 to 40 hours/week, thus resulting in a 67 per cent increased event risk (Trudel et al. 2021). To summarize core features of the four regression models discussed, an overview in Table 5.1 may be instructive.

5.1.1.1 Confounding

Confounding represents a major challenge in observational study designs. In occupational health research, health outcomes are often determined by a number of risk and protective factors, in addition to the specific occupational exposures of interest. Therefore, the contribution of these factors to the elevated probability of disease manifestation has to be assessed, applying stepwise multivariable regression analysis. Table 5.2 gives an example of this procedure, based on a multi-cohort study of 90,164 individuals analysing the risk of incident ischaemic heart disease (IHD) among workers exposed to stressful work vs non-exposed workers (Dragano et al. 2017).

Table 5.2 Summary hazard ratios from random effects meta-analysis of serially adjusted association between effort-reward imbalance and incident coronary heart disease (1985–2010)

Adjustment	N (total)[a]	N (events)	HR (95% CI)
Age, sex	90,164	1,078	1.16 (1.01, 1.34)
Age, sex, SES	90,164	1,089	1.19 (1.04, 1.38)
Age, sex, SES, BMI, physical activity	85,778	1,031	1.20 (1.04, 1.39)
Age, sex, SES, BMI, physical activity, smoking, alcohol consumption	83,564	999	1.18 (1.02, 1.37)
Age, sex, SES, BMI, physical activity, smoking, alcohol consumption, job strain	63,484	997	1.16 (1.00, 1.35)

[a]The numbers of participants vary because of missing data in covariates.

BMI, body mass index; CI, confidence interval; HR, hazard ratio; SES, socioeconomic status.

Source: Reproduced with permission from Dragano, N., Siegrist, J., Nyberg, S. T., et al. (2017), 'Effort-reward imbalance at work and incident coronary heart disease: a multicohort study of 90,164 individuals', *Epidemiology,* 28 (4), 619–26. [Table 2, p. 623]; License no.: 5506970013791.

Data from eleven individual cohort studies were combined in a series of Cox proportional hazard regression models, where the most parsimonious model included age and sex as covariates. Work stress, as measured by the effort-reward imbalance model (ERI; described in Chapters 3 and 4) was associated with a HR of 1.16. This effect was minimally increased after taking into account the influence of socioeconomic position. When additionally adjusting for two important risk factors, body mass index and physical inactivity, no substantial change in the HR was observed, and the same holds true for smoking and alcohol consumption, additionally adjusted for. It is therefore unlikely that the association of stressful work with incident IHD is due to a mediating role of adverse health behaviours. In the final regression model displayed in Table 5.2, the impact of a complementary theoretical concept of work stress, job strain, is included (see Chapters 3 and 4). This is important because job strain was linked to incident IHD in several previous cohort studies (Kivimäki et al. 2012). Of interest, the effect size of the parsimonious model persisted after completion of several adjustment procedures in this stepwise regression analysis, indicating that ERI at work represents an independent risk factor of IHD, with a moderately elevated HR (Dragano et al. 2017).

The analysis of covariates in regression analysis represents a major challenge for at least two relevant reasons. Firstly, the number of potential factors that may confound an observed effect is often large, and few studies can extend their data collection to include an exhaustive list. Therefore, unobserved confounding is a limitation of generalization of study findings in epidemiological cohort studies. Secondly, covariates can have different functions in explanatory analyses. Mediation is an important function. For instance, referring to Table 5.2, if the third and fourth adjustment had substantially reduced the HR of the parsimonious model, this would indicate that the association of work stress with IHD is partly mediated by health-adverse behaviours. Effect modification is a further function of covariates. For instance, socioeconomic position (SEP) can modify the effect of stressful work on IHD, such that this effect is particularly strong among low SEP workers. Dominant versions of tackling these challenges are briefly described here, while we point to innovative statistical approaches in the next section (5.2).

5.1.1.2 Mediation, effect modification, and interaction

All three terms mentioned identify crucial procedures of statistical analysis in socio-behavioural epidemiological research.

- Mediation analysis aims to explain relationships between independent and dependent variables by introducing one or several 'third' variables that are statistically associated with both conditions. To this end, the quantitative contribution of this (or these) mediator(s) to the effect of an independent variable on a dependent variable is estimated. A reduction of the size of the direct effect by an indirect effect is interpreted as an explanatory contribution of the mediator(s) to the underlying association (see Figure 5.1 (A)).

In occupational health research mediation analysis as a strategy of searching for causal links is of high relevance. Based on the conventional statistical procedure of mediation analysis, termed 'difference method', multivariable analysis of the three-way relationship between independent, mediating, and dependent variable is conducted using this sequence: Firstly, a direct effect of the independent on the dependent variable is estimated, adjusting for relevant confounders. Secondly, the mediating variable is introduced to the analysis, and if the size of this new, indirect effect on the dependent variable is substantially smaller than the original effect, this indicates a contributing

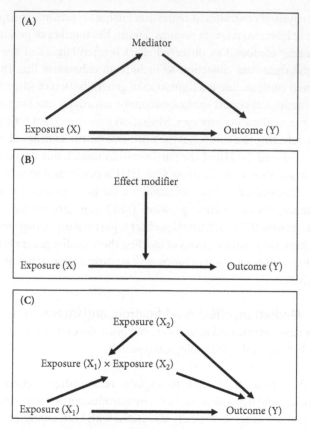

Figure 5.1 Graphical representation of mediation (A), effect modification (B), and interaction (C).

factor of the mediator on the outcome (Baron and Kenny 1986). Thirdly, in contrast, a regression analysis with the mediator as independent variable and the independent as mediating variable is not expected to result in a substantial difference of the effect size. As an example, in an influential paper based on the British Whitehall II study, low SEP was related to elevated IHD risk, and a low level of job control was introduced as mediator in this analysis (Marmot et al. 1997). The direct effect of low SEP on IHD risk, estimated as OR in multivariable regression analysis, was around 1.4. After introducing 'low control' in the analysis, this OR was reduced to around 1.2, thus accounting for almost half the difference of the size of the direct effect. In contrast, the relationship of low job control with IHD was not removed by adjusting for SEP as a mediator (Marmot et al. 1997). This finding was interpreted as support of a partial mediating role of low job control. However, as two causal effects are assumed in this interpretation, one from low SEP to low job control, and one from low job control to elevated IHD risk, it may be difficult to reach a definite conclusion. In other examples of mediation analysis conducted in occupational health research, the causality assumptions are perhaps less problematic. For instance, a direct effect in the association of belonging to the occupational group of construction workers with an elevated risk of lung cancer was largely accounted for by an indirect effect operating through exposure to asbestos fibres. In this case, both causal pathways are substantiated by pathophysiological evidence (Siemiatycki and Xu 2020). These examples illustrate the relevance of mediation analysis, but at the same time, a methodological critique identifying several shortcomings of the 'difference method' resulted in new statistical developments (see Section 5.2).

- Effect modification (also termed 'moderation') analyses the differential strength of the association of an independent variable on a dependent variable according to a 'third' variable. Such a moderator variable identifies a distinct characteristic that is unequally distributed across a population. Stratifying population groups according to this characteristic reveals different effect sizes, either as reduced risk ('protective effect') or as increased risk ('vulnerability effect') (see Figure 5.1 (B)).

Again, occupational health research has repeatedly applied this approach, given the policy implications of respective findings, demonstrating a particularly high adverse effect of an occupational stressor on the health of workers who are characterized by a distinct 'vulnerability factor'. Such results are considered a compelling reason of targeting intervention measures primarily to this vulnerable group. Moderator variables in occupational health research include a wide spectrum, ranging from genetic and health-related factors to the availability of individual and socioeconomic resources of coping with adversity (Diderichsen et al. 2019). Moderators may also focus on psychosocial work characteristics. For instance, work-unit social support was found to moderate the strength of the effect of high physical demands at work on risk of incident IHD in a study in Belgium (Clays et al. 2016). In a Japanese longitudinal investigation, the association of occupational position with risk of stroke incidence was particularly high among blue-collar and non-managerial workers exposed to job strain (Tsutsumi et al. 2011). As mentioned, stratified analyses are conducted to test effect modification, examining additive or multiplicative interaction. Yet, both methods, conventional mediation analysis and moderation analysis, were often performed as distinct approaches, rather than being combined in a more comprehensive analytical framework that decomposes direct effects into components evolving from mediation and interaction (VanderWeele 2015) (see Section 5.2).

- Interaction is calculated in order to examine the joint effect of two (or more) exposures on an outcome. This effect is expected to exceed the sum of individual effects. Interaction analysis is performed on an additive or on a multiplicative scale. In the former case, the relative excess risk due to the interaction (RERI) is estimated, where values beyond zero indicate the presence of a synergistic effect. In order to test the interaction of two or more variables in addition to their main effects on a multiplicative scale, a large sample size is required, in view of the statistical power needed for estimation of reliable effects (Knol and VanderWeele 2012) (see Figure 5.1 (C)).

The analysis of interaction and of other forms of co-manifestation of two variables has been a challenging task in research on psychosocial occupational health. Importantly, in theoretical terms, the demand-control (DC) and the ERI models both assume that a combination of their two core variables exerts a stronger effect on the health outcome under study than their single variables. For either concept a measure reflecting this co-manifestation was developed. In case of the DC model, 'job strain' was constructed as a variable combining scores above the median of the 'demand' scale with scores below the median of the 'control' scale (Karasek et al. 1998). Within the ERI concept, an 'effort-reward ratio' was defined, quantifying the match/mismatch between adjusted scores on the 'effort' and the 'reward' scale at individual level (Siegrist et al. 2004). After adjustment for their single components these summary estimates are expected to maintain their statistical significance. However, these assumptions were not always met in empirical studies, thus calling for alternative approaches. Conventional interaction analysis on an additive scale offers an obvious solution. In this case, separate effects of grouped variables are analysed. These grouped variables represent four constellations ranging from lowest to highest level of exposure (e.g. low demand/high control; high demand/

high control; low demand/low control; high demand/low control), allowing a test of statistical significance of differences in ORs or RRs between the four constellations (for an early example of both models, see De Jonge et al. 2000). Interaction analysis on a multiplicative scale was less often performed in view of the prerequisite of a large sample size (for an example, see Wahrendorf et al. 2012).

The analysis of mediation, effect modification, and interaction represents one of the main tasks of hypothesis-testing empirical research. Conventional statistical approaches still dominate the research although several shortcomings and uncontrolled assumptions were identified and gave rise to new developments (Rijnhart et al. 2021). Some of these developments are briefly described below with a focus on causal analysis (Section 5.2).

5.1.2 Structural equation modelling

The structural equation modelling (SEM) concept was developed in social and behavioural science research as a more complex approach, and it is now increasingly applied to health research as well (Tu 2009). It is best described as a set of statistical techniques to analyse relationships of observed and latent variables (Beran and Violato 2010). As established by factor analysis, latent variables are calculated from measured variables, representing unobserved constructs. Each latent variable consists of at least two interrelated observed variables. In addition to factor analysis, SEM integrates path analysis. Here, equations define the hypothesized relationships between variables. They can be either unidirectional or bidirectional, direct, and indirect. The construction of a structural model to be empirically tested by SEM is a core, intellectually challenging task for the researcher. With the construction of a measurement model, the relations between observed and latent variables are specified. As a special strength of this approach, linear relationships between variables are estimated while accounting for measurement error. By specifying a structural and measurement model in a path diagram, SEM analysis is performed, based on established estimation procedures provided by SEM software. Once a model is identified, it has to be estimated in order to determine how well the model fits the data. As defined by Beran and Violate, 'fitting the latent variable path model involves minimizing the difference between the sample covariances and the covariances predicted by the model' (Beran and Violato 2010, p. 4). The different estimation procedures (e.g. maximum likelihood or least squares) and the tests of evaluating goodness of fit are not described here, as a more extended analysis would be required (see Kline 2016). However, readers interested in applying SEM should be aware of several strengths and restrictions of this approach. Strengths include the complexity of testing relationships between variables, specifically by distinguishing observed from latent variables. Moreover, by testing a hypothesized theoretical model with empirical data, and by assessing the goodness of model fit, this approach can significantly advance scientific insights. At a practical level, strengths concern the integration of continuous and binary variables, application in cross-sectional and longitudinal studies, and the simultaneous, not sequential inclusion of all endogenous variables in calculations. As a particular advantage, simultaneous calculation path coefficients are mutually adjusted. There are also some limitations. For instance, application of SEM requires a relatively large sample size (preferably several hundred participants) to reduce the likelihood of random variation. Furthermore, its mathematical operations require that data are provided at interval-scale level, a prerequisite that is often violated by data derived from social and behavioural science methods. Caution is also needed when assuming causal associations. Although suggested by the term 'causal modelling', a proof of causality cannot be directly deduced from SEM, as it requires that additional criteria are met. Finally, as SEM is based on a number of statistical assumptions and requires advanced statistical expertise, its application should be restricted to well-trained researchers.

5.1.3 Multilevel analysis

Multilevel analysis (also labelled as 'hierarchical modelling') represents an extension of standard regression analysis that deals with correlated observations. In the above-mentioned regression analyses, individual observations are treated as independent facts. Here, correlated individual observations are nested within groups. For instance, an analysis interested in effects of work characteristics on workers' health can study these associations not only at the lowest level of individual data but can additionally collect data from a larger population, such as work groups or companies. These larger groups represent clusters that exert their own effects on health, thus offering a second 'higher' level of analysis. This two-level structure of data analysis is the most commonly used approach, but additional levels (e.g. countries) can be incorporated. An additional application of multi-level analysis concerns repeated measurements of same persons in longitudinal studies. Here, observations assessed at different time points within the same persons are correlated, thus representing a distinct level of analysis.

Starting from the simplest linear regression mentioned above $E(Y) = a + b \times X$, we saw that an independent variable X (e.g. job insecurity of workers at individual level) is related to a dependent variable Y (e.g. quality of life, measured at continuous level), where a is the intercept of the line, and b is its slope (or regression coefficient). If the total sample of workers whose job insecurity is being studied, has been recruited from thirty different work groups, and if we want to take into account this work group effect, linear regression analysis would need to correct for different intercepts across work groups, that is, to estimate twenty-nine additional regression intercept coefficients. This complicated procedure is avoided by multilevel analysis which requires only one single random effect parameter representing the twenty-nine intercepts. As essential information for this statistical approach, the intraclass correlation coefficient (ICC) indicates the correlation between individual observations nested within a group (e.g. job insecurity within workers in a work group). ICC is calculated as the variance between workgroups divided by the total variance including the variance between workgroups and variance within workgroups. Thus, ICC refers to the proportion of the total variance attributed to differences between the level units (i.e. workgroups).

Moving further, as intercepts are assumed to differ between workgroups, the relationship between job insecurity (X) and quality of life (Y) is also assumed to vary across workgroups. To this end, interaction terms between X and workgroups are integrated in the regression equation, estimating different slopes of the regression line for each workgroup. Thus, in addition to random intercepts, random slopes are estimated, based on one variance parameter for the different slopes of the regression lines for the different workgroups.

To sum up, multilevel analysis is an efficient approach of handling data with a hierarchical structure where individuals are nested in higher level categorical variables (such as workgroups) (see also Sinclair et al. 2013). Statistical models enable the analysis of within- and between-cluster variability, where between-cluster variability is modelled with random effect. Sometimes, contextual variables are constructed to disentangle individual-level and organization-level effects within the framework of a proportional hazard Cox regression model. For instance, the contribution of work stress, assessed at individual level and at work-unit level, towards explaining the risk of disability pension due to depression was analysed in a remarkable study in Finland (Juvani et al. 2014). With the availability of useful statistical software, an increasing number of epidemiological studies in the field of occupational health rely on multilevel analysis. Importantly, as this approach represents an extension of standard regression analyses, multilevel analysis should follow all assumptions inherent in standard regression analyses. As an additional assumption to be observed, random intercepts and random slopes are expected to be normally distributed (Diez-Roux 2000; Gelman and Hill 2006; Greenland 2000).

Applying the different types of regression analysis, including multilevel analysis, in occupational health research has advanced the knowledge on the complexity of associations between multiple variables affecting health. Further substantial insights are expected from research using innovative statistical approaches to causal analysis.

5.2 Causal analysis

Randomized controlled trials (RCTs) are considered the 'gold standard' for establishing causal inference. Unfortunately, such randomized studies are often impractical or too costly. Thus, causal inference derived from observational studies provides a challenge when randomized research evidence is difficulty to obtain. Unlike a strictly designed RCT, the different conditions of exposure in observational studies are not randomized, and they are subject to change over time. In addition, the analysis has to deal with confounders, mediators, effect modifiers, and colliders. Despite efforts of meeting the well-known Hill-criteria of a causal relationship in observational epidemiological studies, causal inference in prospective study designs remains a critical issue. Even if reverse causation can be excluded and sources of bias can be controlled, the usual extended time interval between exposure assessment and disease onset, and the many factors potentially interfering with this association complicate clear-cut conclusions. In consequence, it is difficult to exclude a relevant impact of unobserved confounding on the final results. Therefore, new statistical techniques, often referred to as causal methods, were developed to tackle these methodological problems (Wen et al. 2021; Williamson and Ravani 2017). One such approach towards examining causal inference, a counterfactual account of causation, is briefly explained here (VanderWeele 2015). In essence, this approach aims at developing a strategy to estimate unobserved counterfactuals. For instance, based on two binary variables X and Y, each variable can take two forms, 1 or 0, thus offering four effects from X to Y. If X measures work stress and Y measures risk of depression in a population, depression outcomes of those exposed to work stress are used to estimate what outcomes would have been for non-exposed people, if they had been exposed. Similarly, depression risk for non-exposed people is used to estimate the depression risk that would have been experienced by exposed people, if they had not been exposed. To contrast counterfactual outcomes, a metric, such as the risk difference between the two estimates, is applied that points to a causal effect (Glymour and Kubzansky 2018). In other words, a coun terfactual approach to causal inference requires that the causal effects are defined in terms of contrasts between the distributions of the outcome under hypothetically different well-defined interventions. This approach includes covariates that aim to estimate unobservable counterfactuals (VanderWeele 2015).

In view of the complexity of causal analysis in psychosocial occupational health research it is essential to specify causal research questions in terms of hypothetical pathways that need to be tested in a counterfactual framework. To this end, a Directed Acyclic Graphs (DAGs) approach was developed as an instructive tool to guide the analytical process (Greenland et al. 1999). It directs the researcher to decide how variables under study are related, using formal logic. Importantly, the direction of effects and the function of covariates need to be defined. For instance, if a covariate is interpreted as a confounder, the decision would be to adjust for its effects on exposure and on outcome. If the covariate is interpreted as collider, affected by exposure and outcome, it would be excluded from analysis. However, a covariate acting as mediator or effect modifier will be introduced in a respective analytical framework. The application of DAGs follows certain conventions and defined signs of notation (e.g. an arrow between two variables represents a proposed causal effect). Often, a stepwise selection process precedes a final representation of the proposed causal structure. Overall, the use of this tool represents a major advance in developing and analysing research plans in epidemiology (Glymour and Kubzansky 2018).

In counterfactual-based mediation analysis, the total effect of an exposure on an outcome is decomposed into a natural direct effect and a natural indirect, mediated effect. Randomized intervention analogues of the natural direct effect and of the natural indirect effect on the outcome are estimated (for an example, see Box 5.1). This analysis aims to minimize unbiased direct and indirect, mediated effects of an exposure on an outcome, as well as effects due to an interaction between exposure and mediator. By additionally integrating time-variant covariates as potential confounders, this approach provides more detailed and reliable information than the conventional mediation analysis. As a major methodological advancement, counterfactual analysis deserves an extended explanation by statisticians. Here, we can only refer to the impressive work of pioneering experts (e.g. Oakes and Kaufman 2017; VanderWeele 2015). Moreover, a set of software packages is available for application in data analysis (see recommended websites at the end of the chapter). To give readers a first impression of the strengths of counterfactual analysis, a recent publication from psychosocial occupational research is briefly described (see Box 5.1).

In many research areas observational measures of exposures are correlated with an error term, most often with an unmeasured (confounding) variable affecting the independent and the dependent variable. This problem may produce a bias in estimating causal relationships. Introducing an instrumental variable represents a strategy towards controlling this bias. An instrumental variable is defined as an independent indicator strongly correlated with the exposure measure, affecting the outcome exclusively via the exposure. As a precondition, it must not be correlated with unmeasured confounders (Hernán and Robins 2006). Instrumental variables are often used in econometrics, but rarely in psychosocial occupational epidemiology.

One example from this latter field may illustrate the advantage of including an instrumental variable analysis into a multivariable regression approach. The study explored associations of self-reported job demand and job control with sickness absence due to a psychiatric diagnosis among a large sample of hospital nurses in Finland (Kivimäki et al. 2010). The self-reported exposure was judged to be correlated with an error term due to potential reporting bias. To control for this bias, an objective measure of high demand and low control at work was introduced, the amount of hospital bed overcrowding on wards. Monthly bed occupancy rates were computed to construct a four-level indicator of overcrowding. Using instrumental probit regression analysis, associations of psychosocial work factors with psychiatric diagnoses were examined in relation to the variation attributable to overcrowding. In the final model, differences in the levels of self-reported job demands, as predicted by overcrowding, were associated with nurses' absence from work due to a psychiatric diagnosis during a twelve-month follow-up in a dose-response relationship. The authors concluded

Box 5.1 Mediation of the association of job insecurity with incident ischaemic heart disease (IHD) by four proposed constructs, applying counterfactual-based mediation analysis.

The study used data on exposures, mediators, and covariates from phase 5 of the prospective British Whitehall II cohort (1997-1999) and incident data of IHD during follow-up (up to 2007-2009). The prospective association of job insecurity with incident IHD was analysed, exploring the potential mediating role of four factors (unhealthy behaviour; sleep disturbances, allostatic load, and psychological distress). First, the prerequisites of mediation were analysed (i.e. whether associations of job insecurity with the four mediators were statistically significant, and whether relationships of mediators with IHD, adjusting for job insecurity, were significant). Next, counterfactual-based mediation analysis was performed separately for each mediator, including a set of covariates as confounders (e.g. age, sex, education). While the total effect of each mediator indicated a moderately increased risk of IHD, two mediators only demonstrated significant direct effects (sleep disturbances and psychological distress, measuring reduced mental health), and a significant indirect effect of job insecurity on IHD was restricted to psychological distress. Here the hazard ratios were 1.32 for the total effect, 1.22 for the direct effect, and 1.08 for the indirect effect. The authors concluded that about 30 per cent of the total relationship of job insecurity with IHD was mediated by psychological distress, whereas the remaining mediating constructs did not contribute to the explanation of the link of job insecurity with IHD (Magnusson Hanson et al. 2020).

that a reporting bias of self-reported job assessment could be partially excluded (for job demands, but not for job control) by applying instrumental variable analysis (Kivimäki et al. 2010).

Among the different ways of identifying instrumental variables, Mendelian randomization received special attention, in particular in response to ground-breaking advances in molecular genetics. This method uses genetic variants as instrumental variables in analyses of causal effects of behavioural or biomedical risk factors on chronic disease manifestation.

In a short review, Davies et al. (2018) explained this procedure with regard to the relationship between alcohol consumption and high blood pressure (BP), as potentially determined by social deprivation. If social deprivation is proposed as a determinant of alcohol consumption with adverse effects on BP, this variable might be correlated with an error term as it equally affects BP independent of alcohol consumption, thus questioning a causal sequence. To resolve this problem, genetic data may be useful. People with a distinct variant in the ALDH2 gene were found to restrain their alcohol consumption quite dramatically, compared to those without this allele. The ALDH2 variant, while being unrelated to BP, is strongly correlated with alcohol consumption. Therefore, differences in outcomes between the two groups of gene variants may provide an explanation of the association under study more convincingly than a reference to social deprivation (Davies et al. 2018). To summarize, in analogy to a natural experiment, Mendelian randomization uses observational data derived from gene-wide association studies for estimation of a causal effect in associations of modifiable risk factors with disease manifestation. To date, it is not known whether and to what extent insights derived from Mendelian randomization studies can enrich knowledge on psychosocial determinants of occupational disorders and diseases.

In conclusion, causal analysis within observational studies has developed into an innovative field of statistical investigation offering more detailed and more reliable insights than those obtained from conventional approaches. Yet, its application asks for advanced methodological expertise, and in all cases, theoretical justification of decisions on how to construct an analytical model is essential. To this end, DAGs are a supportive tool that deserves wide use in epidemiological research. This section of the chapter has shed light on just a small part of an extended field of analysis, and even this small part was restricted to some basic descriptions and explanations. Consultation of standard literature will be required to advance knowledge of this field of analysis. Some important additional approaches were not even mentioned although they might be of interest to occupational health research. Natural experiments are one such approach. Here, a major societal or organizational ('exogenous') innovation (e.g. implementation of preschool programmes; extension of years of schooling; legal introduction of four-day working week) is defined as an experimental 'treatment' whose effects on specific outcomes are compared with outcomes under non-experimental conditions. For instance, robust effects of extended education time on health and mortality were demonstrated with this method

(Galama et al. 2018). With our exclusive focus on quantitative methods, the contributions of mixed methods (e.g. combining quantitative and qualitative methods) and of triangulation to causal analysis remained unnoticed. Triangulation is particularly important as it combines findings on an identical research question that are derived from different study designs and different disciplines. Integrating evidence from different design-based approaches extends and enriches knowledge that is often constraint by disciplinary boundaries, thus opening new insights into the web of causation. Taken together, a rich inventory of methods and statistical approaches is now available for new investigations into the multiple determinants of occupational health.

5.3 Systematic review and meta-analysis

In times of exponential growth of scientific information, it is increasingly difficult to overview the state of art in almost all disciplines and fields of inquiry. Even in highly specialized areas new findings emerge almost daily, and keeping up with most recent evidence requires never-ending effort. Certainly, to this end, a range of excellent search tools and links to online literature are available, providing extensive information on published work. Yet, retrieving literature in a systematic way is a time-consuming activity, requiring some formal skills. Probably more challenging than being up to date in one's area of research is the problem of judging the quality and significance of published information. In times of openly released fake news and of collective efforts to discredit scientific work, it is particularly important to be able to distinguish between solid research findings and irrelevant or erroneous information. Consulting international handbooks and textbooks, and reading articles in high-quality scientific journals, as documented by a high impact score and complex peer review system, are strategies to successfully tackle this challenge. As an additional highly useful strategy, systematic reviews and meta-analyses of published research evidence on a specific topic or field of inquiry are becoming increasingly popular and widely acknowledged. Over the last few decades, the Cochrane Collaboration established high standards in conducting systematic reviews (Higgins et al. 2019). In this section, we describe some essentials of systematic reviews, their procedures, and the interpretation of their findings.

Our first questions are as follows: What is a hierarchy of scientific evidence? And why are systematic reviews an important contribution to such a hierarchy? In Figure 5.2 an attempt is made to stratify sources of scientific evidence according to their strength of providing information on causal associations. This stratification reflects the degree of certainty of assuming a causal association, based on the ability to exclude and control for sources of bias and error. The classical experiment, the RCT as an interventional study, is considered to provide the most conclusive source of scientific evidence. Even higher rated than results from single RCTs are systematic reviews and meta-analyses that combine and analyse information from several RCTs on a single topic. Meta-reviews range at the top of the hierarchy as they offer a synthesis derived from available systematic reviews of RCTs, thus summarizing and analysing findings at the highest level of generalization. Observational studies are placed below experimental investigations, and the first place is accorded to prospective epidemiological (cohort) studies.

Again, systematic reviews and meta-analyses combining information from several studies on a topic are rated higher than single studies, and again, meta-reviews dominate this range of evidence. There is a zone of intersection between experimental and observational studies not indicated in Figure 5.2, consisting of quasi-experimental (including

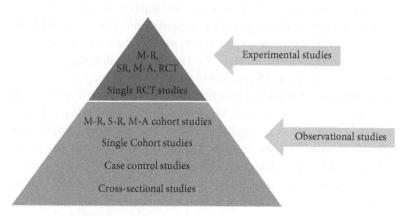

Figure 5.2 Hierarchy of scientific evidence in experimental and observational studies. M-A, meta-analysis; M-R, meta-review; RCT, randomized controlled trials; S-R, Systematic review.

Counterfactual models (e.g. using instrumental variables or Mendelian randomization) and quasi-experimental studies are located at the interface between experimental and observational studies.

Source: Adapted with permission from Davies, N.M., Holmes, M.V., and Davey Smith, G.D. (2018), 'Reading Mendelian randomisation studies: a guide, glossary, and checklist for clinicians', *BMJ*, 362, k601. [Figure 4, p. 8]; license no.: 5497001367711.

non-randomized) study findings and of results derived from new statistical techniques of causal inference (counterfactual models, including application of instrumental variables, Mendelian randomization, etc.) (see also Davies et al. 2018). Future classifications of levels of scientific evidence may develop this intersection in more detail. Downstream, the next stage is defined by case–control studies, again preceded by systematic reviews, meta-analyses, and meta-reviews, while the lowest level of evidence is attributed to cross-sectional investigations either at individual-data level or at aggregate (ecological)-data level. As mentioned, systematic reviews and meta-analyses provide a higher level of certainty than findings from single studies because they collect and evaluate research evidence on a specific topic, identifying consistencies and inconsistencies, and enabling generalization beyond single studies. A large majority of systematic reviews and meta-analyses focus on RCTs and on cohort studies as these designs range at the top of this hierarchy of evidence.

Next, we provide answers to these questions: What types of reviews have been established in scientific research, and what are the specific features of systematic reviews? Reviews represent any effort of collecting and comparing scientific information on a specified research topic within a fixed time interval. Reviews are usually restricted to original research articles published in accessible scientific journals and to scientific books. The number of languages (and countries) included is limited, and consideration of 'grey literature' varies widely. In Box 5.2 the main types of reviews are briefly described.

Systematic reviews represent a comprehensive, transparent, standardized search, identification, analysis, and appraisal of available scientific evidence on a specified research question. Several chapters of this book, most notably Chapter 6, rely heavily on evidence derived from systematic reviews as well as the few meta-reviews already available (e.g. Niedhammer et al. 2021). Systematic reviews usually focus on published scientific reports, but they may include unpublished study findings. The main sources are scientific journals and books, eventually including grey literature and other sources of information. Systematic reviews are based on a written protocol (which is registered in PROSPERO or related sites). The methods to be applied are expected to follow the guidelines of PRISMA (Preferred Reporting Items for Systematic Review and Meta-Analysis: Liberati et al. 2009). These guidelines contain a checklist of twenty-seven items instructing researchers about what information needs to be collected in what form. Items concern the Introduction, Methods, Results, and Discussion parts of scientific

Box 5.2 **Types of reviews of published scientific information**

- Scoping Review: It provides a summary of the current state on a topic or on different approaches towards its analysis. It is useful as an orientation and potential basis for more systematic inquiry. Although based on a protocol defining aims, selection criteria and search strategy, it is not exhaustive as it often lacks specificity. No attempt is made to evaluate the methodological quality of study findings. However, attempts were developed for standardization of the process (Tricco et al. 2018).

- Rapid Review: It aims to summarize evidence on a detailed research topic with the intention of informing decision-making by practitioners and policy makers. Main information is derived from systematic reviews and meta-analysis, supplemented by primary level evidence. Produced as rigorous and critical appraisal in a short time (one or two months), it is nevertheless based on a protocol that defines aims, inclusion criteria of sources, and search strategy (data bases, search terms). Distinct from the scoping review, it proposes preliminary conclusions on the quality and relevance of evidence (Martin et al. 2020).

- Narrative Review: Combining features of scoping and rapid review, this type offers a more extensive, in-depth inquiry into the state of art on a specific research topic or field of interest. While its topical range is broader than that of systematic reviews it does not follow a standardized methodology of literature search, analysis, and evaluation. It aims to compensate these restrictions by identifying open questions, new ideas and directions of further analysis.

- Systematic Review: It provides the results of a transparent process of information synthesis on a detailed research question, based on a pre-defined methodology of literature search, data analysis and appraisal. Its procedures are highly specified and need to meet defined quality criteria. As far as comparable quantitative data are available, a meta-analysis of results is additionally performed. A detailed description of this type of review is given below.

- Meta-Review: If a research area produces abundant new information in a short time, resulting in a number of updated systematic reviews, scientists may be motivated to summarize the most recent state of art in terms of a meta-review. This procedure offers a synthesis of findings derived from comparable systematic reviews on an identical topic performed either as a qualitative or a quantitative analysis. In this latter case, a meta-analysis based on pooled estimates available from the systematic reviews included offers the most robust empirical answer to the research question under study.

reports. As a first step, the research question has to be specified and framed in a scientific context, followed by a series of relevant decisions that are usually listed as PECO. P refers to populations to be studied, and E points to the exposures of interest. In occupational epidemiology, exposures are of main interest, whereas in intervention studies, E is replaced by I (PICO). C refers to comparators, that is, to groups with different levels of exposures or exposed vs unexposed populations, and O stands for outcome (e.g. disease category). Additionally, the different study designs or study types are listed, as well as the types of effect measures to be considered. As defined in the protocol, electronic databases are enumerated and accessed for systematic literature search. They usually include PubMed, Medline, Scopus, PsycINFO, Web of Science, and Cochrane Library, among others. Hand-searching and expert consultation as well as grey literature searches provide further sources of information. As a crucial step, search terms need to be devised and defined as they structure the selection process of study records. Once these study records are identified through the search process titles and abstracts are screened by two independent reviewers, followed by full-text reading of the studies that are finally included. The study selection process is visualized in a flow chart, again instructed by Guidelines for Accurate and Transparent Health Estimating Reporting (GATHER; Stevens et al. 2016).

Based on a standard data extraction form, relevant data from each study are listed, providing the substance for subsequent data analysis. As an important quality criterion risk of bias needs to be assessed. To this end, different approaches were developed, and one of these approaches, the Navigation Guide (Woodruff and Sutton 2014) is particularly suitable for occupational and environmental health research. Its assessment criteria are (i) source population representation; (ii) blinding; (iii) exposure assessment; (iv) outcome assessment; (v) confounding; (vi) incomplete outcome data; (vii) selective outcome reporting; (viii) conflict of interest; and (ix) other sources of bias. The results of bias assessment are summarized in a table, indicating the level of bias (from 'low' to 'high').

Once extracted data are ready for quantitative exploration, a meta-analysis is conducted. This approach is defined as statistical analysis combining comparable data from different studies on a common topic in order to estimate an overall effect size of the association under study. In addition, differences between study findings are investigated. Results of a meta-analysis are presented as pooled estimates in graphical form, indicating elevated or reduced risk estimates (HR, RR) and 95 per cent confidence intervals for single studies and for the total effect. The two main statistical models applied in meta-analysis are labelled 'fixed-effect models' and 'random-effects models'. In the former case, a common effect underlying all single studies is assumed, and differences in observed effects between studies are attributed to sampling errors. In contrast, the random-effects model assumes that variations in observed effects between studies reflect an objective heterogeneity of associations between studies.

In comparative epidemiological investigations, the random-effects model is often an appropriate choice accounting for between-studies heterogeneity. Figure 5.3 gives an example of a random-effects meta-analysis. In a collaborative meta-analysis of individual participant data from thirteen European cohort studies, the effect of job strain, assessed as a binary exposure variable, on risk of incident IHD was estimated (Kivimäki et al. 2012). The figure indicates the study acronyms, the number of IHD events, the size of the study population (to calculate weights), and the HRs with 95 per cent confidence intervals. A combined effect from all studies resulted in an elevated IHD risk of 23 per cent due to exposure to job strain versus no exposure. This analysis further examined the association of job strain with IHD in relation to study follow-up periods, additional adjustments, publication status, and geographical region of studies, corroborating the evidence presented in the figure (Kivimäki et al. 2012).

In a final step, the results of a meta-analysis are judged with respect to the quality and strength of evidence. Again, a tool termed GRADE (Grading of Recommendations Assessment, Development and Evaluation) supports this task accomplishment that is usually performed independently by two review authors (Morgan et al. 2019). For instance, the quality of evidence is downgraded if there is indication of a high risk of bias as well as publication

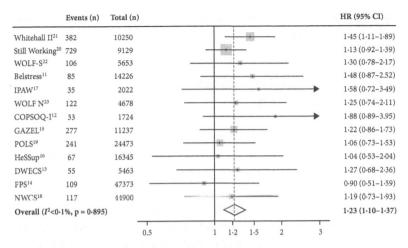

	Events (n)	Total (n)		HR (95% CI)
Whitehall II[21]	382	10250		1·45 (1·11–1·89)
Still Working[20]	729	9129		1·13 (0·92–1·39)
WOLF-S[22]	106	5653		1·30 (0·78–2·17)
Belstress[11]	85	14226		1·48 (0·87–2.52)
IPAW[17]	35	2022		1·58 (0·72–3·49)
WOLF N[23]	122	4678		1·25 (0·74–2·11)
COPSOQ-I[12]	33	1724		1·88 (0·89–3·95)
GAZEL[15]	277	11237		1·22 (0·86–1·73)
POLS[19]	241	24473		1·06 (0·73–1·53)
HeSSup[16]	67	16345		1·04 (0·53–2·04)
DWECS[13]	55	5463		1·27 (0·68–2·36)
FPS[14]	109	47373		0·90 (0·51–1·59)
NWCS[18]	117	44900		1·19 (0·73–1·93)
Overall (I^2<0·1%, p = 0·895)				1·23 (1·10–1·37)

Figure 5.3 Random-effects meta-analysis of the association between job strain and incident coronary heart disease. Estimates are adjusted for age and sex. WOLF-S, Work, Lipids, Fibrinogen-Stockholm; IPAW, Intervention Project on Absence and Well-being; WOLF-N, Work, Lipids, Fibrinogen-Norrland; COPSOQ-I, Copenhagen Psychosocial Questionnaire version I; GAZEL, Electricité De France-Gaz De France; POLS, Permanent Onderzoek Leefsituatie; HeSSup, Health and Social Support; DWECS, Danish Work Environment Cohort Study; FPS, Finnish Public Sector Study; NWCS, Netherlands Working Conditions Survey.

Source: Reproduced with permission from Kivimäki, M., Nyberg, S. T., Batty, G. D., et al. (2012), 'Job strain as a risk factor for coronary heart disease: a collaborative meta-analysis of Individual Participant Data', *Lancet*, 380 (9852), 1491–7. [Figure 1, p. 1493].

bias. Recent statistical methods for meta-analysis help researchers to automatically downgrade studies at high level of risk of bias (Verde 2021).

In summary, carefully conducted systematic reviews and meta-analyses, as well as meta-reviews, are considered a gold standard for presenting and discussing scientific evidence derived from epidemiological research. Performing this task requires a collaborative effort and substantial time (usually between six months and two years). This work provides an essential contribution to scientific progress. With the high quality of guidelines and prescribed standards, it strengthens the credibility and significance of scientific achievements. At the same time, there is room for further development, specifically within observational research (Menon et al. 2022). The following chapters demonstrate the strengths and promises of systematic reviews in the field of psychosocial occupational health research, and they highlight their importance in the crucial process of transmitting scientific evidence to policy measures.

5.4 The ethical dimension of scientific research

Scientific research represents a collective interpersonal activity that can be characterized as the search for new valid knowledge. Individual researchers participate in this collective activity by their—often long-lasting, even life-long—contributions in a process of competitive striving for scientific—and personal—advancement. With their contributions they are part of a transgenerational project that transcends their own lives. As a universal, transgenerational societal activity of outstanding significance, the project of science essentially depends on the validity of distinct binding norms and procedural rules, and on continued institutional support. Integrity of research is the supreme binding norm. It posits that scientific work remains free from personal interests and external pressures, solely committed to the prescribed standards and procedures within scientific communities. Among others, these standards prevent the promotion of unethical projects and methods, the lack of awareness of ethical requirements, and the violation of rules of data collection, analysis, presentation, and discussion. Moreover, they require full transparency of funding conditions and the prevention of their impact on the research process itself. They ask scientists to present and discuss their work in a self-critical way, to accept fair criticism of their work, to support independent analysis or replication of their research results, and to respect alternative views and positions within their scientific community. Adherence to these principles is expected to reduce the risks of disseminating faulty findings, of distorting, manipulating, or falsifying data, and of causing harm by violating ethical norms.

Results derived from solid scientific knowledge represent an essential element of societal progress. The protection of independent, quality-assured scientific work is therefore a crucial task. From its very beginning, the production of scientific knowledge was faced with the challenge of its 'dual use'. On one hand, research findings are applied to promote human well-being and societal progress; on the other hand, they can be applied to damage human well-being, to prevent societal progress, or even to produce far-reaching detrimental effects. To date, with a globalized process of scientific productivity, risks evolving from this dual use continue to raise concerns. Even worse, with the expansion of internet communication and of virtual social media, social movements are gaining impact that aim at discrediting science by promoting 'alternative facts' that consist of distorted or faked information. How can science be protected against these internal and external risks? Although not exhaustive, the following list of measures identifies some particularly relevant requirements that need to be observed .

- Respecting essential the human and civil rights that enable the freedom of research, including the right to discuss, disseminate, and publish results;
- Observing the codes of conduct in scientific research, in particular research on human health and well-being (World Medical Association 2013);
- Ensuring that all research involving human subjects is submitted to, and approved by ethical committees established within, or collaborating with, research institutions;
- Applying independent peer review procedures in decision-making on relevant scientific matters, such as academic appointments, provision of research grants, publication of scientific findings, and evaluation of academic achievements;
- Providing substantial public funding for scientific research to guarantee the independence of research and its avoidance of interest-driven sponsorship;
- Educating and training people involved in scientific research at early stages of their careers; providing supervision by senior leaders, and promoting fair teamwork in scientific collaboration;
- Increasing transparency of procedures and outcomes of scientific work;
- Punishing misconduct of scientists, their supporting peers, and organizations.

In everyday life, scientists are exposed to a variety of pressures and contexts that may interfere with the norms of scientific integrity. First of all, as there is recurrent competition for, and shortage of, funding from public agencies, there is a risk that researchers are tempted to look for—and find—resources from market-related funding agencies with economic interests. In fact, in some areas, close collaboration between scientists and corporations, enterprises, or specific interest groups was established, opening possibilities of suppressing undesired research evidence or of manipulating scientific data and results. The tobacco industry is a well-documented example (Bero 2005). Yet, such collaboration was also observed in occupational medical research dealing with toxic occupational substances (Markowitz and Rosner 1991). The problem of dual use is aggravated if research institutions are under direct control of market-related funding agencies, or of private or public funding agencies that exert political control of the direction of research. Freedom and independence of research carried out at universities as public, independent institutions may be weakened by the appearance of entrepreneurial, privately funded universities striving for short-term success and practical utility of research outcomes. Within a globalized development of scientific competition, incentives for careerism and the promotion of individual excellence undermine a spirit of trustful cooperation and solidarity among peers. A pressure towards 'publish or perish' is omnipresent, often linked to bonus payments and career promotion prospects within universities.

One is not surprised to learn that competition in academic settings results in unequal treatment of colleagues and subordinates, giving rise to attempts of privileging certain members and of disadvantaging or excluding others. Those in the early stage of careers, those with fixed-term contracts, or those working in the periphery are at risk of being treated unfairly in their research development, that is, being victims of procedural and distributive injustice within their organization. A pioneering study of a large, representative sample of publicly funded US scientists revealed that those early-career and mid-career scientists who experienced organizational injustice at their work placee were more often engaged in some form of scientific misconduct than those treated with fairness (Martinson et al. 2006). Violating scientific norms, even by committing a minor deviance from established standards, can be interpreted as a compensation for experienced injustice, a measure of retaliation that may damage the integrity of the institution. These study findings support practical measures to monitoring and foster good scientific conduct and to prevent practices of distributive and procedural injustice in everyday settings of scientific work (Martinson et al. 2006).

The problem of personal responsibility of scientists lies at the core of the dual use challenge of research findings. While the codes of conduct and other measures mentioned may prevent or at least reduce misuse and intended damage, it remains an open question to what extent scientists are obliged to commit themselves to transmission of their findings into practical action. Although opportunities for transmission vary across scientific disciplines, topics, and socio-political contexts of research, two basic normative positions offer different answers to this question. One position maintains that the task of science is restricted to the production of high-quality research findings, and that researchers should not compromise their unique social capital of independence, objectivity, and integrity by confounding their role through dependence from external constraints by offering advice and being engaged in practical applications of research findings. According to another position, the contribution of scientific research to the promotion of human welfare, well-being, and global sustainability is considered the supreme goal, and to the extent that scientific knowledge contributes to this goal, researchers are expected to be proactively engaged in this promotion. Of course, this engagement should not conflict with the basic standards and principles of scientific conduct. Scientists have to deliberately decide on the direction they are following in their research contributions. In times of global crises, such as climate change and environmental destruction, the COVID-19 pandemic, or increasing social inequalities in health and well-being, influential scientific associations, organizations, and networks started to take an active role in the transmission of scientific evidence into political action. The Intergovernmental Panel on Climate Change is an instructive example of extensive, continued scientific engagement with political impact, while maintaining a high level of scientific expertise throughout this process (Intergovernmental Panel on Climate Change 2022). The outbreak of the COVID-19 pandemic not only boosted international collaboration among scientists, but it broadened the impact of scientific advice to policy in unprecedented ways at local, national, and international levels. Another example concerns the initiative of the World Health Organization in setting up a scientific Commission on Social Determinants of Health to synthesize global evidence on social inequalities in health, and to develop recommendations for action (CSDH 2008). These recommendations were not only endorsed by the WHO General Assembly, but they contributed to a number of national health policy agendas. Within the field of occupational health research, the International Committee on Occupational Health (ICOH) represents a global scientific association with potential policy impact, mainly through collaboration with the International Labour Organization and WHO. Although this organization produced several relevant declarations (e.g. elimination of asbestos-related diseases; development of occupational health services for all) its impact on political developments so far remains rather modest. The challenges of improving occupational health at national and transnational level are briefly discussed in the final chapter of this book (Chapter 11). An in-depth discussion of the ethical dimension of scientific research is not feasible without expert knowledge derived from philosophy, law, sociology, and those scientific disciplines that are most directly confronted with ethical risks (e.g. molecular genetics, physics). Nevertheless, to conclude, compliance with scientific codes and standards, and awareness of the pressing problem of dual use of research results are universal normative duties for scientists in any field of research. Moreover, every individual researcher has to decide whether or not to be proactively engaged in the transmission of new scientific knowledge into policy and practical action.

5.5 Summary

Data analysis is a core task of scientific research. This chapter presented some basic introductory information on essential approaches of analytic statistics, starting with regression including mediation, effect modification, and interaction analysis. Subsequently, structural equation and multilevel analysis were introduced, and the challenge of causal analysis in observational studies was briefly discussed. In times of excessive flow of scientific information systematic reviews and meta-analyses are useful tools of updating, structuring, and evaluating current knowledge. Readers have been acquainted with the principles of these tools. In a final part, ethical aspects of scientific research were addressed, emphasizing basic principles of scientific integrity, and pointing to the dangers of scientific misconduct as well as the role of personal responsibility.

5.6 Relevant questions

- Can you explain the differences between mediation, effect modification, and interaction by using an example from the field of occupational health?
- If you are expected to solve an urgent problem and are urged to rely on evidence from scoping and rapid reviews, what are the main disadvantages of using this information, compared to a systematic review and meta-analysis? Why is it nevertheless useful to rely on these tools?

- Competition and pressure in scientific research open possibilities for scientific misconduct, at least in less severe forms. Which measures are most efficient in preventing this behaviour?

Recommended reading

❖ Gelman, A., and Hill, J. (2006), *Data analysis using regression and multilevel/ hierarchical models*. Cambridge: Cambridge University Press.
❖ Sinclair, R. R., Wang, M., and Tetrick, L. E. (eds.) (2013), *Research methods in occupational health psychology. Measurement, design, and data analysis*. New York, NY, London: Routledge.
❖ VanderWeele, T. J. (2015), *Explanation in causal inference: methods for mediation and interaction*. Oxford: Oxford University Press.

Useful websites

❖ Analysing and Interpreting Data https://www.cdc.gov/eis/field-epi-manual/chapters/analyze-Interpret-Data.html
❖ Programme R: Calculation of descriptive statistics and production of graphs: https://statsandr.com/blog/descriptive-statistics-in-r/https://socialsciences.mcmaster.ca/jfox/Misc/Rcmdr/
❖ Mediation https://davidakenny.net/cm/mediate.htm
❖ Causal Analysis in Theory and Practice http://causality.cs.ucla.edu/blog/

References

Baron, R. M., and Kenny, D. A. (1986), 'The moderator-mediator variable distinction in social psychological research: conceptual, strategic, and statistical considerations', *J Pers Soc Psychol*, 51 (6), 1173–82.

Bender, R., and Grouven, U. (1997), 'Ordinal logistic regression in medical research', *J R Coll Physicians Lond*, 31 (5), 546.

Beran, T. N., and Violato, C. (2010), 'Structural equation modeling in medical research: a primer', *BMC Res*, 3 (1), 1–10.

Bero, L. A. (2005), 'Tobacco industry manipulation of research', *Public Health Rep*, 120 (2), 200.

Borritz, M., Rugulies, R., Christensen, K. B., et al. (2006), 'Burnout as a predictor of self-reported sickness absence among human service workers: Prospective findings from three year follow up of the PUMA study', *Occup Environ Med*, 63 (2), 98–106.

Celentano, D. D., and Szklo, M. (2018), *Gordis epidemiology* 6th edn. Philadelphia: Elsevier.

Checkoway, H., Pearce, N., and Kriebel, D. (2004), *Research methods in occupational epidemiology* 2nd ed. New York: Oxford University Press.

Clays, E., Casini, A., Van Herck, K., et al. (2016), 'Do psychosocial job resources buffer the relation between physical work demands and coronary heart disease? A prospective study among men', *Int Arch Ocup Environ Health*, 89, 1299–307.

CSDH (2008), 'Closing the gap in a generation: health equity through action on the social determinants of health. Final report of the Commission on Social Determinants of Health', Geneva: WHO.

Davies, N. M., Holmes, M. V., and Davey Smith, G. (2018), 'Reading Mendelian randomisation studies: a guide, glossary, and checklist for clinicians', *BMJ*, 362, k601.

De Jonge, J., Bosma, H., Peter, R., et al. (2000), 'Job strain, effort-reward imbalance and employee well-being: a large-scale cross-sectional study', *So Sci Med*, 50 (9), 1317–27.

Denzin, N. K., and Lincoln, Y. S. (2011), *Handbook of qualitative research*. Thousand Oaks, CA: Sage Publications.

Diderichsen, F., Hallqvist, J., and Whitehead, M. (2019), 'Differential vulnerability and susceptibility: how to make use of recent development in our understanding of mediation and interaction to tackle health inequalities', *Int J Epidemiol*, 48 (1), 268–74.

Diez-Roux, A. V. (2000), 'Multilevel analysis in public health research', *Annu Rev Public Health*, 21 (1), 171–92.

Dragano, N., Siegrist, J., Nyberg, S. T., et al. (2017), 'Effort-reward imbalance at work and incident coronary heart disease: a multicohort study of 90,164 individuals', *Epidemiology*, 28 (4), 619–26.

Galama, T., Lleras-Muney, A., and van Kippersluis, H. (2018), *The effect of education on health and mortality: a review of experimental and quasi-experimental evidence*. Cambridge, MA: National Bureau of Economic Research.

Gelman, A., and Hill, J. (2006), *Data analysis using regression and multilevel/hierarchical models*. Cambridge: Cambridge University Press.

Glymour, M. M., and Kubzansky, L. D. (2018), 'Causal inference in psychosocial epidemiology'. In M. Kivimäki, G. D. Batty, A. Steptoe, and I. Kawachi (eds.), *The Routledge international handbook of psychosocial epidemiology*. Abingdon, New York, NY: Routledge/Taylor & Francis Group, 21–45.

Greenland, S. (2000), 'Principles of multilevel modelling', *Int J Epidemiol*, 29 (1), 158–67.

Greenland, S., Pearl, J., and Robins, J. M. (1999), 'Causal diagrams for epidemiologic research', *Epidemiology*, 10 (1), 37–48.

Hayat, M. J., and Higgins, M. (2014), 'Understanding poisson regression', *J Nurs Educ*, 53 (4), 207–15.

Hernán, M. A., and Robins, J. M. (2006), 'Instruments for causal inference: an epidemiologist's dream?', *Epidemiology*, 17 (4), 360–72.

Higgins, J. P. T., Thomas, J., Chandler, J., et al. (eds.) (2019), *Cochrane handbook for systematic reviews of interventions* 2nd edn. Chichester: John Wiley & Sons.

Hosmer, D., Lemeshow, S., and May, S. (2008), *Applied survival analysis: regression modeling of time-to-event data* 2nd ed. Hoboken, NJ: John Wiley & Sons.

Intergovernmental Panel on Climate Change (2022), *Climate change 2022*. Geneva: IPCC.

Juvani, A., Oksanen, T., Salo, P., et al. (2014), 'Effort-reward imbalance as a risk factor for disability pension: the Finnish Public Sector Study', *Scand J Work Environ Health*, 40 (3), 266–77.

Karasek, R. A., Brisson, C., Kawakami, N., et al. (1998), 'The Job Content Questionnaire (JCQ): an instrument for internationally comparative assessments of psychosocial job characteristics', *J Occup Health Psychol*, 3 (4), 322–55.

Kivimäki, M., Vahtera, J., Kawachi, I., et al. (2010), 'Psychosocial work environment as a risk factor for absence with a psychiatric diagnosis: an instrumental-variables analysis', *Am J Epidemiol*, 172 (2), 167–72.

Kivimäki, M., Nyberg, S. T., Batty, G. D., et al. (2012), 'Job strain as a risk factor for coronary heart disease: a collaborative meta-analysis of individual participant data', *Lancet*, 380 (9852), 1491–7.

Kline, R. B. (2016), *Principles and practice of structural equation modelling* 4th ed. New York, NY: The Guilford Press.

Knol, M. J., and VanderWeele, T. J. (2012), 'Recommendations for presenting analyses of effect modification and interaction', *Int J Epidemiol*, 41 (2), 514–20.

Liberati, A., Altman, D. G., Tetzlaff, J., et al. (2009), 'The PRISMA statement for reporting systematic reviews and meta-analyses of studies that evaluate health care interventions: explanation and elaboration', *PLoS Med*, 6 (7), e1000100.

Magnusson Hanson, L. L., Rod, N. H., Vahtera, J., et al. (2020), 'Job insecurity and risk of coronary heart disease: Mediation analyses of health behaviors, sleep problems, physiological and psychological factors', *Psychoneuroendocrinology*, 118, 104706.

Markowitz, G., and Rosner, D. (1991), *Deadly dust: silicosis and the politics of occupational disease in twentieth century America*. Princeton, NJ: Princeton University Press.

Marmot, M. G., Bosma, H., Hemingway, H., et al. (1997), 'Contribution of job control and other risk factors to social variations in coronary heart disease incidence', *Lancet*, 350 (9073), 235–9.

Martin, A., Shann, C., and LaMontagne, A. D. (2020), 'Promoting workplace mental wellbeing: a rapid review of recent intervention research'. In U. Bültmann and J. Siegrist (eds.), *Handbook of disability, work and health*. Cham: Springer, 289–308.

Martinson, B. C., Anderson, M. S., Crain, A. L., et al. (2006), 'Scientists' perceptions of organizational justice and self-reported misbehaviors', *J Empir Res Hum Res Ethics*, 1 (1), 51–66.

Matthews, T. A., Robbins, W., Preisig, M., et al. (2021), 'Associations of job strain and family strain with risk of major depressive episode: a prospective cohort study in US working men and women', *J Psychosom Res*, 147, 110541.

Menon, J. M. L., Struijs, F., and Whaley, P. (2022), 'The methodological rigour of systematic reviews in environmental health', *Crit Rev Toxicol*, 52 (3), 167–87.

Morgan, R. L., Beverly, B., Ghersi, D., et al. (2019), 'GRADE guidelines for environmental and occupational health: a new series of articles in *Environment International*', *Environ Int*, 128, 11–12.

Niedhammer, I., Bertrais, S., and Witt, K. (2021), 'Psychosocial work exposures and health outcomes: a meta-review of 72 literature reviews with meta-analysis', *Scand J Work Environ Health*, 47 (7), 489–508.

Oakes, J. M., and Kaufman, J. S. (eds.) (2017), *Methods in social epidemiology* 2nd ed. San Francisco, CA: Jossey-Bass & Pfeiffer.

Rijnhart, J. J. M., Lamp, S. J., Valente, M. J., et al. (2021), 'Mediation analysis methods used in observational research: a scoping review and recommendations', *BMC Med Res Methodol*, 21 (1), 226.

Schreier, M. (2012), *Qualitative content analysis in practice*. London: Sage Publications.

Siegrist, J., Starke, D., Chandola, T., et al. (2004), 'The measurement of effort-reward imbalance at work: European comparisons', *Soc Sci Med*, 58 (8), 1483–99.

Siemiatycki, J., and Xu, M. (2020), 'Occupational causes of cancer'. In U. Bültmann and J. Siegrist (eds.), *Handbook of disability, work and health*. Cham: Springer, 127–51.

Sinclair, R. R., Wang, M., and Tetrick, L. E. (eds.) (2013), *Research methods in occupational health psychology: measurement, design, and data analysis*. New York, NY, London: Routledge.

Stevens, G. A., Alkema, L., Black, R. E., et al. (2016), 'Guidelines for Accurate and Transparent Health Estimates Reporting: the GATHER statement', *Lancet*, 388 (10062), e19–e23.

Tricco, A. C., Lillie, E., Zarin, W., et al. (2018), 'PRISMA Extension for Scoping Reviews (PRISMA-ScR): Checklist and Explanation', *Ann Intern Med*, 169 (7), 467–73.

Trudel, X., Brisson, C., Talbot, D., et al. (2021), 'Long working hours and risk of recurrent coronary events', *J Am Coll Cardiol*, 77 (13), 1616–25.

Tsutsumi, A., Kayaba, K., and Ishikawa, S. (2011), 'Impact of occupational stress on stroke across occupational classes and genders', *Soc Sci Med*, 72 (10), 1652–8.

Tu, Y.-K. (2009), 'Commentary: is structural equation modelling a step forward for epidemiologists?', *Int J Epidemiol*, 38 (2), 549–51.

VanderWeele, T. J. (2015), *Explanation in causal inference: methods for mediation and interaction*. Oxford: Oxford University Press.

Verde, P. E. (2021), 'A bias-corrected meta-analysis model for combining, studies of different types and quality', *Biom J*, 63 (2), 406–22.

Wahrendorf, M., Sembajwe, G., Zins, M., et al. (2012), 'Long-term effects of psychosocial work stress in midlife on health functioning after labor market exit: results from the GAZEL study', *J Gerontol B Psychol Sci Soc Sci*, 67 (4), 471–80.

Wege, N., Li, J., and Siegrist, J. (2018), 'Are there gender differences in associations of effort-reward imbalance at work with self-reported doctor-diagnosed depression? Prospective evidence from the German Socio-Economic Panel', *Int Arch Occup Environ Health*, 91 (4), 435–43.

Wen, L., Young, J. G., Robins, J. M., et al. (2021), 'Parametric g-formula implementations for causal survival analyses', *Biometrics*, 77 (2), 740–53.

Williamson, T., and Ravani, P. (2017), 'Marginal structural models in clinical research: when and how to use them?', *Nephrol Dial Transplant*, 32 (suppl_2), ii84–ii90.

Woodruff, T. J., and Sutton, P. (2014), 'The Navigation Guide systematic review methodology: a rigorous and transparent method for translating environmental health science into better health outcomes', *Environ Health Perspect*, 122 (10), 1007–14.

World Medical Association (2013), 'World Medical Association Declaration of Helsinki: ethical principles for medical research involving human subjects', *JAMA*, 310 (20), 2191–4.

Zou, G. (2004), 'A modified poisson regression approach to prospective studies with binary data', *Am J Epidemiol*, 159 (7), 702–6.

PART III

EFFECTS OF WORK ON HEALTH

6
Evidence from cohort studies

6.1 Social distribution of psychosocial work environments

Having introduced the main theoretical concepts of psychosocial work en vironments with relevance to health and their measurement (Chapters 3 and 4), it is of interest to learn how exposure to these conditions varies across different working populations. For two reasons it is not easy to give a straight answer to this question. Firstly, there is an unequal number of studies collecting data on the social distribution of the work stress models mentioned. For instance, comparative data on the demand-control (DC) and the effort-reward imbalance (ERI) models, based on proxy measures, are available from a European-wide survey (see Figure 6.1), whereas comparable information on the Organizational Justice (OJ) and Job Demands-Resources (JD-R) models was available from fewer countries. Secondly, there are no uniform cut-off points for the scales measuring these models that define an identical exposure threshold for all populations. Often, exposure is measured either as a continuous variable or cut-off points depending on the distribution of scores. It is now common practice to define the highest (or lowest) quartile of the score distribution of scales in a study population as risk exposure. In cross-national studies, this exposure is identified at country level, and in cohort studies at the level of each study population. In general, scale means compare well across studies, thus supporting this approach (Karasek et al. 1998; Montano et al. 2016; Siegrist et al. 2004).

To illustrate the social distribution of adverse psychosocial work across European countries, an analysis of the prevalence of job strain and effort-reward imbalance was conducted, using data on twenty-nine countries from the European Working Conditions Survey obtained in 2015. To assess socio-economic status, four groups of occupational positions based on the ISCO-88 classification were defined with a focus on skill level: (1) high-skilled clerical (HC); (2) low-skill clerical (LC); (3) high-skill manual (HM); (4) low-skill

Psychosocial Occupational Health. Johannes Siegrist and Jian Li, Oxford University Press.
© Oxford University Press 2024. DOI: 10.1093/oso/9780192887924.003.0006

manual (LM). The core scales of the two models were measured with an abbreviated number of validated items, and two summary indices were constructed, 'job strain' as the ratio of 'demand and 'control', and 'effort-reward imbalance' as the ratio of 'effort' and 'reward', with continuous data ranging from 0.5 to 2 (see Rigó et al. 2021). In Figure 6.1, results of multilevel regression analysis are depicted, with countries as levels and adjusted for age group and gender. Higher means indicate a higher level of stressful work. Means with confidence intervals clearly differ according to occupational group, confirming a steep social gradient in exposure for both work stress models.

In addition to socioeconomic position, the distribution of work stress was analysed between men and women and between three age groups (below 30, 30–50, beyond 50). Gender differences were small, with a somewhat higher level of effort-reward imbalance among women. Concerning age, exposure was higher in the younger and middle-aged than in the older group (not shown). These data underline some relevant variations in the prevalence of adverse psychosocial working conditions across European countries, most importantly their social inequality along the occupational hierarchy. More information will be needed from other regions and from analyses based on additional concepts of critical working conditions.

6.2 Effects on major chronic diseases

6.2.1 Basic notions

As prospective cohort studies are the best available approach to causal inference within an observational study design, this chapter focuses mainly on this type of knowledge generation. It informs readers on essentials of the current state of the art in research on psychosocial work environments and their effects on health. This ambitious aim cannot be realized without several limitations. Firstly, given our interest in providing scientific explanations, theoretical models offer the best approach to this end. Therefore, our analysis is essentially based on the theoretical models introduced in Chapter 3. Secondly, no attempt is made to provide a systematic review or meta-review of the whole field of research. Many such systematic reviews are available and will be mentioned below, including an excellent meta-review of systematic reviews and meta-analyses (Niedhammer et al. 2021). Rather, we present empirical evidence related to four major chronic disorders selected by two criteria, the quantity and quality of available research

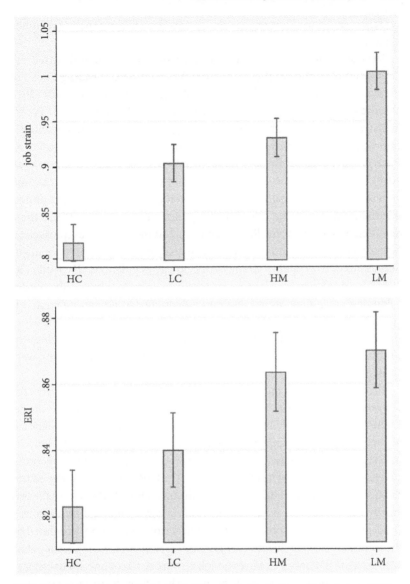

Figure 6.1 Prevalence of job strain (A) and of effort-reward imbalance (ERI) (B) according to occupational position in European countries (EWCS data 2015). HC, high-skilled clerical; LC, low-skilled clerical; HM, high-skilled manual; LM, low-skilled manual.

Source: Data from Rigó, M., et al. (2021), 'Work stress on rise? Comparative analysis of trends in work stressors using the European working conditions survey', *Int Arch Occup Environ Health*, 94 (3), 459–74.

evidence, and the relevance of these disorders for occupational public health.

The outstanding public health relevance of cardiovascular diseases and depression is obvious as these two disorders are globally leading causes of premature mortality and reduced disability-free life expectancy (GBD 2017 Disease and Injury Incidence and Prevalence Collaborators 2018). Type 2 diabetes mellitus, a health problem growing rapidly worldwide, contributes significantly to this burden of disease (World Health Organization 2016). Synergies between cardiovascular and metabolic disorders (De Rosa et al. 2018), between cardiovascular diseases and depression (Hare 2021), and between type 2 diabetes and depression (Graham et al. 2020) further underline their importance for global health policy and prevention. While these disorders matter most for life expectancy and mortality, musculoskeletal disorders cause substantial reductions in quality of life, and they are major limitations of work ability among working-age populations (Driscoll et al. 2014). In addition to these chronic diseases, we include some promising developments regarding other, less frequently studied health outcomes in this chapter, illustrating the potential range of this explanatory approach. More specifically, addictive disorders, sleep disturbances, cognitive decline (including dementia), and infectious diseases, in particular COVID-19, were chosen to this end.

The four theoretical models introduced in Chapter 3 are unequally represented in this analysis. The overarching representation of the DC model is due to its leading role in current research on psychosocial occupational health. Although less frequently applied than the DC model, the ERI model has often been studied as a complementary concept in these investigations, covering a wide range of health outcomes. The JDR model was analysed less frequently in cohort studies dealing with main chronic diseases, as it was largely used to explain burnout and work engagement, with burnout as a concept that—despite some overlap—differs from depression, as defined by the International Classification of Diseases (see Section 6.3) (Lesener et al. 2019). As the JDR model focuses on job resources, it is of interest to observe a growing recent research activity related to health-protective working conditions (e.g. Xu et al. 2022a; Xu et al. 2022b). Yet, at the theoretical level, these resources are conceptualized in terms of the OJ model rather than in terms of the JDR model. Specifically, as leadership quality, procedural and relational justice, and co-worker support are indicators of job resources in these analyses (Nielsen et al. 2017), we decided to integrate separate research findings into the review of evidence related to the OJ model. In conclusion, we are aware that this unequal weight of empirical substance related to the four theoretical models reflects a transient stage in the production of scientific knowledge, and that changes are likely in future assessments of the state of the art. As a further limitation it should be mentioned that the theoretical models illustrated in this chapter are not always assessed in their complexity. Many analyses of the three-dimensional job strain model are restricted to 'demand' and 'control', thus neglecting the contribution of 'social support'. Equally so, a majority of studies examining the ERI model focus on the two extrinsic components, thus neglecting the additional explanatory role of individual coping in terms of 'over-commitment'. Finally, in the OJ model, most results focus on 'relational and procedural justice', thus bypassing a potential explanatory role of 'distributive justice'.

In this chapter, the results of analyses demonstrating associations of psychosocial working conditions with health outcomes are displayed as relative risks, hazard ratios or odds ratios (ORs) with 95 per cent confidence intervals (given in brackets). Readers should be aware that the precision of these estimates is restricted. Firstly, the impact of confounding factors was not controlled for in identical ways across the different studies. While main confounders, such as age, gender, or socioeconomic status, were often included in the final multivariable model of analysis, this heterogeneity of adjustments prevents a strict comparison of risk estimates. A second source of restricted precision of risk estimates is due to the heterogeneity of measurement of theoretical models. Although psychometrically validated scales were developed to standardize and compare research findings, many studies used abbreviated measures ('proxies') that do not fully reflect the underlying theoretical constructs. The following text should be read with these reservations in mind.

6.2.2 Cardiovascular diseases (ischaemic heart disease, stroke, hypertension)

The history of research on psychosocial occupational determinants of health started with the paradigmatic health outcome of ischaemic heart disease (IHD) (see Chapter 1). In 1981, the first prospective study documenting an elevated IHD risk among Swedish working men exposed to job strain (DC model) was published (Karasek et al. 1981). Several years later, a study demonstrated that components of the effort-reward imbalance (ERI) model were associated with elevated IHD risks in a German blue-collar cohort (Siegrist et al. 1990). The independent role of these two models in predicting elevated IHD risks was first examined in the British Whitehall II study (Bosma et al. 1998). Finally, the first report on a prospective association of organizational injustice (OJ model) with IHD was published in 2006 (Elovainio et al. 2006). Up to now, dozens of investigations were conducted on this topic, and a short summary of the current state of art is provided here.

Strongest evidence on an explanatory role of psychosocial adversity at work for incident IHD comes from research using Karasek's Job Strain or DC model (Karasek 1979). With a landmark study published in the Lancet in 2012, Mika Kivimäki and colleagues analysed data from thirteen European cohort studies integrated in the individual-participant-data meta-analysis in working populations (IPD-Work) consortium (Kivimäki et al. 2012). This analysis included published and unpublished studies, and during a mean follow-up time of 7.5 years first non-fatal acute myocardial infarction (AMI) and coronary death were primary outcomes. A validated measure of job strain was the predicting variable. After adjustment for confounders, the hazard ratio for job strain versus no job strain was 1.23 (1.10; 1.37). These results were compared with findings from several other reviews and meta-analyses summarized in a recent meta-review that integrated information from up to twenty- seven cohort studies (Niedhammer et al. 2021). Here, pooled risk estimates varied between 1.17 and 1.50, irrespective of whether the model was assessed with a summary measure or with its single components. As the confidence intervals in these estimates were beyond 1.0 in most cases, a moderately increased relative risk of IHD due to job strain is considered a robust, repeatedly validated finding. Of interest, this risk may be particularly pronounced if a cardiometabolic disease is already manifest, thus increasing the vulnerability of cardiovascular events and mortality. This hypothesis was tested in a further analysis of data from the IPD-work consortium, based on seven cohort studies. In fact, among men, but not among women with cardiometabolic disease, the hazard ratio due to job strain was further increased (HR = 1.68 (1.19; 2.35) (Kivimäki et al. 2018). A test of this hypothesis with respect to the ERI model yielded negative results, but this latter model was associated with an elevated mortality risk in the disease-free male sample (see Table 6.1). Some reports observed strong effects of the component of low control, specifically with regard to coronary and all-cause mortality (e.g. Taouk et al. 2020). Additional support comes from studies using proxy measures of single components of the model, specifically those assessing continued

Table 6.1 Risk estimates of IHD or mortality according to different psychosocial exposures at work, based on systematic reviews (SR) and individual studies (IS)

First author (year)	Study type	Exposure	Health outcome	RR (95% CI)
Kivimäki et al., (2012)	SR	Job strain	Incident IHD	1.23 (1.10; 1.37)
Dragano et al., (2017)	SR	Effort-reward	Incident IHD	1.16 (1.00; 1.35)
Dragano et al., (2017)	SR	Job strain + Effort reward	Incident IHD	1.41 (1.12; 1.76)
Niedhammer et al., (2021)	SR	Job insecurity	Incident IHD	1.32 (1.09: 1.59)
Li et al., (2015)	SR	Job strain + Effort reward	Recurrent IHD	1.65 (1.23; 2.22)
Trudel et al., (2021)	IS	Job strain + LWH	Recurrent IHD	2.55 (1.30; 4.98)
Kivimäki et al., (2018)	IS	Job strain (with CMD)	Mortality (men)	1.68 (1.19; 2.35)
Kivimäki et al., (2018)	IS	Effort reward (without CMD)	Mortality (men)	1.22 (1.06; 1.41)
Niedhammer et al. (2021)	SR	Organisational justice	Cardiovascular mortality	1.62 (1.24; 2.13)

CMD = cardiometabolic disease; LWH = long working hours; RR = relative risk.

high demands at work in terms of long working hours. Based on several cohort studies and meta-analyses a recent systematic review concluded that working 55 or more hours per week was associated with a modestly increased risk of fatal or non-fatal IHD (J. Li et al. 2020). This new occupational risk factor was also predictive of recurrent IHD among employees who returned to work after their first myocardial infarction. Importantly, in a Canadian study, the hazard ratio of combined exposure to long working hours (≥55 h/week) and job strain was 2.55 (1.30; 4.98) compared to non-exposed employees (Trudel et al. 2021).

Substantially less findings are available from the ERI model (six studies) and the OJ model (two studies), with pooled risk estimates of similar magnitude as those already reported. Few studies only combined theoretical models to increase their explanatory contribution. However, there is preliminary evidence of an additive effect of the DC and ERI measures on incident IHD (Dragano et al. 2017). Further investigations discovered that effort-reward imbalance, in addition to job strain, increased the risk of recurrent IHD among people who returned to work after surviving a first AMI (J. Li et al. 2015). Single components of the model were also associated with elevated risk. Job insecurity, while an occupational exposure on its own (Niedhammer et al. 2021), is a sub-component of the 'reward' factor within the ERI model. Further evidence is available from the OJ model, specifically if bullying is considered a critical aspect of interpersonal injustice (e.g. Niedhammer et al. 2021; Xu et al. 2019). Table 6.1 gives an overview of selected risk estimates of IHD related to the psychosocial exposures mentioned, reflecting an updated state that is likely to be modified by future research. Of notice, similar reviews are available (e.g. Sara et al. 2018; Theorell 2020a). In the publication by Sara et al. (2018) reviewing prospective associations of the DC, ERI, and OJ models with ischaemic heart disease, five underlying pathways were suggested: adverse health behaviours, coagulation, inflammation, enhanced autonomic nervous system, and endocrine activation (see also Chapter 7).

Stroke was the second cardiovascular disease analysed along this line of research, but few cohort studies were performed with this outcome. The meta-review of Isabelle Niedhammer and co-authors listed two systematic reviews that indicated a moderately increased risk of ischemic, but not haemorrhagic stroke among people exposed to high demand/low control jobs (Niedhammer et al. 2021). In addition, a meta-analysis of the relationship between long working hours and stroke revealed an increased risk among those working 55 hours and more per week (HR = 1.35 (1.13; 1.81) (Descatha et al. 2020b). High blood pressure and its clinical manifestation of hypertension is an important risk factor of stroke. In occupational research, hypertension is not only analysed as a risk factor of stroke and IHD, but also as a further health outcome related to adverse working conditions. However, findings from prospective studies on associations of exposure to psychosocial work environments and risk of hypertension are conflicting, showing more consistent associations among men, specifically with regard to job strain, but also an association among women with regard to effort-reward imbalance (Gilbert-Ouimet et al. 2014; Trudel et al. 2016). Several studies analysed changes in blood pressure over time in relation to stressful work, but this research is more closely discussed below (see Chapter 7).

To summarize, a substantial part of new knowledge on the contribution of psychosocial work environments towards explaining cardiovascular disease risks is related to IHD as stroke and hypertension were less often included in respective cohort studies. Job strain resulted as the risk factor with strongest confirmation across studies. Effort-reward imbalance was also associated with elevated disease risk of similar magnitude, and combining the two models further increased the risk. A remarkable effect of organizational justice on cardiovascular mortality was reported, although based on fewer studies. Findings resulting from single components, such as job insecurity (Virtanen et al. 2013) or long working hours (J. Li et al. 2020), support the available evidence. However, it should be mentioned that gender differences in these associations need further exploration. Although effects were comparable in the study by Kivimäki et al. (2012), other studies reported inconsistent findings or pointed to an additional explanatory contribution of social stressors outside of work among women (Wang et al. 2021). To conclude, overall, the current knowledge on the impact of psychosocial work characteristics on cardiovascular diseases is quite far advanced, thanks to intense cumulative research efforts, and it offers several options for primary and secondary prevention. Further evidence supporting this conclusion is discussed in later chapters of this book (see also an instructive report commissioned by the European Agency for Safety and Health at Work (Ervasti and Kivimäki 2023; Theorell 2020b).

6.2.3 Depression

Depression is the second chronic disorder to be reviewed with regard to the role of psychosocial occupational health. In working-age populations, depression is prominent due to its prevalence, its duration, its recurrence, its comorbidity risks, and its role as a leading cause of disability pension (Liu et al. 2020). Given the multi-dimensionality of this disorder, there are different diagnostic entities and degrees of severity of symptoms, as evident from the International Classification of Diseases. In occupational epidemiology, a majority of studies focussed on depressive episodes as health outcomes. These outcomes are defined by three core symptoms (depressed mood; loss of interest and enjoyment; reduced energy) and several additional symptoms, including ideas of guilt, suicidal ideation, sleep disturbances, and diminished appetite. They are assessed by experts based on standardized clinical interviews (e.g. CIDI; World Health Organization

1990) or alternatively by psychometrically validated scales (e.g. CES-D; Radloff 1977). Many investigations link their data with diagnostic information obtained from official disease registries. Other studies use self-reported information of participants indicating the presence or absence of a doctor-diagnosed depression.

Although the number of studies analysing associations of work characteristics with depression is steadily increasing in occupational epidemiology, even more investigations use 'burnout' as a health outcome. This outcome was originally defined by the following three dimensions: 'an overwhelming exhaustion, feelings of cynicism and detachment from the job, and a sense of ineffectiveness and lack of accomplishment' (Maslach and Leiter 2017, p. 37). Recent discussions resulted in an updated definition, based on a systematic review and consensus procedure (Guseva Canu et al. 2021). Burnout is assessed by several psychometrically validated scales, following the early Maslach Burnout Inventory (Maslach et al. 1996). There are clear differences between burnout and depression. A state of pronounced exhaustion is the only major symptom that is common to both conditions, whereas the remaining symptoms show little overlap (Bakker et al. 2000). Moreover, burnout is closely linked to the work context, while depression occurs in a broader social context. Some studies demonstrated that burnout precedes the onset of depression, but in a Finnish study, less than half of those with severe burnout were suffering from depression (Ahola 2007). Concerning prospective association, burnout turned out to be a risk factor of a broad spectrum of disorders, not specifically depression (Salvagioni et al. 2017). A further distinction between the two conditions concerns the severity of symptoms and the risk of comorbidity of physical diseases. In both cases, depression is considered a disorder with more severe consequences for health and survival (Bertolote et al. 2004; De Rosa et al. 2018; Hare 2021). Mainly for these reasons, this section of the chapter is limited to studies with depression as health outcome. It should nevertheless be noted that burnout has been explored as a relevant cause of absenteeism and disability pension and as a direct consequence of exposure to stressful working conditions. In this latter respect, all four theoretical models were included in respective studies, but the JDR model exceeds the other models if extent of evidence and strength of study design (in particular studies containing three waves of data collection) are considered. A recent meta-analysis based on twenty-nine high-quality longitudinal studies offers convincing evidence of a positive effect of job demands and of a negative effect of job resources on future burnout symptoms (Lesener et al. 2019).

During the past ten years, results of cohort studies analysing associations of the core theoretical models (or their components) of psychosocial work environments with depression were evaluated in several systematic reviews and meta-analyses, most recently those by Madsen et al. (2017), Rugulies et al. (2017), Mikkelsen et al. (2021), and Seidler et al. (2022). Before considering this research, a note of caution is again required. In the reviewed studies, exposures were assessed in different ways, using original scales or proxies, applying self-report information or job exposure data. Moreover, depression was measured by different instruments, and the risk estimates were based on different number of confounding factors included in multivariable models. Most studies linked baseline exposure level to prospective risk of depression onset. Although depression at baseline was controlled for in a majority of cases, bi-directional associations between exposure and outcome were not adequately explored. Against these limitations, the evidence of risk estimates derived from recent systematic reviews and meta-analyses is summarized in Table 6.2. The table lists the first author of the review with publication date, the theoretical model, the number of cohort studies, and the pooled risk estimate with 95 per cent confidence intervals. The fact that risk estimates differ between two or more systematic reviews of the same model may be due to a different number of studies included.

Table 6.2 documents a moderately elevated risk of depression for each one of the three work stress models. The strength of associations varies slightly between the models. It also varies considerably between the estimates of the DC model if the review by Mikkelsen et al. (2021) is compared to the other three reviews. This discrepancy calls for further analysis. In part, it may be due to different criteria for study selection, inclusion of work-unit and job exposure assessments, or differential adjustment for covariates. We do not claim that these moderately elevated relative risks represent evidence of a causal association as bias control and residual confounding still offer methodological challenges (see Chapter 5). Yet, the amount of independent empirical confirmation provided from a wide range of occupations and countries lends support to the main research hypothesis.

The results summarized in Table 6.2 can be supplemented by pooled estimates of single components of the models or their proxies (not shown). Importantly, in addition to these models, the psychosocial risk factor 'bullying' was shown to be strongly associated with risk of depression (Mikkelsen et al. 2021). A further systematic review on psychosocial work characteristics and stress-related mental disorders based on fourteen

Table 6.2 Pooled risk estimate of depression according to different theoretical models, based on meta-analyses from systematic reviews

Reference (year)	Model	No. of studies	Pooled risk estimate 95 % CI
Theorell et al. (2015)[1]	Job strain	14	1.74 (1.53; 1.96)
Madsen et al. (2017)[2]	Job strain	7	1.77 (1.47; 2.13)
Madsen et al. (2017)[3]	Job strain	14	1.27 (1.04; 1.55)
Mikkelsen et al. (2021)[4]	Job strain	9	1.14 (1.05; 1.25)
Seidler et al. (2022)[5]	Job strain	8	1.99 (1.68; 2.35)
Rugulies et al. (2017)[6]	Effort-reward	8	1.49 (1.23; 1.80)
Mikkelsen et al. (2021)[4]	Effort-reward	6	1.53 (1.21; 1.92)
Seidler et al. (2022)[5]	Effort-reward	4	1.72 (1.50; 1.97)
Mikkelsen et al. (2021)[4]	Procedural justice	4	1.23 (1.02; 1.47)
Mikkelsen et al. (2021)[4]	Relational justice	4	1.60 (1.14: 2.24)

[1] This review analysed also subcomponents of the demand-control model (not shown).

[2] This review was based on studies with depression measured by clinical interviews.

[3] This review was based on unpublished data from 14 cohort studies using data from hospital treatment of depressive disorders.

[4] This review was based on a rigid study selection procedure. Additionally analysed subcomponents of the DC model are not shown. Details on the measurement of procedural and relational justice were not given.

[5] This review presents additionally findings for different operationalisations of the model, according to gender, and it includes results on other psychosocial occupational risk factors. It includes only four cohort studies for Effort-Reward Imbalance.

[6] An updated meta-analysis including 5 more studies resulted in a pooled risk ratio of 1.81 (1.54; 2.13) (Siegrist and Li 2020).

longitudinal studies supports the findings in Table 6.2 (van der Molen et al. 2020). Here, we briefly expand the discussion of relationships between psychosocial work characteristics and depression by three aspects, the role of sickness absence due to depression, the question of gender-specific differences in this research, and the proposition that cumulative effects resulting from a combination of the theoretical models improves their explanatory contribution.

From an economic point of view, it is important to estimate the impact of adverse working conditions on sickness absence due to depression. Costs of related productivity loss are substantial (Evans-Lacko and Knapp 2016), and it was estimated that about every third worker with depression will be granted sick leave (Duchaine et al. 2020). A systematic review with meta-analysis was recently published on this topic, analysing thirteen cohort studies with data on the DC, ERI, and OJ models as exposures and data on sickness absence due to a diagnosed mental disorder as health outcome. Chronic stressful work was associated with significantly elevated risk estimates, with an effect size of 1.66 (1.37; 2.00) for the ERI model (Duchaine et al. 2020). A further study examined the protective effect of interactional justice on risk of sickness absence due to anxiety disorder, observing a significant risk reduction (Elovainio et al. 2013). Concerning the role of gender differences in these studies, an interesting finding revealed that despite a higher prevalence of depression among women the relative risks of work stress on depression were not substantially different between men and women (Seidler et al. 2022; Theorell et al. 2015; Wege et al. 2018). Nevertheless, further research should explore more carefully gender differences in exposure to stressful work as potential determinants of inequalities in depression (Milner et al. 2021).

So far, most publications examining theoretical concepts of psychosocial work environments focussed on one specific model. Yet, attempts were made to combine these models in order to increase the explanatory power resulting from their additive or synergistic effects. We demonstrate one instructive example of this latter approach. A Finnish research team examined the clustering of the three models DC, ERI, and OJ as risk factors of cause-specific disability pensions. Of interest in the current context is the association with risk of disability pension from depressive disorders (Juvani et al. 2018). Survey data from 41,862 Finnish employees aged 30 to 63 obtained in 2008 were linked to national records of disability pensions until 2011. Exposure was defined as scores of DC and ERI in the highest quartile, and of OJ in the lowest quartile. An eight-category variable was constructed to assess all possible combinations of the three models. Figure 6.2 demonstrates cumulative hazard curves of depression-related disability pension for the different combinations, derived from Cox proportional hazard marginal models adjusted for several covariates. While about half of the sample was free from any type of work stress, twenty-seven per cent experienced one stressor, eighteen per cent reported two stressors, and six per cent indicated exposure to all three stressors. Hazard ratio of depression-caused work disability was more than four times higher in the group exposed to all three stressors compared to the risk in the stress-free group. Respective risks were substantially lower if employees were exposed to only one of the three work stressors.

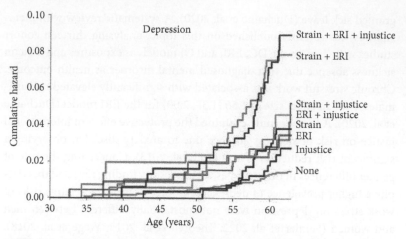

Figure 6.2 Cumulative hazard curves of disability pension due to depression by combination of self-reported work stressors (ERI, effort-reward imbalance). N = 41,862 Finnish employees.

Source: Reproduced with permission from Juvani, A., Oksanen, T., Virtanen, M., et al. (2018), 'Clustering of job strain, effort-reward imbalance, and organizational injustice and the risk of work disability: a cohort study', *Scand J Work Environ Health*, 44 (5), 485–95. [Figure 2b, p. 489] (Creative Commons Attribution 4.0 International License, https://crea tivecommons.org/licenses/by/4.0/).

In conclusion, there is substantial empirical support for an association of three models of a psychosocial work environment with relevance to health (DC, ERI, and OJ) with a moderately elevated risk of depression. Even if further research on causal inference of this association is required, the policy implication of available evidence cannot be ignored. Two statistical analyses of the population-attributable fraction of work stress (in terms of the DC and the ERI models) estimate that, theoretically, about 25 per cent of all cases of incident depression in working-age populations are attributed to this psychosocial risk factor (Niedhammer et al. 2022; Pena-Gralle 2022).

6.2.4 Metabolic disorders (metabolic syndrome, type 2 diabetes mellitus)

Type 2 diabetes mellitus (T2DM) is a further chronic disease with world-wide impact on morbidity and mortality (Lin et al. 2020). Its rapid growth in ageing societies is closely related to an unhealthy lifestyle, specifically an augmented proportion of adult people with obesity (World Health Organization 2016). Among several risk factors for T2DM, metabolic syndrome is particularly relevant. This syndrome represents a cluster of abdominal obesity, atherogenic dyslipidaemia, high blood pressure, and reduced glucose tolerance (Alberti et al. 2005). In addition to increasing diabetes risk, this syndrome is associated with elevated cardiovascular morbidity and mortality (Mottillo et al. 2010). As a condition of allostatic load, metabolic syndrome is characterized by a dysregulation of endocrine, inflammatory, and autonomic nervous system activity, specifically by elevated levels of prothrombotic and proinflammatory states, altered cardiac autonomic function, and increased cortisol output (Chandola et al. 2006; see Chapter 7). Both health outcomes, T2DM and metabolic syndrome, were targets of prospective cohort studies in occupational research although the majority of studies and of systematic reviews relate to the former outcome.

6.2.4.1 Metabolic syndrome

Up to now, several prospective studies explored associations of psychosocial work characteristics with the metabolic syndrome, using the DC, ERI, or OJ model. Sometimes, additional work characteristics, such as shift work or blue-collar work, were included (Watanabe et al. 2018). The findings of these studies are not consistent. The best evidence is available from the British Whitehall II study where a repetitive score of high demand, low control, and low social support was associated with a two-fold risk of future metabolic syndrome (Chandola et al. 2006). Modest support comes from a study combining the DC and ERI models (Garbarino and Magnavita 2015) and from an investigation testing the OJ model (Gimeno et al. 2010), but negative results prevail (De Bacquer et al. 2009; Edwards et al. 2012). To strengthen potential links with stressful work, as suggested by experimental findings using psychobiological markers of metabolic regulation, additional epidemiological evidence is required (Hackett and Steptoe 2017; Kelly and Ismail 2015; see Chapter 7). A more consistent link of stressful work with T2DM as health outcome has been documented (see next section).

6.2.4.2 Type 2 diabetes mellitus

In recent years, three systematic reviews and meta-analyses on associations of psychosocial job characteristics with risk of T2DM were published, based on 7 (Sui et al. 2016), 9 (W. Li et al. 2021b), and 18 original reports (Pena-Gralle et al. 2022). The studies included were largely overlapping in

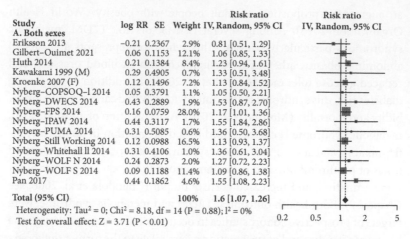

Figure 6.3A Effect of job strain on type 2 diabetes mellitus. Both sexes; only cohorts without critical risk of bias were included. CI, confidence interval at 95%; RR, risk ratio; SE, standard error. For study references, see original source.

Source: Reproduced with permission from Pena-Gralle, A. P. B., Talbot, D., Duchaine, C. S., et al. (2022), 'Job strain and effort-reward imbalance as risk factors for type 2 diabetes mellitus: A systematic review and meta-analysis of prospective studies', *Scand J Work Environ Health*, 48 (1), 5. [Figure 1A, p. 13] (Creative Commons Attribution 4.0 International License, https://creativecommons.org/licenses/by/4.0/).

these reviews, but whereas the first two reviews focussed on the DC model, the third one was more comprehensive. A rather modest, statistically significant effect of job strain on risk of T2DM results from this latter meta-analysis, as indicated in Figure 6.3A (reproduced from Pena-Gralle et al. 2022). Figure 6.3B displays the pooled risk estimate for the ERI model, based on four studies, where two publications provide gender-specific estimates. Again, a statistically significant effect size is observed. This knowledge needs to be extended to the OJ model as beneficial long-term effects of experienced justice on metabolic trajectories were reported from the British Whitehall II study (Varga et al. 2022).

These and additional results (Nordentoft et al. 2020) may be generalizable to high-income countries, but more research is needed from rapidly developing countries. Moreover, the gender-specific risk of T2DM deserves more in-depth analysis, and additional concepts of health-adverse working conditions deserve an examination. For instance, based on the Finnish Public Sector cohort study, protective job-related resources were

Study	log (RR)	SE	Weight	Risk ratio IV, Random, 95% CI	Risk ratio IV, Random, 95% CI
Kumari 2004 (M)	0.51	0.2438	8.0%	1.66 [1.03, 2.68]	
Kumari 2004 (F)	−0.08	0.3802	3.3%	0.92 [0.44, 1.94]	
Mutambudzi 2018	0.17	0.1141	36.7%	1.18 [0.94, 1.48]	
Nordentoft 2020	0.24	0.1116	38.4%	1.27 [1.02, 1.58]	
Souza Santos 2020 (F)	0.30	0.2584	7.2%	1.35 [0.81, 2.24]	
Souza Santos 2020 (M)	0.08	0.2734	6.4%	1.08 [0.63, 1.85]	
Total (95% CI)			100.0%	1.24 [1.08, 1.42]	

Heterogeneity: $Tau^2 = 0$; $Chi^2 = 2.65$, $df = 5$ $(P = 0.75)$; $I^2 = 0\%$
Test for overall effect: $Z = 3.14$ $(P < 0.01)$

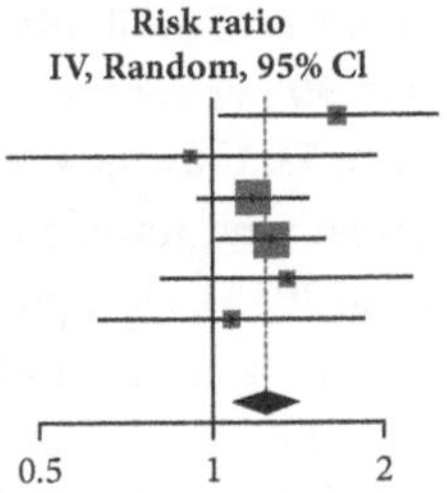

Figure 6.3B Effect of effort-reward imbalance on type 2 diabetes mellitus. Male and female subjects were considered separately. All effect measures (OR HR) were transformed into rate ratios. CI, confidence interval at 95%; SE, standard error. For study references, see original source.

Source: Reproduced with permission from Pena-Gralle, A. P. B., Talbot, D., Duchaine, C. S., et al. (2022), 'Job strain and effort-reward imbalance as risk factors for type 2 diabetes mellitus: A systematic review and meta-analysis of prospective studies', *Scand J Work Environ Health*, 48 (1), 5. [Figure 3, p. 14] (Creative Commons Attribution 4.0 International License, https://creativecommons.org/licenses/by/4.0/).

prospectively investigated, applying components of the OJ model. The hazard ratio of incident T2DM was 0.77 (0.60; 0.86) among employees experiencing these resources, compared to the less protected employees (Xu et al. 2022a; see also Xu et al. 2022b).

To conclude, on balance, a body of new knowledge derived from cohort studies in a number of high-income countries demonstrates a moderately elevated risk of T2DM among employed people exposed to high demand and low control, or high effort and low reward at work. Conversely, tangible psychosocial job resources seem to protect against this risk. The effect size of these associations is often larger among women, and there is little evidence that relevant known risk factors of diabetes account for the observed effects.

6.2.5 Musculoskeletal disorders

Unlike the major chronic diseases discussed so far, musculoskeletal disorders (MSD) are not main contributors to premature mortality, but they play an important role in absenteeism as well as 'presenteeism' at work, early exit from work, and prevalence of disability in midlife and early old age (Driscoll et al. 2014). In OECD countries, MSD represent the second most frequent diagnosis of disability benefit claims (OECD 2010). Prevalence rates of MSD up to 30 per cent were reported in several European countries (Farioli et al. 2014). Due to their wide prevalence among employed populations, a substantial amount of the cost of lost productivity is attributable to MSD (e.g. Bevan 2015). Occupational determinants of MSD are of primary importance although non-occupational influences due to lifestyle factors (e.g. sports) and medical risk factors (e.g. obesity, genetic disposition) were documented as well (Descatha et al. 2020a). Distinct biomechanical exposures are main occupational determinants of MSD, affecting soft tissue structures (mainly muscles, joint bones, nerves) (Hulshof et al. 2021). In addition to the classical biomechanical model psychosocial work-related factors were identified as risk factors for MSD. Stress-related musculoskeletal pain was defined as an interaction of biomechanical load, tissue alterations, neurohormonal imbalance, and related pain perception (McFarlane 2007). There is a wide spectrum of symptoms and disorders related to MSD affecting shoulder, elbow, hand/wrist, cervical spine (neck, low back pain), hip, and knee. Non-specific back pain, upper extremity disorders, and hip and knee disorders are more frequent than other manifestations, and some of these disturbances are clinically well defined, based on imaging or laboratory tests, whereas others rely on symptom descriptions (Descatha et al. 2020a).

The prevalence of MSDs is particularly high among working people in lower socioeconomic positions. Excess risks were reported for elementary occupations, craft workers, service and sales workers, and more generally for manual workers in lowest occupational positions. Although men are overrepresented in these latter occupations, associations of work characteristics with MSD are at least as strong among women (Montano 2014). In these occupations, cumulative exposure to biomechanical and psychosocial adversity at work is expected to contribute to the burden of disease. A large amount of empirical data on psychosocial work environments and MSD has been collected in recent years, but knowledge based on prospective cohort studies is largely restricted to the DC model. Overall, high demand, low decision latitude, and low social support, are associated with a moderately elevated risk of future reports of MSD (Amiri and Behnezhad 2020; Niedhammer et al. 2021; Taibi et al. 2021).

Future studies should include complementary work stress models to estimate the burden of MSD attributable to these conditions. In fact, several prospective studies examined the ERI model in this context, with comparable risk estimates (Krause et al. 2010; Lapointe et al. 2013; Lee et al. 2015; Rugulies and Krause 2008). More recently, a Swedish cohort study reported elevated relative risks of neck-shoulder and low back pain among those with high effort and low reward at work (Halonen et al. 2018). To our knowledge, no prospective study was conducted testing the role of the OJ or JDR models in explaining MSD risk. However, a cross-sectional study comparing the three models of DC, ERI and OJ with respect to a sum score of MSD symptoms observed that OJ and ERI were related to significantly elevated risks of MSD among white-collar works, whereas DC and ERI were associated with significantly elevated risks of MSD among blue-collar workers (Herr et al. 2015).

In conclusion, moderate support for an association of the DC model with increased musculoskeletal pain and disorder was found. A higher burden of MSD was also observed among workers scoring high on effort-reward imbalance, based on a small number of reports. While data on this association with further models are still missing, a combined analysis of their cumulative effects seems a promising option of future research.

6.3 Effects on other health outcomes

6.3.1 Addictive disorders (alcohol, drugs)

Addictive disorders result from at-risk use of toxic substances, such as alcohol, nicotine, and psychotropic drugs. Apart from acute intoxication, chronic excessive use of these substances triggers a state of dependence and the development of a series of chronic diseases. Most prominent examples are lung cancer and liver cirrhosis, but cardiovascular and neuropsychiatric disorders are further important outcomes. Dependence is defined by a set of criteria that include craving, limited control of substance use, neglect of interests due to substance use, development of tolerance, and a physiological state of withdrawal. Risky substance use is quite prevalent in working populations. It was estimated that more than two thirds of illicit drug users and heavy alcohol consumers belong to the workforce or are unemployed in consequence (Veltrup and John 2020). This figure indicates the adverse long-term consequences of substance misuse for social functioning, in addition to the burden of disease attributable to these behaviours.

Substance use is a complex behaviour varying according to its frequency, intensity, and duration; its development in a life course perspective; and the resources and vulnerabilities preventing or promoting this behaviour. Whereas a more sophisticated concept may be required for its analysis (e.g.

the moderated mediation model proposed by Frone 1999), available cohort studies mainly used established work stress models. If alcohol dependence is considered, with a noticeable exception (Head et al. 2004), stressful work was not found to increase this risk (Niedhammer et al. 2021).

Information on a critical aspect of addiction, the misuse of drugs, was rarely reported in these studies. We looked for additional investigations exploring this aspect. Among the prospective studies addressing this behaviour the following deserve special attention. Firstly, in a large study of German workers, the intrinsic component of the ERI model (overcommitment) was significantly associated with a higher misuse frequency (Sattler and von dem Knesebeck 2022). Secondly, a study of young adults entering the labour market in the US reported a significant relationship between low level of job control at work and increased risk of incident drug dependence after one year (Reed et al. 2006). Another investigation based on the French CONSTANCES study included data from 31,077 employed men and women. Work stress was measured by the psychometrically validated scales of the ERI model, and benzodiazepine long-term use was determined by the drug reimbursement administrative database. After a two-year follow-up about one per cent of the sample were identified as long-term users of this drug. A dose-response relationship was observed between quartiles of the effort-reward (E-R) ratio and drug risk. In the adjusted multivariable model scoring in the highest quartile of the E-R ratio was associated with an OR of 2.18 (1.50; 3.16) of benzodiazepine use (Airagnes et al. 2019).

Opioid misuse, a particularly harmful condition, has been reported among different groups of employees in the US, where mortality rates increased subsequently. Interpreted as an important determinant of deaths from despair, this excess mortality was associated with severe disadvantage at work, job loss, and poverty (Shaw et al. 2020). So far, the analysis of psychosocial adversity at work in relation to opioid misuse was restricted to cross-sectional studies. Nevertheless, their findings are noteworthy. Two reports used data from a nationally representative US sample of employed men and women (MIDUS study) (Choi 2020; J. Li et al. 2021a). In the first study, the risk of opioid misuse was more than twice as high among those working in jobs with high physical and mental demand and low control if compared to those with higher quality jobs (Choi 2020). In the second study, use of up to ten types of drugs or substances during the previous twelve months was assessed, focusing on use without a doctor's prescription. When applying the established definition of misuse, stressful work in terms of the ERI model was associated with increased risks of any substance misuse, and specifically of opioid misuse (J. Li et al. 2021a). Both studies lend preliminary support to the notion that opioid misuse may be increased by chronic psychosocial stress at work. This research needs to be extended to prospective investigations, using administrative data on drug consumption, and including distinct vulnerability and protective factors. If corroborated by subsequent results, this new knowledge can serve as a basis for a targeted implementation of preventive worksite programmes.

To summarize, despite wide use of addictive substances in working populations, relatively little research has been devoted to the analysis of the impact of adverse psychosocial occupational factors on this behaviour. Findings were less consistent than in the case of major chronic diseases, and elevated risks, where documented, were rather modest. Investigations focussing on drug misuse (e.g. benzodiazepine, opioids) deserve special attention for preventive reasons, although the evidence base needs to be extended.

6.3.2 Sleep disturbances

Disturbed sleep is a frequent experience in working populations. In high-income countries, at least every fourth adult person reports sleep disturbances involving difficulties initiating or maintaining sleep, and waking up too early in the morning (Linton et al. 2015). Although only a small proportion suffers from clinically certified insomnia, recurrent difficulties of sleeping go along with impaired functioning in everyday life and reduced well-being. Disturbed sleep can also be a marker of subclinical disease development, signalling disturbed physiological functioning with a growing imbalance between the sympathetic and parasympathetic nervous system. In large-scale surveys, difficult working conditions were often identified as causes of disturbed sleep, and this association has stimulated a series of research projects in occupational health. To date, two systematic reviews (Linton et al. 2015; Yang et al. 2018) and a meta-review (based on these two reviews) (Niedhammer et al. 2021) are available. Of interest, interpersonal aspects, such as bullying (Niedhammer et al. 2021), organizational injustice (Elovainio et al. 2009), and over-commitment at work (Yoshioka et al. 2013) seem to matter as much as job-content related features.

Two neglected aspects deserve some attention at this point: the role of social inequalities in studies on work stress and disturbed sleep, and the

Box 6.1 **The role of social inequalities and time frame in studies on work stress and disturbed sleep**

Social inequalities

In a cross-sectional study on male civil servants in Japan, the moderation of associations of stressful work (demand-control (DC) and the effort-reward imbalance (ERI), models) with sleep disturbances by level of employment hierarchy was analysed (Yoshioka et al. 2013). Employment hierarchy was defined by higher-level non-manual workers, lower-level non-manual workers, and manual workers. At some 23 per cent, the prevalence of sleep disturbances was high in this sample, leaving those in the lowest occupational position at highest risk.

For either work stress model, associations were strongest in the low employment group, with a significant synergy index in case of the ERI model, where odds ratios varied from 3.9 in the highest to 9.4 in the lowest employment group.

Unlike many other investigations, this study also included the intrinsic component 'over-commitment' of the ERI model and observed a strong independent contribution towards explaining disturbed sleep (Yoshioka et al. 2013).

Time frame

Few studies explored the duration of effects of stressful work on health outcomes. A Danish cohort studies tackled this question by applying a three-wave design with repetitive measures of work stress (ERI) and disturbed sleep, collected in two-year intervals (Nordentoft et al. 2020).

An increased level of work stress from wave one to wave two was associated with an elevated risk of onset of sleep disturbances at wave two (adjusted odds ratio: 3.16 (2.56; 3.81)). However, after four years, this association was no longer significant.

The finding may indicate that the observed association is time-dependent, with a short- to medium-term effect, but not a longer-term effect (Nordentoft et al. 2020).

methodological problem of the time dimension of this association (see Box 6.1).

Despite a restricted number of longitudinal studies, current research on psychosocial work environments and sleep disturbances documents associations of interest with components of established work stress models. Further aspects, such as bullying, violence at work, and work-family conflicts, point to promising additions that deserve more in-depth inquiry.

6.3.3 Reduced cognitive functioning (including dementia)

Aging is associated with alterations of cognitive functioning and structural changes in the brain. A mild decline of executive functions of fluid intelligence and working memory occurs during midlife, long before the appearance of manifest symptoms of cognitive impairment (Salthouse 2009). As a long-term consequence, dementia may evolve from this decline, representing a growing challenge as a leading cause of dependency and disability in old age (Livingston et al. 2020). Several risk and protective factors for dementia were identified in clinical and epidemiological research. Hypertension, dyslipidaemia, and T2DM are vascular risk factors, complemented by genetic susceptibility factors. Moreover, low socioeconomic status, and specifically low educational level, is a strong predictor of dementia in old age. Conversely, a healthy lifestyle and the availability of a 'cognitive reserve' act as protective factors (Livingston et al. 2020). Cognitive reserve was defined as a set of cognitive capabilities acquired during life including intelligence, continued learning, and stimulation that provides a resource compensating functional loss. This compensation is due to an enhanced plasticity of neuronal circuits in the cognitively enriched brain (Stern 2009). It is therefore of interest to examine the role of occupational factors that promote or prevent cognitive reserve and its neurodegenerative consequences.

Early findings explored physical and chemical risk factors for cognitive decline that act through neurotoxic effects. Evidence is relatively advanced in the case of long-term exposure to organic solvents at work (Berr and Letellier 2020). More recently, harmful and beneficial effects of psychosocial work environments were analysed, offering new insights. In a systematic review of prospective studies, mental work and jobs with high complexity were associated with reduced risk of mild cognitive decline, while passive jobs and high strain jobs increased the risk of cognitive decline (Huang et al. 2020). This conclusion was supported by long-term results on a deleterious effect of low stimulation at work for cognitive functioning (Duchaine et al. 2021). Importantly, in a European-wide investigation among retired men and women, the combination of previous exposure to low demand and low control at work (passive job) with sleep disturbances was predictive of an elevated risk of dementia onset over a mean 4.1-year observation period (Tan et al. 2023).

Less evidence is available on the impact of organizational justice and of ERI on cognitive function. Yet, in the frame of the Whitehall II study some support for a beneficial role of organizational justice on prospective cognitive functioning was found, specifically for short-term memory and phonemic and semantic fluency (Elovainio et al. 2012). The ERI model is linked to a neuro-affective rather than a neuro-cognitive approach. With a focus on reward-based learning, it may point to brain reward circuits involved in cognitive performance (Rowe et al. 2008). A prospective study in Germany analysed the combined effect of high effort and high reward at baseline on changes in cognitive functioning over a six-year period (Riedel et al. 2017). Significant improvements of perceptual speed and verbal fluency were observed among employed men and women with a high level of effort in combination with high reward, compared to those with low effort and low reward. An analysis of subcomponents revealed that 'promotion reward' contributed most to this finding. In a large Canadian cohort study, low reward at work was associated with poorer cognitive performance (Duchaine et al. 2023).

Despite their merits, these scientific advances may not convincingly demonstrate a causal link between a favourable psychosocial work environment and a reduced risk of developing dementia in later life. Such a demonstration requires a very large study population a long follow-up time, as well as reliable diagnostic information. With their publication in the BMJ in 2021, a research team led by Mika Kivimäki demonstrated this link in a landmark collaborative study (Kivimäki et al. 2021; see Box 6.2 and Figure 6.4).

It seems unlikely that more evidence on a causal link of work characteristics with dementia risk will be obtained within the restrictions of observational study designs. Combined with previous findings on the impact of favourable working conditions on improved cognitive functioning, this robust knowledge can be used for future strategies of preserving an ageing workforce from cognitive decline, early exit from work, and increased neuropsychiatric morbidity and mortality.

Box 6.2 Cognitive stimulation at work and risk of dementia

The individual participant data work consortium integrated data from seven cohort studies conducted in Europe and the US with a baseline sample of more than 100,000 participants and a mean follow-up time of 16.7 years. Largely based on hospital admission data, 1143 cases of dementia were documented. A favourable, cognitively stimulating work environment was defined by the quadrant of 'active job' in the DC-model (high demand and high control), compared to 'passive job' (low demand, low control) and intermediary profiles (Kivimäki et al. 2021).

In the 'active job' group incidence of dementia per 10,000 person years was 4.3, compared to 6.8 in the intermediary group and 7.3 in the passive job group. Respective hazard ratios in multivariable analysis confirmed a significant protective effect of active job on dementia risk. This effect was modified by level of education. Figure 6.4 demonstrates a dose-response relationship with increasing protection from low education in combination with passive job to high education in combination with active job.

In this publication, supporting evidence was presented by two complementary analyses from single cohort studies. In a random sample of one study (the British Whitehall II study) a large number of plasma proteins was analysed in relation to active versus passive jobs, and six proteins were found to exhibit lower levels in the group with active versus passive jobs.

Subsequently, in a third set of analyses performed in two of the seven cohorts, these six proteins were defined as predictors of dementia risk, and the results found support of an association of three such proteins with elevated dementia risk (Kivimäki et al. 2021).

6.3.4 Infectious diseases (COVID-19)

In the past, acute infectious diseases were less well studied than chronic disorders in psychosocial occupational health research. With the global outbreak of the COVID-19 epidemic this situation changed quite markedly. The direct and indirect worldwide consequences of this health crisis for working people are dramatic. Direct consequences, first of all, concern the

Cognitive stimulation		Total	Dementia	Incidence per 10 000 person years	Hazard ratio (95% CI)	Hazard ratio (95% CI)
Education	At work	No	No			
Low	Low	55 540	768	8.1	◆	1.00
Low	High	14 005	138	5.9	—◆—	0.80 (0.66 to 0.97)
High	Low	24 984	162	4.1	—◆—	0.73 (0.61 to 0.89)
High	High	13 367	75	3.5	◀—◆—	0.63 (0.49 to 0.82)

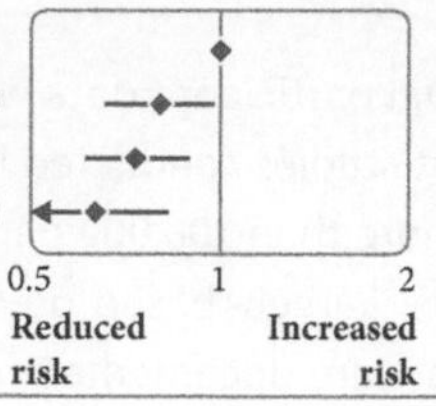

0.5   1   2
Reduced risk   Increased risk

Figure 6.4 Association of cognitive stimulation ('active job') and educational level with risk of dementia

Source: Reproduced with permission from Kivimaki, M., Walker, K. A., Pentti, J., et al. (2021), 'Cognitive stimulation in the workplace, plasma proteins, and risk of dementia: three analyses of population cohort studies', *BMJ*, 374, n1804. [Figure 4, p. 11] (Creative Commons Attribution 4.0 International License, https://creativecommons.org/licenses/by/4.0/).

morbidity and mortality toll resulting from transmitted infections at work. Frontline workers were at highest risk of being infected. People working in service jobs, health-care workers, and those involved in transport and direct communication with clients suffered most. A social gradient of morbidity and mortality was documented, leaving those in more disadvantaged positions at higher risk (see Chapter 1). Many employees were forced to work from home, with positive and negative consequences for their well-being. More importantly, job insecurity, reduced working time and in-work poverty, and job loss and long-term unemployment due to downsizing and closure of whole business sectors threatened millions of people at a global scale (International Labour Organization 2022). Chronic stressful experience was particularly pronounced among those who continued to work during the different waves of the infection.

Health-care workers in hospitals belong to the most seriously exposed professional groups. The first systematic reviews and meta-analyses have already been performed to document the negative health consequences of this exposure. For instance, Batra et al. reviewed sixty-five cross-sectional studies on the prevalence of mental health problems in this context (Batra et al. 2020). Within high-quality-rated studies, the prevalence of anxiety disorders and of depressive symptoms was thirty-one and thirty-five per cent respectively. In a majority of cases, the level of depression was moderate, and nurses were more often affected than physicians. Of interest, with twenty-four per cent, the prevalence of depression among frontline workers in hospitals was somewhat lower than among other professional groups. It is possible that those who were retained at work were more resistant against these threats. A further review largely confirmed these findings, but it additionally explored risk and protective factors at work. Among the latter, good training and leadership, strong social support, recognition at work, and high self-efficacy contributed to resilience (De Kock et al. 2021). Among the former, work stress was significantly increased during the pandemic (Taş et al. 2021), and it was associated with increased depression and anxiety (Zhang et al. 2021). In addition to elevated levels of poor mental health, turnover intentions raised significantly among health professionals during the COVID-19 crisis (Tolksdorf et al. 2022). There are now many more original studies and reviews worldwide on direct and indirect effects of this pandemic on health and well-being of health-care workers. Given overwhelming empirical evidence, the WHO started a global initiative to preserve and promote mental health at work (World Health Organization 2022) (see also Chapters 1 and 11).

In view of the amount of suffering of patients with severe complications of COVID-19 infection, and in view of the recurrent experience of helplessness among health-care workers who are deprived of successful treatment options, it may be important to extend the analysis beyond workers' negative emotions and their impact on mental health. If vital resources in life-threatening situations are lacking, as often experienced in crowded intensive care units during a COVID-19 crisis, this condition evokes moral conflicts among health-care professionals as their ethical principles and values are violated. The experience of moral injury aggravates the emotional burden of care, and it exacerbates the stress-induced arousal. In an innovative study the prevalence of experiences of moral injury among frontline health-care workers during the third wave of the COVID-19 crisis was analysed by a Canadian team (Gilbert-Ouimet et al. 2022). Importantly, the main psychosocial stressors at work were included in this analysis in order to explore their potentially aggravating role. The findings of this cross-sectional study among several hundred participants demonstrated that the risk of experiencing moral injury was strongly elevated if the clinical work setting was characterized by a poorly developed ethical culture, an atmosphere of incivility, a lack of appreciation within the organization, and a heavy workload borne by the personnel. According to the authors, these findings should encourage decision makers and managers to improve the quality of psychosocial work environments in hospitals as a strategy to prevent moral injury and to improve the well-being of their highly committed workforce.

Further research evidence on the detrimental effects of the pandemic on workers' health, well-being, and moral integrity will augment the pressure of intensifying preventive measures at the macro-, meso- and microstructural level.

6.4 Work and unequal health: mediation and moderation

At the beginning of this chapter, we demonstrated the socially unequal distribution of health-adverse psychosocial working conditions across employed populations, using the example of European survey data. A social gradient of this exposure was observed, with higher frequencies among those in lower socioeconomic positions (see Section 6.1). It is important to ask whether, and to what extent, social inequalities in health can be attributed to this unequal exposure. To this end mediation analysis is applied. For a long time, this statistical approach was performed by the so-called difference method where two subsequent estimates are compared (Baron and Kenny 1986). In the first estimate, the contribution of socioeconomic position towards explaining a health outcome is quantified before controlling for the 'mediating' variable measuring adverse psychosocial work. For instance, using multivariable logistic regression, an elevated relative risk of poor health according to low socioeconomic position is observed and interpreted as 'effect'. A subsequent estimate statistically adjusts for this 'mediating' variable, expecting a reduction or attenuation of the 'effect' size. A quantification of the difference between the two estimates is interpreted as the contribution of the mediating variable towards explaining health inequalities. Many analyses were performed with this method, and the results usually confirmed attenuation to some extent (for review, see Hoven and Siegrist 2013). The mediating role of low job control in the association of socioeconomic position with IHD in the British Whitehall II study was mentioned as an example (see Chapter 5). In this case, low job control accounted for about half the social gradient of IHD (Marmot et al. 1997). Similarly, a French study documented a significant reduction of the 'effect' of socioeconomic position on mortality after adjusting for adverse psychosocial and physical working conditions (Niedhammer et al. 2011).

Yet, more recently, the 'difference method' of mediation analysis was criticized on methodological grounds, and a more elaborated statistical analysis based on a counterfactual model was developed (VanderWeele 2015) (see Chapter 5). Up to now, only a few empirical tests based on this approach are available (e.g. Laine et al. 2020; Pena-Gralle 2022). It seems therefore premature to judge whether this new approach invalidates findings from conventional mediation analysis (Mackenbach 2019).

Analysing the social gradient of health raises a second relevant question: Is the higher burden of disease among employed people in lower socioeconomic position due to their reduced availability of resources that are needed to successfully cope with adversity at work? In other words, does an increased vulnerability or susceptibility of those in more disadvantaged socioeconomic circumstances provide an explanation of observed health inequalities? This question is answered by the statistical approach of 'moderation' or 'effect modification' analysis. By estimating differences in the effect size of the moderating variable (adverse health) on the health outcome according to socioeconomic position, one can examine whether this effect is particularly strong in the most disadvantaged socioeconomic group. Such analysis to estimate moderation effects was less often applied in social epidemiology dealing with work and health inequalities (e.g. Hallqvist et al. 1998). We have discussed one example of such an analysis when we referred to a Japanese study on social inequalities in sleep disturbances (Section 6.3). In this study, ORs of sleep disturbances due to high ERI at work were several times higher in the lowest compared to the highest socioeconomic group (Yoshioka et al. 2013). New statistical approaches allow a combined analysis of moderation and mediation (VanderWeele 2015). Apart from focusing on complex statistical approaches, analyses combining categories of both socioeconomic position and psychosocial work factors provide further evidence of a contributing role of low socioeconomic position to reduced health (see Fig. 6.4 as an example). The results of a combined analysis of socioeconomic position and adverse psychosocial work environments can have strong practical implications. For instance, higher vulnerability of socially disadvantaged workers suggests that preventive resources are prioritized according to need, following the principle of proportionate universalism (Marmot et al. 2010). Whether distinct national labour and social policies can reduce work-related social inequalities and their effects on health is a challenging, still open question (Wahrendorf et al. 2023; see Chapter 11).

6.5 Summary

This chapter provided accumulated evidence on the impact of adverse psychosocial work environments on elevated risks of several major, widely prevalent chronic diseases and of additional conditions of poor health. Taken together, it documented a considerable burden of disease attributable to these newly examined risk factors. Yet, these epidemiological findings need to be supplemented by research achievements derived from experimental and quasi-experimental studies (Chapter 7). Moreover, to do justice to the complexity of associations, the impact of reduced health on work deserves attention (Chapters 8 and 9). Against this background the benefits of preventive activities are highlighted (Chapters 10 and 11).

6.6 Relevant questions

- Which results of this chapter were most convincing for you, and why? And what relevant questions remain to be answered by further research?
- Given a rich amount of scientific information on adverse health effects of stressful psychosocial work, how would you select and present relevant data to motivate decision-makers to take some preventive action?

Recommended reading

- ❖   Niedhammer, I., Bertrais, S., and Witt, K. (2021), 'Psychosocial work exposures and health outcomes: a meta-review of 72 literature reviews with meta-analysis', *Scand J Work Environ Health*, 47 (7), 489–508.
- ❖   Theorell, T. (ed.), (2020), *Handbook of socioeconomic determinants of occupational health*. Cham: Springer.
- ❖   Wahrendorf, M., Chandola, T., and Descatha, A. (eds.) (2023), *Handbook of life course occupational health*. Cham: Springer

Useful websites

- ❖   Occupational and Environmental Medicine https://oem.bmj.com/
- ❖   Scandinavian Journal of Work, Environment & Health https://www.sjweh.fi/
- ❖   American Journal of Industrial Medicine: https://onlinelibrary.wiley.com/journal/10970274
- ❖   Journal of Occupational Health Psychology https://www.apa.org/pubs/journals/ocp/index

References

Ahola, K. (2007), 'Occupational burnout and health. People and Work Research Reports 81', (Helsinki: Finnish Institute of Occupational Health).

Airagnes, G., Lemogne, C., Kab, S., et al. (2019), 'Effort-reward imbalance and long-term benzodiazepine use: longitudinal findings from the CONSTANCES cohort', *J Epidemiol Community Health*, 73 (11), 993–1001.

Alberti, K. G., Zimmet, P., Shaw, J., et al. (2005), 'The metabolic syndrome: a new worldwide definition', *Lancet*, 366 (9491), 1059–62.

Amiri, S., and Behnezhad, S. (2020), 'Is job strain a risk factor for musculoskeletal pain? A systematic review and meta-analysis of 21 longitudinal studies', *Public Health*, 181, 158–67.

Bakker, A. B., Schaufeli, W. B., Demerouti, E., et al. (2000), 'Using equity theory to examine the difference between burnout and depression', *Anxiety Stress Coping*, 13 (3), 247–68.

Baron, R. M., and Kenny, D. A. (1986), 'The moderator-mediator variable distinction in social psychological research: conceptual, strategic, and statistical considerations', *J Pers Soc Psychol*, 51 (6), 1173–82.

Batra, K., Singh, T. P., Sharma, M., et al. (2020), 'Investigating the psychological impact of COVID-19 among healthcare workers: a meta-analysis', *Int J Environ Res Public Health*, 17 (23), 9096.

Berr, C., and Letellier, N. (2020), 'Occupational determinants of cognitive decline and dementia'. In U. Bültmann and J. Siegrist (eds.), *Handbook of disability, work and health*. Cham: Springer, 235–49.

Bertolote, J. M., Fleischmann, A., De Leo, D., et al. (2004), 'Psychiatric diagnoses and suicide: revisiting the evidence', *Crisis*, 25 (4), 147–55.

Bevan, S. (2015), 'Economic impact of musculoskeletal disorders (MSDs) on work in Europe', *Best Pract Res Clin Rheumatol*, 29 (3), 356–73.

Bosma, H., Peter, R., Siegrist, J., et al. (1998), 'Two alternative job stress models and the risk of coronary heart disease', *Am J Public Health*, 88 (1), 68–74.

Chandola, T., Brunner, E., and Marmot, M. G. (2006), 'Chronic stress at work and the metabolic syndrome: prospective study', *BMJ*, 332 (7540), 521–25.

Choi, B. (2020), 'Opioid use disorder, job strain, and high physical job demands in US workers', *Int Arch Occup Environ Health*, 93 (5), 577–88.

De Bacquer, D., Van Risseghem, M., Clays, E., et al. (2009), 'Rotating shift work and the metabolic syndrome: a prospective study', *Int J Epidemiol*, 38 (3), 848–54.

De Kock, J. H., Latham, H. A., Leslie, S. J., et al. (2021), 'A rapid review of the impact of COVID-19 on the mental health of healthcare workers: implications for supporting psychological well-being', *BMC Public Health*, 21 (1), 104.

De Rosa, S., Arcidiacono, B., Chiefari, E., et al. (2018), 'Type 2 diabetes mellitus and cardiovascular disease: genetic and epigenetic links', *Front Endocrinol (Lausanne)*, 9, 2.

Descatha, A., Evanoff, B. A., Leclerc, A., et al. (2020a), 'Occupational determinants of musculoskeletal disorders'. In U. Bültmann and J. Siegrist (eds.), *Handbook of disability, work and health*. Cham: Springer, 169–88.

Descatha, A., Sembajwe, G., Pega, F., et al. (2020b), 'The effect of exposure to long working hours on stroke: a systematic review and meta-analysis from the WHO/

ILO Joint Estimates of the Work-related Burden of Disease and Injury', *Environ Int*, 142, 105746.

Dragano, N., Siegrist, J., Nyberg, S. T., et al. (2017), 'Effort-reward imbalance at work and incident coronary heart disease: a multicohort study of 90,164 individuals', *Epidemiology*, 28 (4), 619–26.

Driscoll, T., Jacklyn, G., Orchard, J., et al. (2014), 'The global burden of occupationally related low back pain: estimates from the Global Burden of Disease 2010 study', *Ann Rheum Dis*, 73 (6), 97581.

Duchaine, C. S., Brisson, C., Talbot, D., et al. (2021), 'Cumulative exposure to psychosocial stressors at work and global cognitive function: the PROspective Quebec Study on Work and Health', *Occup Environ Med*, 78 (12), 884–92.

Duchaine, C. S., Aube, K., Gilbert-Ouimet, M., et al. (2020), 'Psychosocial stressors at work and the risk of sickness absence due to a diagnosed mental disorder: a systematic review and meta-analysis', *JAMA Psychiatry*, 77 (8), 842–51.

Duchaine, C. S., Brisson, C., Diorio, C., et al. (2023), 'Work-related psychosocial factors and global cognitive function: are telomere length and low-grade inflammation potential mediators of this association?', *Int J Environ Res Public Health*, 20 (6), 4929.

Edwards, E. M., Stuver, S. O., Heeren, T. C., et al. (2012), 'Job strain and incident metabolic syndrome over 5 years of follow-up: the coronary artery risk development in young adults study', *J Occup Environ Med*, 54 (12), 1447–52.

Elovainio, M., Leino-Arjas, P., Vahtera, J., et al. (2006), 'Justice at work and cardiovascular mortality: a prospective cohort study', *J Psychosom Res*, 61 (2), 271–4.

Elovainio, M., Linna, A., Virtanen, M., et al. (2013), 'Perceived organizational justice as a predictor of long-term sickness absence due to diagnosed mental disorders: results from the prospective longitudinal Finnish Public Sector Study', *Soc Sci Med*, 91, 39–47.

Elovainio, M., Ferrie, J. E., Gimeno, D., et al. (2009), 'Organizational justice and sleeping problems: the Whitehall II study', *Psychosom Med*, 71 (3), 334–40.

Elovainio, M., Singh-Manoux, A., Ferrie, J. E., et al. (2012), 'Organisational justice and cognitive function in middle-aged employees: the Whitehall II study', *J Epidemiol Community Health*, 66 (6), 552–6.

Ervasti, J., and Kivimäki, M. (2023), *The links between exposure to work-related psychosocial risk factors and cardiovascular disease. Discussion paper*. Bilbao: European Agency for Safety and Health at Work (EU-OSHA).

Evans-Lacko, S., and Knapp, M. (2016), 'Global patterns of workplace productivity for people with depression: absenteeism and presenteeism costs across eight diverse countries', *Soc Psychiatry Psychiatr Epidemiol*, 51 (11), 1525–37.

Farioli, A., Mattioli, S., Quaglieri, A., et al. (2014), 'Musculoskeletal pain in Europe: the role of personal, occupational, and social risk factors', *Scand J Work Environ Health*, 40 (1), 36–46.

Frone, M. R. (1999), 'Work stress and alcohol use', *Alcohol Res Health*, 23 (4), 284.

Garbarino, S., and Magnavita, N. (2015), 'Work stress and metabolic syndrome in police officers: a prospective study', *PLoS One*, 10 (12), e0144318.

GBD 2017 Disease and Injury Incidence and Prevalence Collaborators (2018), 'Global, regional, and national incidence, prevalence, and years lived with disability for 354 diseases and injuries for 195 countries and territories, 1990-2017: a systematic analysis for the Global Burden of Disease Study 2017', *Lancet*, 392 (10159), 1789–858.

Gilbert-Ouimet, M., Trudel, X., Brisson, C., et al. (2014), 'Adverse effects of psychosocial work factors on blood pressure: systematic review of studies on demand-control-support and effort-reward imbalance models', *Scand J Work Environ Health*, 40 (2), 109–32.

Gilbert-Ouimet, M., Zahiriharsini, A., Biron, C., et al. (2022), 'Predict, prevent and manage moral injuries in Canadian frontline healthcare workers and leaders facing the COVID-19 pandemic: protocol of a mixed methods study', *SSM Ment Health*, 2, 100124.

Gimeno, D., Tabák, Á. G., Ferrie, J. E., et al. (2010), 'Justice at work and metabolic syndrome: the Whitehall II study', *Occup Environ Med*, 67 (4), 256–62.

Graham, E. A., Deschenes, S. S., Khalil, M. N., et al. (2020), 'Measures of depression and risk of type 2 diabetes: a systematic review and meta-analysis', *J Affect Disord*, 265, 224–32.

Guseva Canu, I., Marca, S. C., Dell'Oro, F., et al. (2021), 'Harmonized definition of occupational burnout: a systematic review, semantic analysis, and Delphi consensus in 29 countries', *Scand J Work Environ Health*, 47 (2), 95–107.

Hackett, R. A., and Steptoe, A. (2017), 'Type 2 diabetes mellitus and psychological stress: a modifiable risk factor', *Nat Rev Endocrinol*, 13 (9), 547–60.

Hallqvist, J., Diderichsen, F., Theorell, T., et al. (1998), 'Is the effect of job strain on myocardial infarction risk due to interaction between high psychological demands and low decision latitude? Results from Stockholm Heart Epidemiology Program (SHEEP)', *So Sci Med*, 46 (11), 1405–15.

Halonen, J. I., Virtanen, M., Leineweber, C., et al. (2018), 'Associations between onset of effort-reward imbalance at work and onset of musculoskeletal pain: analyzing observational longitudinal data as pseudo-trials', *Pain*, 159 (8), 1477–83.

Hare, D. L. (2021), 'Depression and cardiovascular disease', *Curr Opin Lipidol*, 32 (3), 167–74.

Head, J., Stansfeld, S. A., and Siegrist, J. (2004), 'The psychosocial work environment and alcohol dependence: a prospective study', *Occup Environ Med*, 61 (3), 219–24.

Herr, R. M., Bosch, J. A., Loerbroks, A., et al. (2015), 'Three job stress models and their relationship with musculoskeletal pain in blue- and white-collar workers', *J Psychosom Res*, 79 (5), 340–7.

Hoven, H., and Siegrist, J. (2013), 'Work characteristics, socioeconomic position and health: a systematic review of mediation and moderation effects in prospective studies', *Occup Environ Med*, 70 (9), 663–9.

Huang, L. Y., Hu, H. Y., Wang, Z. T., et al. (2020), 'Association of occupational factors and dementia or cognitive impairment: a systematic review and meta-analysis', *J Alzheimers Dis*, 78 (1), 217–27.

Hulshof, C. T. J., Pega, F., Neupane, S., et al. (2021), 'The effect of occupational exposure to ergonomic risk factors on osteoarthritis of hip or knee and selected other musculoskeletal diseases: a systematic review and meta-analysis from the WHO/ILO Joint Estimates of the Work-related Burden of Disease and Injury', *Environ Int*, 150, 106349.

International Labour Organization (2022), *World employment and social outlook – trends 2022*. Geneva: ILO.

Juvani, A., Oksanen, T., Virtanen, M., et al. (2018), 'Clustering of job strain, effort-reward imbalance, and organizational injustice and the risk of work disability: a cohort study', *Scand J Work Environ Health*, 44 (5), 485–95.

Karasek, R. A. (1979), 'Job demands, job decision latitude, and mental strain: implications for job redesign', *Adm Sci Q*, 24 (2), 285–308.

Karasek, R. A., Baker, D., Marxer, F., et al. (1981), 'Job decision latitude, job demands, and cardiovascular disease: a prospective study of Swedish men', *Am J Public Health*, 71 (7), 694–705.

Karasek, R. A., Brisson, C., Kawakami, N., et al. (1998), 'The Job Content Questionnaire (JCQ): an instrument for internationally comparative assessments of psychosocial job characteristics', *J Occup Health Psychol*, 3 (4), 322–55.

Kelly, S. J., and Ismail, M. (2015), 'Stress and type 2 diabetes: a review of how stress contributes to the development of type 2 diabetes', *Annu Rev Public Health*, 36, 441–62.

Kivimäki, M., Walker, K. A., Pentti, J., et al. (2021), 'Cognitive stimulation in the workplace, plasma proteins, and risk of dementia: three analyses of population cohort studies', *BMJ*, 374, n1804.

Kivimäki, M., Pentti, J., Ferrie, J. E., et al. (2018), 'Work stress and risk of death in men and women with and without cardiometabolic disease: a multicohort study', *Lancet Diabetes Endocrinol*, 6 (9), 705–13.

Kivimäki, M., Nyberg, S. T., Batty, G. D., et al. (2012), 'Job strain as a risk factor for coronary heart disease: a collaborative meta-analysis of individual participant data', *Lancet*, 380 (9852), 1491–7.

Krause, N., Burgel, B., and Rempel, D. (2010), 'Effort-reward imbalance and one-year change in neck-shoulder and upper extremity pain among call center computer operators', *Scand J Work Environ Health*, 36 (1), 42–53.

Laine, J. E., Baltar, V. T., Stringhini, S., et al. (2020), 'Reducing socio-economic inequalities in all-cause mortality: a counterfactual mediation approach', *Int J Epidemiol*, 49 (2), 497–510.

Lapointe, J., Dionne, C. E., Brisson, C., et al. (2013), 'Effort-reward imbalance and video display unit postural risk factors interact in women on the incidence of musculoskeletal symptoms', *Work*, 44 (2), 133–43.

Lee, S. J., You, D., Gillen, M., et al. (2015), 'Psychosocial work factors in new or recurrent injuries among hospital workers: a prospective study', *Int Arch Occup Environ Health*, 88 (8), 1141–8.

Lesener, T., Gusy, B., and Wolter, C. (2019), 'The job demands-resources model: a meta-analytic review of longitudinal studies', *Work Stress*, 33 (1), 76–103.

Li, J., Zhang, M., Loerbroks, A., et al. (2015), 'Work stress and the risk of recurrent coronary heart disease events: a systematic review and meta-analysis', *Int J Occup Med Environ Health*, 28 (1), 8–19.

Li, J., Matthews, T. A., Chen, L., et al. (2021a), 'Effort-reward imbalance at work and drug misuse: evidence from a national survey in the U S', *Int J Environ Res Public Health*, 18 (24), 13334.

Li, J., Pega, F., Ujita, Y., et al. (2020), 'The effect of exposure to long working hours on ischaemic heart disease: a systematic review and meta-analysis from the WHO/

ILO Joint Estimates of the Work-related Burden of Disease and Injury', *Environ Int*, 142, 105739.

Li, W., Yi, G., Chen, Z., et al. (2021b), 'Is job strain associated with a higher risk of type 2 diabetes mellitus? A systematic review and meta-analysis of prospective cohort studies', *Scand J Work Environ Health*, 47 (4), 249–57.

Lin, X., Xu, Y., Pan, X., et al. (2020), 'Global, regional, and national burden and trend of diabetes in 195 countries and territories: an analysis from 1990 to 2025', *Sci Rep*, 10 (1), 14790.

Linton, S. J., Kecklund, G., Franklin, K. A., et al. (2015), 'The effect of the work environment on future sleep disturbances: a systematic review', *Sleep Med Rev*, 23, 10–9.

Liu, Q., He, H., Yang, J., et al. (2020), 'Changes in the global burden of depression from 1990 to 2017: findings from the Global Burden of Disease study', *J Psychiatr Res*, 126, 134–40.

Livingston, G., Huntley, J., Sommerlad, A., et al. (2020), 'Dementia prevention, intervention, and care: 2020 report of the Lancet Commission', *Lancet*, 396 (10248), 413–46.

Mackenbach, J. P. (2019), *Health inequalities*. Oxford: Oxford University Press.

Madsen, I. E. H., Nyberg, S. T., Magnusson Hanson, L. L., et al. (2017), 'Job strain as a risk factor for clinical depression: systematic review and meta-analysis with additional individual participant data', *Psychol Med*, 47 (8), 1342–56.

Marmot, M. G., Bosma, H., Hemingway, H., et al. (1997), 'Contribution of job control and other risk factors to social variations in coronary heart disease incidence', *Lancet*, 350 (9073), 235–9.

Marmot, M. G., Allen, J., Goldblatt, P., et al. (2010), *Fair society, healthy lives: strategic review of health inequalities in England post 2010*. The Marmot Review (London: Institute of Health Equity).

Maslach, C., and Leiter, M. P. (2017), 'Understanding burnout'. In C. L. Cooper and J. C. Quick (eds.), *The handbook of stress and health* Chichester: Wiley Blackwell, 36–56.

Maslach, C., Jackson, S. E., and Leiter, M. P. (1996), *The Maslach Burnout Inventory*. Palo Alto, CA: Consulting Psychologists Press

McFarlane, A. C. (2007), 'Stress-related musculoskeletal pain', *Best Pract Res Clin Rheumatol*, 21 (3), 549–65.

Mikkelsen, S., Coggon, D., Andersen, J. H., et al. (2021), 'Are depressive disorders caused by psychosocial stressors at work? A systematic review with metaanalysis', *Eur J Epidemiol*, 36 (5), 479–96.

Milner, A., Scovelle, A. J., King, T., et al. (2021), 'Gendered working environments as a determinant of mental health inequalities: a systematic review of 27 studies', *Occup Environ Med*, 78 (3), 147–52.

Montano, D. (2014), 'Upper body and lower limbs musculoskeletal symptoms and health inequalities in Europe: an analysis of cross-sectional data', *BMC Musculoskelet Disord*, 15, 285.

Montano, D., Li, J., and Siegrist, J. (2016), 'The measurement of effort-reward imbalance (ERI) at work'. In J. Siegrist and M. Wahrendorf (eds.), *Work stress and health in a globalized economy*. Cham: Springer, 21–42.

Mottillo, S., Filion, K. B., Genest, J., et al. (2010), 'The metabolic syndrome and cardiovascular risk a systematic review and meta-analysis', *J Am Coll Cardiol*, 56 (14), 1113–32.

Niedhammer, I., Bertrais, S., and Witt, K. (2021), 'Psychosocial work exposures and health outcomes: a meta-review of 72 literature reviews with meta-analysis', *Scand J Work Environ Health*, 47 (7), 489–508.

Niedhammer, I., Bourgkard, E., Chau, N., et al. (2011), 'Occupational and behavioural factors in the explanation of social inequalities in premature and total mortality: a 12.5-year follow-up in the Lorhandicap study', *Eur J Epidemiol*, 26 (1), 1–12.

Niedhammer, I., Sultan-Taieb, H., Parent-Thirion, A., et al. (2022), 'Update of the fractions of cardiovascular diseases and mental disorders attributable to psychosocial work factors in Europe', *Int Arch Occup Environ Health*, 95 (1), 233–47.

Nielsen, K., Nielsen, M. B., Ogbonnaya, C., et al. (2017), 'Workplace resources to improve both employee well-being and performance: a systematic review and meta-analysis', *Work Stress*, 31 (2), 101–20.

Nordentoft, M., Rod, N. H., Bonde, J. P., et al. (2020), 'Effort-reward imbalance at work and risk of type 2 diabetes in a national sample of 50,552 workers in Denmark: a prospective study linking survey and register data', *J Psychosom Res*, 128, 109867.

OECD (2010), *Sickness, disability and work: breaking the barriers: a synthesis of findings across OECD countries*. Paris: OECD.

Pena-Gralle, A. P. B. (2022), 'Inégalités socioéconomiques, contraintes psychosociales aú travail et données administratives sur la depression: résultats du PROspective Québec. Dissertation', (Université Laval, Québec, Canada). https://corpus.ulaval.ca/server/api/core/bitstreams/5bbde76c-e9a7-450e-8be8-8ddc73ca4bce/content.

Pena-Gralle, A. P. B., Talbot, D., Duchaine, C. S., et al. (2022), 'Job strain and effort-reward imbalance as risk factors for type 2 diabetes mellitus: a systematic review and meta-analysis of prospective studies', *Scand J Work Environ Health*, 48 (1), 5.

Radloff, L. S. (1977), 'The CES-D scale: a self-report depression scale for research in the general population', *Appl Psychol Meas*, 1 (3), 385–401.

Reed, P. L., Storr, C. L., and Anthony, J. C. (2006), 'Drug dependence enviromics: job strain in the work environment and risk of becoming drug-dependent', *Am J Epidemiol*, 163 (5), 404–11.

Riedel, N., Siegrist, J., Wege, N., et al. (2017), 'Do effort and reward at work predict changes in cognitive function? First longitudinal results from the representative German Socio-Economic Panel', *Int J Environ Res Public Health*, 14 (11), 1390.

Rigó, M., Dragano, N., Wahrendorf, M., et al. (2021), 'Work stress on rise? Comparative analysis of trends in work stressors using the European working conditions survey', *Int Arch Occup Environ Health*, 94 (3), 459–74.

Rowe, J. B., Eckstein, D., Braver, T., et al. (2008), 'How does reward expectation influence cognition in the human brain?', *J Cogn Neurosci*, 20 (11), 1980–92.

Rugulies, R., and Krause, N. (2008), 'Effort-reward imbalance and incidence of low back and neck injuries in San Francisco transit operators', *Occup Environ Med*, 65 (8), 525–33.

Rugulies, R., Aust, B., and Madsen, I. E. (2017), 'Effort-reward imbalance at work and risk of depressive disorders: a systematic review and meta-analysis of prospective cohort studies', *Scand J Work Environ Health*, 43 (4), 294–306.

Salthouse, T. A. (2009), 'When does age-related cognitive decline begin?', *Neurobiol Aging*, 30 (4), 507–14.

Salvagioni, D. A. J., Melanda, F. N., Mesas, A. E., et al. (2017), 'Physical, psychological and occupational consequences of job burnout: a systematic review of prospective studies', *PLoS One*, 12 (10), e0185781.

Sara, J. D., Prasad, M., Eleid, M. F., et al. (2018), 'Association between work-related stress and coronary heart disease: a review of prospective studies through the job strain, effort-reward imalance, and organizational justice models', *J Am Heart Assoc*, 7 (9), e008073.

Sattler, S., and von dem Knesebeck, O. (2022), 'Effort-reward imbalance at work and prescription drug misuse: prospective evidence from Germany', *Int J Environ Res Public Health*, 19 (13), 7632.

Seidler, A., Schubert, M., Freiberg, A., et al. (2022), 'Psychosocial occupational exposures and mental illness', *Dtsch Arztebl Int*, 119 (42), 709–15.

Shaw, W. S., Roelofs, C., and Punnett, L. (2020), 'Work environment factors and prevention of opioid-related deaths', *Am J Public Health*, 110 (8), 1235–41.

Siegrist, J., and Li, J. (2020), 'Effort-reward imbalance and occupational health'. In T. Theorell (ed.), *Handbook of socioeconomic determinants of occupational health: from macro-level to micro-level evidence*. Cham: Springer, 355–82.

Siegrist, J., Peter, R., Junge, A., et al. (1990), 'Low status control, high effort at work and ischemic heart disease: prospective evidence from blue-collar men', *Soc Sci Med*, 31 (10), 1127–34.

Siegrist, J., Starke, D., Chandola, T., et al. (2004), 'The measurement of effort-reward imbalance at work: European comparisons', *Soc Sci Med*, 58 (8), 1483–99.

Stern, Y. (2009), 'Cognitive reserve', *Neuropsychologia*, 47 (10), 2015–28.

Sui, H., Sun, N., Zhan, L., et al. (2016), 'Association between work-related stress and risk for type 2 diabetes: a systematic review and meta-analysis of prospective cohort studies', *PLoS One*, 11 (8), e0159978.

Taibi, Y., Metzler, Y. A., Bellingrath, S., et al. (2021), 'A systematic overview on the risk effects of psychosocial work characteristics on musculoskeletal disorders, absenteeism, and workplace accidents', *Appl Ergon*, 95, 103434.

Tan, X., Lebedeva, A., Akerstedt, T., et al. (2023), 'Sleep mediates the association between stress at work and incident dementia: study from the Survey of Health, Ageing and Retirement in Europe', *J Gerontol A Biol Sci Med Sci*, 78 (3), 447–53.

Taouk, Y., Spittal, M. J., LaMontagne, A. D., et al. (2020), 'Psychosocial work stressors and risk of all-cause and coronary heart disease mortality: a systematic review and meta-analysis', *Scand J Work Environ Health*, 46 (1), 19–31.

Taş, B. G., Ozceylan, G., Ozturk, G. Z., et al. (2021), 'Evaluation of job strain of family physicians in COVID-19 pandemic period: an example from Turkey', *J Community Health*, 46 (4), 777–85.

Theorell, T. (2020a), 'Occupational determinants of cardiovascular disorders including stroke'. In U. Bültmann and J. Siegrist (eds.), *Handbook of disability, work and health*. Cham: Springer, 189–206.

Theorell, T., Hammarstrom, A., Aronsson, G., et al. (2015), 'A systematic review including meta-analysis of work environment and depressive symptoms', *BMC Public Health*, 15, 738.

Theorell, T. (ed.), (2020b), *Handbook of socioeconomic determinants of occupational health: from macro-level to micro-level evidence*. Cham: Springer.

Tolksdorf, K. H., Tischler, U., and Heinrichs, K. (2022), 'Correlates of turnover intention among nursing staff in the COVID-19 pandemic: a systematic review', *BMC Nurs*, 21 (1), 174.

Trudel, X., Brisson, C., Milot, A., et al. (2016), 'Adverse psychosocial work factors, blood pressure and hypertension incidence: repeated exposure in a 5-year prospective cohort study', *J Epidemiol Community Health*, 70 (4), 402–8.

Trudel, X., Brisson, C., Talbot, D., et al. (2021), 'Long working hours and risk of recurrent coronary events', *J Am Coll Cardiol*, 77 (13), 1616–25.

van der Molen, H. F., Nieuwenhuijsen, K., Frings-Dresen, M. H. W., et al. (2020), 'Work-related psychosocial risk factors for stress-related mental disorders: an updated systematic review and meta-analysis', *BMJ Open*, 10 (7), e034849.

VanderWeele, T. J. (2015), *Explanation in causal inference: methods for mediation and interaction*. Oxford: Oxford University Press.

Varga, T. V., Xu, T., Kivimäki, M., et al. (2022), 'Organizational justice and long-term metabolic trajectories: a 25-year follow-up of the Whitehall II Cohort', *J Clin Endocrinol Metab*, 107 (2), 398–409.

Veltrup, C., and John, U. (2020), 'Addictive disorders: problems and interventions at workplace'. In U. Bültmann and J. Siegrist (eds.), *Handbook of disability, work and health* Cham: Springer, 505–24.

Virtanen, M., Nyberg, S. T., Batty, G. D., et al. (2013), 'Perceived job insecurity as a risk factor for incident coronary heart disease: systematic review and meta-analysis', *BMJ*, 347, f4746.

Wahrendorf, M., Chandola, T., and Descatha, A. (eds.) (2023), *Handbook of life course occupational health*. Cham: Springer.

Wang, C., Le-Scherban, F., Taylor, J., et al. (2021), 'Associations of job strain, stressful life events, and social strain with coronary heart disease in the Women's Health Initiative Observational Study', *J Am Heart Assoc*, 10 (5), e017780.

Watanabe, K., Sakuraya, A., Kawakami, N., et al. (2018), 'Work-related psychosocial factors and metabolic syndrome onset among workers: a systematic review and meta-analysis', *Obes Rev*, 19 (11), 1557–68.

Wege, N., Li, J., and Siegrist, J. (2018), 'Are there gender differences in associations of effort-reward imbalance at work with self-reported doctor-diagnosed depression? Prospective evidence from the German Socio-Economic Panel', *Int Arch Occup Environ Health*, 91 (4), 435–43.

World Health Organization (1990), *Composite International Diagnostic Interview (CIDI)*. Geneva: WHO.

World Health Organization (2016), 'Global report on diabetes', (Geneva: WHO).

World Health Organization (2022), *WHO guidelines on mental health at work*. Geneva: WHO.

Xu, T., Clark, A. J., Pentti, J., et al. (2022a), 'Characteristics of workplace psychosocial resources and risk of diabetes: a prospective cohort study', *Diabet Care*, 45 (1), 59–66.

Xu, T., Rugulies, R., Vahtera, J., et al. (2022b), 'Workplace psychosocial resources and risk of cardiovascular disease among employees: a multi-cohort study of 135 669 participants', *Scand J Work Environ Health*, 48 (8), 621–31.

Xu, T., Magnusson Hanson, L. L., Lange, T., et al. (2019), 'Workplace bullying and workplace violence as risk factors for cardiovascular disease: a multi-cohort study', *Eur Heart J*, 40 (14), 1124–34.

Yang, B., Wang, Y., Cui, F., et al. (2018), 'Association between insomnia and job stress: a meta-analysis', *Sleep Breath*, 22 (4), 1221–31.

Yoshioka, E., Saijo, Y., Kita, T., et al. (2013), 'Effect of the interaction between employment level and psychosocial work environment on insomnia in male Japanese public service workers', *Int J Behav Med*, 20 (3), 355–64.

Zhang, J., Wang, Y., Xu, J., et al. (2021), 'Prevalence of mental health problems and associated factors among front-line public health workers during the COVID-19 pandemic in China: an effort-reward imbalance model-informed study', *BMC Psychol*, 9 (1), 55.

7

Evidence on psychobiological pathways

7.1 Study designs with stress-related biomarkers

In Chapter 6, an impressive amount of new knowledge on work-related psychosocial determinants of a range of health outcomes was presented. This knowledge is important as it is based on the best available level of evidence in this field of research, the prospective epidemiological co-hort study design. Yet, in a majority of investigations, essential information is restricted to two distant time points, the baseline assessment with exposure data, and the health outcome assessment. It is true that high-quality studies include additional measurement waves to analyse changes of exposure over time and bi-directional associations between exposure and health (see Chapter 8). Nevertheless, mainstream information in published epidemiological reports is derived from the two measurement waves mentioned that are usually separated by several years. This leaves an important question: What happens in between? What do we know about the processes linking exposure with health? In earlier parts of the book, we discussed three main pathways, (1) people's adverse health behaviour; (2) exposure to adverse material environments and living conditions, including poverty; and (3) exposure to stressful psychosocial environments. We also briefly mentioned interactions with genetic and epigenetic factors, but our main emphasis was on the third pathway. How can this pathway be analysed? An initial answer points to the temporal structure of the association. Psychosocial work environments exert their effects on health via chronic, repetitive stimuli rather than via an acute traumatic event. Of course, major threatening life events occur in occupational contexts, such as a plant closure, an economic crisis, or an assault or betrayal in interpersonal relationships at work. Such events, however, are often exacerbations of chronically occurring conflicts and difficulties. The main way this exposure affects health is through recurrent low-level physiological arousal

Psychosocial Occupational Health. Johannes Siegrist and Jian Li, Oxford University Press.
© Oxford University Press 2024. DOI: 10.1093/oso/9780192887924.003.0007

enduring for months, years, or even decades. This arousal is best described as a psychobiological process (see Box 7.1).

When we discussed the problem of causality in epidemiological research, one of the main criteria to be met in favour of the causality assumption was biological plausibility of pathways linking exposure with disease development (see Section 3.1). Information on psychobiological processes

---

Box 7.1 Psychobiological processes

- 'Psychobiological processes are the pathways through which psychosocial factors stimulate biological systems via central nervous system activation of autonomic, neuroendocrine, immune and inflammatory responses... Structures in the limbic system (notably the amygdala) operate in conjunction with the prefrontal cortex to control lower brain processes regulating peripheral physiological activity' (Steptoe 2006, p. 103).
- Information from central nervous system to the periphery is transmitted mainly through two stress axes, the sympathetic-adrenal-medullary axis and the hypothalamic-pituitary-adrenocortical axis (see Section 3.3). Their biological responses include a release of hormones (such as adrenaline, noradrenaline, cortisol) and a differential stimulation of the sympathetic and vagal components of the autonomic nervous system.
- Stress responses are elicited by stimuli that threaten a person's essential desiderata (such as survival, social status, close relationships, core resources) and that require coping efforts, even under conditions of uncertainty. Intensity, duration, and probability of mastering the threat are major determinants of the features of biological responses (Section 3.3).
- Recurrent psychobiological processes trigger discrete disturbances and dysregulation of physiological systems. Repeated increases in blood pressure and heart rate, chronic cortisol-induced release of free fatty acids and glucose, or recurrent dampening of immune system activity are examples. As long-term outcomes, these dysregulations produce structural lesions and pathological developments (e.g. sustained blood pressure resulting in hypertension).

represents the main plausible pathway linking psychosocial work environments to the development of stress-related disorders. Fundamentally, three study designs offer this crucial type of information:

- Experiment: This design includes laboratory mental stress testing as a main form of collecting and analysing psychobiological data in relation to a standardized challenge. Due to the strict control of independent, dependent, and confounding factors this design offers high-quality information;
- Naturalistic study: With this design, psychobiological data are continuously collected in real life settings, using ambulatory monitoring devices (e.g. blood pressure; salivary cortisol). While this information offers a high degree of external validity, its quality is nevertheless impaired due to limited control of confounding factors;
- Biomonitoring within a cohort study: This design enables a linkage of exposure data with psychobiological data. However, this linkage is restricted to statistical correlations, as no mediating processes can be studied. Moreover, due to logistic and economic constraints, biomonitoring is often performed in subsamples of cohorts, thus limiting generalizability.

Experiments represent the classical approach towards studying causal associations. Their strengths include a standardized exposure that is identical for all subjects, and a systematic registration of psychobiological responses, with a time frame enabling the assessment of reactivity to, as well as recovery from, the challenge. Relevant confounding factors are controlled within the experimental design. It is the aim of a laboratory mental stress test to challenge a person by eliciting those cognitive and affective responses that trigger physiological arousal through the activation of stress axes. Resolving difficult tasks under time pressure, coping with conflicting information, or performing a task threatened by interruptions are examples of such challenges. Resolving arithmetic tasks and providing correct answers to a colour/word interference test are frequently used procedures. The Trier Social Stress Test (TSST) represents a powerful, well-validated tool: Two challenges have to be met in front of an audience, a free speech task and a mental arithmetic task. Participants are given ten minutes for preparation, and they are expected to resolve the tasks within another ten minutes. Performing in front of anonymous experts is a particularly stressful condition, as evident from strong elevations of psychobiological markers from baseline to peak during the test. For instance, two- to four- fold elevations of salivary cortisol above baseline were observed during this challenge (Kirschbaum et al. 1993). It is often not easy to assess the main components of stress-theoretical models in a laboratory design. In case of high mental effort or low control this seems easier than in the case of organizational injustice or effort-reward imbalance (ERI). Researchers often stratify participants in laboratory experiments according to their degree of work stress exposure such that a group with high exposure (e.g. scoring high on job strain, ERI or OJ measures), a group with moderate exposure (scoring in a medium range on these measures), and a group with low exposure (scoring low on these measures) are differentiated. As all participants undergo the same experimental procedure, differential physiological responsiveness according to degree of exposure can be tested (see Section 7.2).

Naturalistic studies collect data in everyday life. To this end, work stress levels of distinct groups of working people are measured by established questionnaires, including event momentary assessments, and their physiological responses during normal daily activities (at work, at home, during sleep) are recorded during a predefined time window (e.g. twenty-four-hour monitoring). The range of biological markers is restricted to those that can be continuously or repeatedly collected by available monitoring devices. With the technological development of mobile phones and wearables, such devices are now easily applicable. Heart rate, heart rate variability, breathing activity, and blood pressure are the main measures. Simultaneous registration of movement and physical activity is important for appropriate interpretation of data. In addition, several hormones are assessed, e.g. by collecting saliva samples at predefined times. This technology has been widely used in stress research, most often with regard to the collection of salivary cortisol (see Section 7.2). Despite the proximity of naturalistic studies to everyday life situations that are free from any research intervention, the interpretation of findings is difficult. The multitude of biological data has to be reduced to meaningful parameters and specific time periods, and it is uncertain whether the observations can be generalized beyond this context. Moreover, the impact of confounding factors needs to be taken into account, and by linking biological data to exposure information, data analysis is often limited to the presentation of group means with standard deviation.

In clinical epidemiology, biomonitoring within cohort studies represent a major approach. The collection of biomarkers is a usual practice, and the same holds true for environmental and traditional, basic-science-oriented occupational epidemiology. Social or psychosocial epidemiological investigations and population surveys less frequently involved or attempted the integration of such data. Data protection regulations as well as expensive and time-consuming procedures prevented their large-scale application. Meanwhile, the situation has changed, with availability of less expensive biomonitoring devices and with growing interest in transdisciplinary research. Scientific breakthroughs in molecular biology and substantial investments in genetic and epigenetic research increased the population-wide availability of a range of biomarkers. As mentioned, the linkage of biomonitoring data with exposure information is restricted in these studies as no information on biological responsiveness to a challenge of interest, on dynamic changes over time, is available. On the other hand, biomonitoring data in cohort studies can be used as predictors of future subclinical or clinical outcomes. The role of low heart rate variability, assessed in a two-minute rhythm strip, in predicting ischaemic heart disease risk is an impressive example (Dekker et al. 2000).

The next section—the main content of this chapter—is divided into four parts. Firstly, selected studies analysing associations of psychosocial work-related exposures with markers of the sympathetic-adreno-medullary (SAM) stress axis (cardiovascular parameters, catecholamines) are demonstrated, followed by investigations dealing with the hypothalamic-pituitary-adrenocortical (HPA) stress axis (mainly cortisol release). A third part is directed to studies with data on immune system functioning and inflammatory responses, while an integrated pattern of biological responsiveness, the allostatic load index, is considered in relation to work stress assessments in a final part (Section 7.2). In all these parts, available investigations in their majority used either the demand-control (DC) model or the ERI model for exposure information. Therefore, the chapter offers a selective view of psychobiological pathways linking stressful work with disease risk. In Section 7.3, some reflections on future directions of research, including a focus on epigenetic markers, are proposed.

7.2 Psychosocial work environments and stress-related biomarkers

7.2.1 The sympathetic-adreno-medullary stress axis

In epidemiological investigations, blood pressure (BP), heart rate, and heart rate variability were analysed in association with level of work stress, as assessed by the DC or the ERI model. The database on work stress and BP is particularly rich, given a significant contribution of high blood pressure to the occurrence of end-stage disease (ischaemic heart disease; stroke). In several reviews, the state of the art on this association was elucidated. The first systematic review, conducted by Landsbergis et al. (2013), was restricted to the DC model and included only few prospective investigations. However, this health indicator was measured by ambulatory blood pressure (ABP) which provides more valid data than the conventional assessment. To this end, the person wears a portable BP monitoring system throughout a regular working day, often over twenty-four hours. Repeated measures both in and outside work give a more ecologically accurate estimate of BP than standard clinical measures. In these studies, a significant link between job strain and increased ABP was observed. A second systematic review focusing on ABP included the ERI model and extended the range of prospective studies (Gilbert-Ouimet et al. 2014). Although relationships of stressful work with ABP were more consistent among men, prospective data from Canada reported higher ABP levels among younger women with high levels of stress, and a higher incidence of hypertension among older women with this exposure, compared to women with low levels of stress. These differences ranged from 1.9 to 11.0 mmHg for systolic (SBP), and from 1.5 to 7.0 mmHg for diastolic blood pressure (DBP) (Gilbert-Ouimet et al. 2014). Differences of this magnitude were shown to be of clinical significance for cardiovascular mortality (Lewington et al., 2002, see also Fuchs and Whelton, 2020). Further reviews confirmed statistically significant BP differences between high and low level of stressful work (for the ERI model, see Eddy et al., 2017), and a higher risk of incident hypertension (for the job strain model, see Babu et al., 2014). Yet, a meta-analysis based on a large sample from several cross-sectional investigations reported no link of job strain with high BP (Nyberg et al. 2013). More recently, relevant further aspects of BP, such as an influence of work stress on masked hypertension or on uncontrolled hypertension, were analysed (Trudel et al. 2018). Masked hypertension is observed if ABP, but not conventional BP values indicate the presence of hypertension, as defined by clinical thresholds. For both work stress models, and specifically for their combination, an increased risk of masked hypertension was observed (Trudel et al. 2018). Of note, even among workers undergoing antihypertensive treatment, chronic stressful work was found to increase the prevalence of uncontrolled hypertension. In one study of several hundred white-collar employees treated for hypertension, scoring high on ERI was associated with a forty-five per cent increase in risk of uncontrolled hypertension, compared to the risk among those scoring low on ERI (Trudel et al. 2017).

Whereas these reviews illustrate the clinical significance of findings from recent occupational research, results from single investigations add further useful knowledge. Two such investigations are briefly mentioned here. In a representative cohort study in the Netherlands, three job exposure matrices were constructed for job strain, effort-reward imbalance, and emotional demands (Faruque et al. 2022). Cross-sectional analyses documented significant associations of high job strain with SBP, DBP, and with a risk ratio of hypertension. ERI was significantly associated with high DBP, while emotional demands were inversely associated with these health measures. Replicating findings with exposure data measured by an objective matrix rather than by self-reports may strengthen their validity. In the large French CONSTANCES cohort, regression analyses of baseline data documented gender-specific associations of ERI with a range of biomarkers obtained from health examinations (Magnusson Hanson et al. 2017). Findings are displayed in Figure 7.1, where regression coefficients, adjusted for age and socioeconomic position, estimate the difference on the standardized ERI-scale between participants scoring high on this work stress measure compared to those scoring low. Among high-scoring men, DBP is significantly elevated, in addition to several other cardiovascular risk factors (BMI, triglycerides, cholesterol, glucose, platelets). Furthermore, white bloods cells count as inflammatory marker and signs of chronic alcohol consumption are significantly increased. Among women, the same holds true for BMI, white blood cells and lipids, but not for other cardiovascular markers (Magnusson Hanson et al. 2017).

Compared to BP, other indicators of an activated SAM axis, such as catecholamines, heart rate (HR), and heart rate variability (HRV), were less frequently analysed in cohort studies. HRV refers to the short-term moment-to-moment variations in HR, where a lower HRV indicates the dominance of the sympathetic nervous system, while high HRV reflects greater vagal control and a less stressed system. As documented by three reviews, links between HRV and work stress have been analysed quite substantially. In a first review, nine out of nineteen studies reported a negative and significant association of vagally mediated HRV with stressful work, where the majority of investigations assessed either the DC or the ERI model (Jarczok et al. 2013). A second review summarized findings from seventeen studies published between 2013 and 2019 (Jarczok et al. 2020). Due to heterogeneous data collection and measurement procedures a

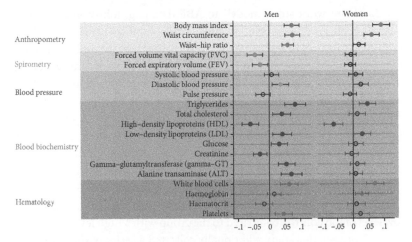

Figure 7.1 Results of regression analyses of work stress (ERI ratio >1) and biomedical markers, adjusted for age and socioeconomic position. Coefficients estimate the difference on the standardized scale between individuals with ERI ratio >1 vs those with a lower score.

Source: Reproduced with permission from Magnusson Hanson, L. L., Westerlund, H., Goldberg, M., et al. (2017), 'Work stress, anthropometry, lung function, blood pressure, and blood-based biomarkers: a cross-sectional study of 43,593 French men and women', *Sci Rep*, 7 (1), 9282. [Figure 1, p. 4] (Creative Commons Attribution 4.0 International License, https://creativecommons.org/licenses/by/4.0/).

meta-analysis of results was not feasible, but seven investigations reported a significant negative association between vagally mediated HRV and work stress. The third review was restricted to the ERI model, reporting associations with a variety of HRV parameters from five studies (Thielmann et al. 2022). Results documented a trend towards decreased parasympathetically mediated HRV parameters in response to high work stress. Single studies provide additional data on these associations (Collins et al. 2005; Hintsanen et al. 2007; Loerbroks et al. 2010; Vrijkotte et al. 2000). To summarize, more standardized, high-quality research in this domain is required, but preliminary evidence suggests that exposure to chronic stress at work is associated with reduced parasympathetically mediated HRV, thus reflecting a compromised capacity of the autonomic nervous system to successfully adapt to environmental challenges.

With the application of ABP monitoring over full working days, a strict differentiation between epidemiological and naturalistic studies in this field is not meaningful. An impressive number of studies applied the dominant work stress models to ABP data (e.g. Johnston et al. 2015; Schnall et al. 1998; Steptoe et al. 2004; Trudel et al. 2013, 2016; Vrijkotte et al. 2000). Instead of reporting their results a striking example of this type of research is demonstrated in Figure 7.2. Performed under the leadership of the internationally renowned pioneer of psychobiological investigations on stressful work, Andrew Steptoe, this naturalistic investigation analysed ABP data throughout a working day in relation to the level of job task control, based on a subsample of the British Whitehall II study participants (Steptoe and Willemsen 2004). In this analysis, the confounding effects of socioeconomic position, age, smoking, and physical activity were taken into account. As can be seen from Figure 7.2, mean levels of SBP and DBP throughout a working day were continuously higher in the group with a low level of job control, compared to the group with a high level of job control. Of interest, this study additionally collected a series of subjective momentary stress ratings during the monitoring phase. It turned out that the group with low job control reported stressful accounts more than twice as often than was the case in the high control group.

Taken together, the hypothesis of an association of stressful psychosocial work with elevated BP and increased risk of hypertension has received some support in epidemiologic and naturalistic studies. Despite some inconsistencies, this conclusion can be applied to both leading work stress models (or at least to their single components). Other markers of the SAM stress axis were less often investigated. To strengthen the current knowledge, results derived from laboratory experiments are required, and novel biomarkers are expected to shed light on underlying causal mechanisms (see 7.2.2 and 7.2.3).

We mentioned that challenging tasks in experimental stress research usually require increased mental effort from participants, and that this effort goes along with control-limiting circumstances (Section 7.1). For instance, in the TSST tool, difficult tasks need to be resolved under time pressure (preparation of a free speech and mental arithmetic solutions within ten minutes), and performing a free speech in front of an anonymous expert group is a threat-provoking, control-limiting experience. Thus, this device to some extent represents the core assumption of the DC model. To receive new insights into basic biological processes linking psychosocial stress with downstream signalling activity at cellular level, innovative research using the TSST tool in combination with molecular biological markers can be instructive. In a now classic experiment, Angelika Bierhaus and colleagues applied the TSST in a group of young adult volunteers (Bierhaus et al. 2003).

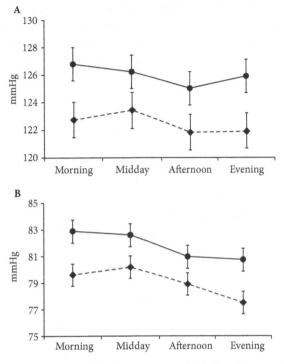

Figure 7.2 (a) Mean systolic blood pressure and (b) diastolic pressure, in the morning, midday, afternoon and evening periods in high (dotted line) and low (solid line) job control groups, adjusted for gender, employment grade, age, body mass index, smoking status and physical activity. Error bars are standard errors of the mean (SEM).

Source: Reproduced with permission from Steptoe, A. and Willemsen, G. (2004), 'The influence of low job control on ambulatory blood pressure and perceived stress over the working day in men and women from the Whitehall II cohort', *J Hypertens*, 22 (5), 915–20. [Figure 1, p. 918]; licence no.: 5497030131951.

It was the main aim of this study to explore how the SAM-induced adrenergic signalling pathway converts stress information into a cellular response. More specifically, the nuclear factor kappa B (NF-κB) is supposed to play a crucial role in transforming this information. Accordingly, a sharp increase of all stress hormones from TSST baseline to TSST peak was paralleled by an augmentation of NF-κB binding activity in peripheral mononuclear cells, confirming that NF-κB links downstream endocrine signals induced by the SAM stress axis to a wide range of crucial cellular responses (Bierhaus et al. 2003). By affecting mitochondrial function and increasing

oxidative stress, cellular responses modulate transcriptional, inflammatory, metabolic, and cardiovascular processes. Subsequently, physiological
dysregulation may occur that augments the susceptibility to a stress-related
disease, such as ischaemic heart disease (Siegrist and Sies 2017). In preliminary studies, psychosocial stress, as elicited by TSST, was shown to directly
increase oxidative stress (Kim et al. 2021). In a further investigation, conducted in Japan, a high level of ERI and a low level of social support at work
were associated with an increase of a marker of oxidative stress among men
(Takaki 2013).

These innovative approaches point to basic biological downstream processes mediating psychosocial stress to cellular activity and physiological
functioning. At the same time, more upstream research seems equally important. With its path-breaking function, the TSST tool can stimulate researchers to develop complementary experimental devices representing
the theoretical models of psychosocial work environments. One such device concerns the ERI model. Informed by basic research in behavioural
economics, Armin Falk and his team developed a laboratory experiment
with an employer-employee relation using the principal-agent framework (Falk et al. 2018). Each participant in the role of agent (employee)
was required to produce revenue by working on a simple task, whereas the
principal (employer) was free to allocate the revenue between himself or
herself and the agent. Randomly matched pairs of one agent and one principal interacted anonymously in the experiment. While agents accomplished their task online, they also received instructions and feedback from
the principal on screen. After twenty-five minutes of work, the agent's acquired revenue was displayed on the agent's screen. As principals were free
to decide they often attempted to maximize their benefit, thus violating the
principle of fair return of revenue to agents. After receiving feedback from
their principal, agents were expected to cope with this judgment during a
time window of fifteen minutes. Physiological responsiveness in terms of
HRV was monitored during the experiment. The difference between HRV
measured after exposure to the unfairness stimuli and the baseline HRV
was defined as outcome measure. Results based on 30 agents and 30 principals documented a sharp contrast between expected fair revenue (mean
about €13 per agent) and actual pay (mean about €9), with considerable
variation in fairness violations. Moreover, regressing the standardized HRV
difference on the standardized degree of unfair pay resulted in a significant
negative effect of the amount of unfairness on HRV. In other words, greater
unfairness of pay went along with lower HRV (Falk et al. 2018). The finding

is of interest in the context of clinical evidence that low HRV increases the probability of future IHD (Dekker et al. 2000).

This brief account of some experimental investigations on effects of recurrent activation of the SAM stress axis following exposure to stressful psychosocial work environments is selective and fragmentary, thus calling for more investigations along these lines. Nevertheless, current knowledge helps disentangling the complex processes underlying the reported statistical associations of work-related exposures with incident disease risk.

7.2.2 The hypothalamic-pituitary-adrenocortical stress axis

The release of glucocorticoids (mainly cortisol) from the HPA axis has far-reaching regulatory effects on metabolism, and inflammatory and immune function (Chrousos and Gold 1992). Moreover, cortisol is a relevant component of the allostatic load concept (see Section 3.2). Its release varies substantially across the day, and relevant intrinsic and extrinsic factors contribute to its concentration in plasma, urine, and saliva. Numerous epidemiological, naturalistic, and experimental studies demonstrated associations of cortisol with measures of psychosocial stress. Among different assessments the cortisol response to waking (cortisol awakening response, CAR) was proposed as a promising marker of adrenocortical activity in relation to stress (Pruessner et al. 1997). However, an elevated level of cortisol during a certain time window may not be the only marker of interest. A flatter slope in cortisol across the day and a reduced, rather than increased, cortisol reactivity were also related to psychosocial stress (Bellingrath and Kudielka 2016). Of note, a systematic review and meta-analysis based on eighty investigations documented a significant association of flatter diurnal cortisol slopes and poorer mental and physical health (Adam et al. 2017). These latter observations can be interpreted as the result of an attenuated HPA axis response reflecting functional adaptation to excessive long-term activation. In addition to short-term assessments, hair cortisol concentration was developed as an indicator of cumulative cortisol excretion over months (Stalder and Kirschbaum 2012). It is therefore evident that the interpretation of results linking psychosocial stress to cortisol release is a challenging task. Here, we illustrate these links with a few examples from psychosocial occupational health research, without an attempt to do justice to a large and diverse field of research.

Thanks to efficient and reliable collection of saliva cortisol samples in real-life settings, including the workplace, several cohort studies in psychosocial occupational epidemiology integrated these measures in their data collection. At least, in subsamples with naturalistic study designs, an in depth analysis of this information was obtained. The Whitehall II study is one such example. In a subgroup of 97 men and 84 women from this cohort, saliva samples assessing CAR as well as the diurnal profile of cortisol secretion over a typical working day were analysed in relation to job demands and job control (Kunz-Ebrecht et al. 2004). This study additionally explored a moderating role of socioeconomic status (SES) in these associations. Concerning CAR, a significant interaction between job demands and SES was observed. This response was greatest among the low SES group of civil servants who reported high job demands. In this analysis, job control showed no association with CAR. Analyses of cortisol profiles over the working day revealed gender differences, where low level of job control was related to a high level of cortisol among men, but not among women (Kunz-Ebrecht et al. 2004). These results demonstrate the benefit of interpreting single components of work stress models in addition to their summary measure. Additionally, they point to gender differences in response to stressful stimuli. A comparable analysis using hair cortisol and measuring the ERI model was performed in a subsample of the Dresden Burnout study (Penz et al. 2019). The study assumed that increasing work stress over time (i.e. from first to second year) may compromise the regulatory mechanisms of the HPA axis, thus down-regulating responses to a state of hypo-responsiveness. Main results of the study were in line with this assumption: A one-year increase in stressful work predicted a decreasing concentration of hair cortisol over two years (Penz et al. 2019).

Blunted cortisol release following severe chronic psychosocial stress was previously reported. For instance, in a study of teachers suffering from burnout, low reward at work was associated with stronger cortisol suppression after low-dose application of dexamethasone. This may indicate a change in sensitivity of a negative feedback loop within the HPA axis (Bellingrath et al. 2008). Another investigation observed inconsistent effects when comparing the DC and ERI models with regard to cortisol responsiveness, documenting dampened diurnal cortisol responsiveness only among those scoring high on ERI (Maina et al. 2009). Taken together, whether chronic work stress is associated with hyper- or hypo-responsiveness of the HPA axis still needs more convincing evidence, specifically from longitudinal studies.

For a long time, research was exclusively interested in HPA axis functioning, thereby neglecting the organism's substantial balance between energy-demanding (catabolic) and regenerative (anabolic) physiological processes. Importantly, a compensating innate system in the organism, the hypothalamo-pituitary-gonadal (HPG) axis, supports regenerative processes, thus counterbalancing health-adverse stress reactions. Töres Theorell, an eminent pioneer of stress research, has emphasized this fundamental interplay of catabolic and anabolic processes (Theorell 2009). Starting from the hypothalamus, this system targets the gonadal glands, the male testes, and the female ovaries. Again, corticosteroids are released from adrenal cortex in this axis, but their composition differs from the one in hormones released through the HPA axis. Here, testosterone, oestrogen, and their precursor DHEA-s (de-hydro-epi-androsterone sulphate) are the main anabolic outputs (Theorell 2020). Given this balance between the two crucial physiological activities, a protective role of the HPG axis under stressful conditions is expected to occur. Equally so, according to this approach, reinforcing regenerative activities in daily life and at work are expected to stimulate the release of these regenerative, restoring, and stress-dampening hormones. In line with this reasoning, interventions that improve work organization, social support, control, and reward, and interventions that strengthen leadership behaviour, may contribute to a pronounced release of protective hormones, in addition to their beneficial mental and behavioural effects.

An innovative Swedish intervention study tested this latter assumption in a randomized trial with managers andemployees both randomly assigned to an innovative and a conventional training programme (49 managers and 74 employees participating in the study) (Romanowska et al. 2011). The intervention consisted of three introductory days and twelve extended group sessions for the managers distributed across one year, aiming to reinforce empathy and emotional and moral experience by confronting managers in the art group with art-based methods of creativity and aesthetics, i.e. sessions with relevant poetry and music followed by group discussions (Romanowska and Theorell 2020). Managers in the control group spent the same amount of time in a respected more conventional management course with seminars and group discussions without any art-based activities. Biological and self-reported data were collected at baseline, after twelve, and after eighteen months. While overall a decrease in DHEA-s concentration over time in the employees was observed, the intervention group employees maintained their initial (protective) level whereas it dropped significantly after eighteen months in the corresponding conventional group (Theorell 2016). The employees whose managers attended the art group improved their psychological well-being and coping questionnaire scores significantly more than did the employees in the comparison group. The art-based programme for the managers was followed by improvement in their agreeableness scores during the intervention year, and this was subsequently followed by improved well-being scores and an advantage in DHEA-s output among their employees, visible eighteen months after the start.

These findings suggest that a combined analysis of the HPA and HPG axis in stress research may deliver new insights in the interplay between damaging and restoring physiological effects of stress-enhancing and stress-reducing working conditions, with an option of identifying health-protective aspects of sustained control and of sustained reward. In a thoughtful contribution, Töres Theorell proposed to combine the following three core psychobiological notions with relevance to stress and recovery into a unifying theoretical model, 'control', 'flow', and 'reward' (Theorell 2016).

7.2.3 Immune function and inflammation

The hypothesis that chronic disorders, such as ischaemic heart disease, hypertension, metabolic syndrome, and type 2 diabetes mellitus, are 'inflammatory diseases' has received increased attention in recent years (Furman et al. 2019). The underlying assumption refers to a shift from normal short-term to long-term low-grade inflammation affecting different tissues and organs (systemic chronic inflammation). Strongly correlated with progressing age, systemic chronic inflammation originates from elevated levels of cytokines, proliferation of senescent cells, and increased expression of genes involved in inflammation (Furman et al. 2019). Reduced immuno-competence evolves from conditions where pro-inflammatory activity (e.g., interleukin (IL-1b, IL-6), tumour-necrosis factor (TNF-α) overrides anti-inflammatory responses (e.g. IL-4, IL-10). Systemic inflammation, as reflected in elevated levels of C-reactive protein (CRP), initiates selective damage in single tissues and organs that gradually develop into distinct organ pathologies.

The research field of psychoneuroimmunology has grown at accelerated pace, demonstrating multiple links with stressful living and working conditions, with a mediating role of activated stress axes, and with a range of clinical outcomes. Associations of psychosocial working conditions, immune function, and inflammation define a small subset within this broad stream of knowledge. To date, to our knowledge, there is only one comprehensive systematic review on the state of the art (Nakata 2012). More recently, a systematic review and meta-analysis focusing on the ERI model was published (Eddy et al. 2016; see also Siegrist and Li 2017). In this section, we give a short overview of the main insights of these two reviews, and we complement this information by illustrating the quality of evidence by findings from a few selected research reports.

In his systematic literature review, Akinori Nakata analysed forty-six cross-sectional and ten prospective studies, with a majority of reports containing immune or inflammatory information derived from blood samples. The main predictors were the DC and ERI models, social support at work, and more objective factors, such as unemployment and job insecurity/downsizing. In addition, distinct risky occupations were included, such as air traffic controllers and nurses (Nakata 2012). Results were categorized according to cellular immune markers and according to humoral immune markers and cytokine concentrations. Twelve studies analysed associations of immune or inflammatory markers with job strain, eleven studies were related to social support at work, five studies to the ERI model, and five studies to unemployment. We summarize the main findings in Box 7.2.

These findings are complemented by a second systematic review with a focus on the ERI model, where the results of seven studies enter a meta-analysis (Eddy et al. 2016). In brief, associations with the extrinsic components of the model were more consistent than those with its intrinsic component. Forest plots of effect sizes indicated significant reductions of cytokines, leukocytes, and mucosal immunity (saliva immunoglobulin A) in association with high work stress. Of interest, in the English longitudinal study on ageing ERI was assessed repeatedly over five measurement waves and linked to an inflammatory index at wave six, covering a nine-year period of observation. This index was composed by white blood cell count, CRP, and fibrinogen. In the subgroup of those exposed to high ERI twice or more often, the inflammatory index was significantly higher than in the group of those never exposed to high ERI (Coronado et al. 2018).

As experimental designs offer more detailed insights into stress-induced psychobiological processes than naturalistic or epidemiological studies, we describe the results from three experimental studies dealing with immunity and inflammation. Firstly, in a British investigation, ninety-two

---

Box 7.2 **Job conditions and immune/inflammatory markers**

- Job strain: While the reports on inflammation revealed no or limited relationships with job strain, relatively consistent effects were found for counts of natural killer (NK) cells. High demand and low control at work were inversely related to counts of NK cells and CD4+T cell subsets.
- Social support at work: Among studies exploring the role of social support at work, seven out of eleven reports documented a beneficial effect on immune markers, in particular CD4+/CD8+ ratio, NK cells, CD8+ T cells, IL-4 and IL-6.
- Effort-reward imbalance (ERI): In a study in Japan, among men, count and toxicity of NK cells were significantly reduced with high ERI. In a German study, low reward and low support at work was associated with increased markers of immuno-senescence. A laboratory stress test revealed elevated inflammatory activity (see Figure 7.3).
- Unemployment: In an early study in Sweden, unemployment was related to decreased cellular immune response, with a considerable time-lagged effect. In a case-control study in the US, unemployed people exhibited lower NK cell activity than employed people did, but in the subgroup of those who became re-employed, immunity increased within one month. Another US study showed a prospective association of unemployment with elevate CRP levels (for details, see Nakata 2012).

---

young, employed men underwent a laboratory experiment with the combined challenge of a free speech task, responding to a stressful situation (e.g. becoming unemployed), and a mirror-tracing task with negative feedback (Hamer et al. 2006). Blood samples were collected before and after the experiment, in addition to continuous BP and HR monitoring. This enabled an analysis of change in reactivity of two important inflammatory markers, C reactive protein (CRP) and von Willebrand factor. This factor induces platelet aggregation in vessel walls and promotes blood coagulation. Based on items measuring the effort-reward ratio, tertiles representing different levels of stressful work experience were computed (ERI tertiles). In Figure

7.3, a positive association of work-related stress with challenge-induced increases of the two inflammatory markers is observed. This effect was adjusted for relevant confounders, such as age, BMI, and baseline levels. Thus, this figure demonstrates greater inflammatory responses with increasing work stress.

In a second laboratory investigation, performed with a group of female and male schoolteachers in Germany, high levels of both the extrinsic and intrinsic components of the ERI model were associated with lower levels of natural killer cells, indicating a dampened immune response, and higher pro-inflammatory activity, as expressed by higher TNF-a production (Bellingrath et al., 2010; see also Bathman et al., 2013 for reduced mucosal immunity). Findings point to a potential impact of stressful work on immune and inflammatory activity (Bellingrath and Kudielka 2016).

This evidence can be extended to fibrinogen as a marker of blood coagulation. A third laboratory experiment, again conducted by the distinguished researcher Andrew Steptoe and his team, examined the responsiveness of fibrinogen to a mental stress test as a function of job stress (low vs high job task control). Analyses were conducted separately for men and women (Steptoe et al. 2003). Figure 7.4 demonstrates the main findings. An interaction term of job control with gender points to a significant effect among men only. Again, it is the component of job control that exerts a significant effect, not the summary index of the DC model (see also Fig. 7.1). Additional findings of this study, documenting an influence of occupational grade, are not discussed in this context.

However, these experimental results are not consistently supported by epidemiological data. For instance, a large prospective investigation from Canada, meeting high quality standards, did not observe direct associations of the two dominant work stress models with CRP, IL-6, and a combined index of chronic low-grade inflammation (Duchaine et al. 2021). Associations were obvious in subgroups only, where among men below age sixty-five, iso-strain (the combination of high demand, low control, low social support) was related to increased inflammation. Similar relationships were found for job strain and for ERI in this age group. Among women below age sixty-five, low reward and moderate social support were linked to increased inflammation (see also Fig. 7.1). In a further epidemiological investigation, the Whitehall II study, low social support at work, but not high demand and/or low control, was prospectively associated with higher levels of IL-6 (Magnusson Hanson et al. 2019). These discordant findings between two different study designs call for further in-depth analysis. It

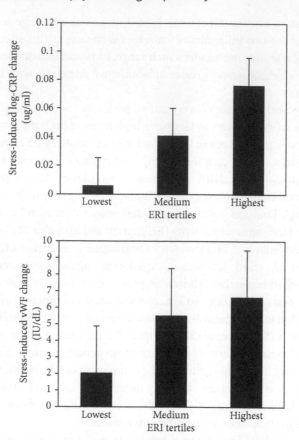

Figure 7.3 The effect of effort-reward imbalance on C-reactive protein and von Willebrand factor responses to mental stress. Values are mean ± SEM adjusted for age, BMI, and baseline levels.

Source: Reproduced with permission from Hamer, M., Williams, E., Vuonovirta, R., et al. (2006), 'The effects of effort-reward imbalance on inflammatory and cardiovascular responses to mental stress', *Psychosom Med*, 68 (3), 408–13. [Figure 2, p. 411]; license no.: 5497031252434.

might be instructive to stratify analyses according to socioeconomic position, given robust evidence of a steep social gradient of low-grade inflammation throughout the life course (Berger et al. 2019).

The findings on work stress and immune/inflammatory markers reported in this section reflect only a small part of the biological consequences of stress-induced alterations in these systems. Knowledge needs

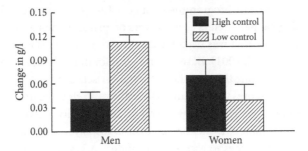

Figure 7.4 Mean changes in plasma fibrinogen (in g/litre) between baseline and stress samples in men and women reporting high or low job control. Error bars are SEM.

Source: Reproduced with permission from Steptoe, A., Kunz-Ebrecht, S., Owen, N., et al. (2003), 'Influence of socioeconomic status and job control on plasma fibrinogen responses to acute mental stress', *Psychosom Med*, 65 (1), 137–44. [Figure 2, p. 141]; license no.: 5497040002820.

to be extended to metabolic, procoagulant, atherosclerotic, auto-immune-related, and cancer-promoting conditions. This task cannot be accomplished in the context of this book. Yet, one strategy of analysis focuses on summary markers of psychobiologic dysregulation. In Chapter 3, we introduced the concept of allostatic load with its primary mediators and secondary outcomes (see Section 3.2). This concept aims at bridging the psychobiological markers discussed so far with processes triggering subclinical and clinical developments of bodily diseases. The next section offers a closer look at this concept.

7.2.4 Allostatic load

Each one of the psychobiological pathways discussed in this chapter produces subtle physiological dysregulation under chronic activation. As these pathways interact in multiple ways, cumulative effects of 'wear and tear' occur that increasingly impair regular functioning and trigger tissue damage in different bodily parts. This process is analysed as 'allostatic load', resulting in 'overload', and ultimately in clinical disease manifestation (see Section 3.2). As a heuristic concept, allostatic load is thought to indicate a vulnerable stage of a physiological stress trajectory characterized by recurrent systemic dysregulation. To measure this concept, a research team of the US MacArthur programme of successful ageing developed a list of ten physiological parameters as indicators of 'primary mediators' and 'secondary outcomes' that was used for constructing an Allostatic Load (AL) index (Seeman et al. 2001). Based on the distribution of these components in each study sample, the quartile with highest scores was defined as 'risk quartile', as high scores were assumed to indicate an elevated morbidity risk. This assumption was examined with respect to mortality risks (Gruenewald et al. 2006). In Table 7.1, this original list is displayed, together with two more recent approaches to assess an AL index. A systematic review of AL measures in epidemiological and experimental research in occupational settings, published in 2015, revealed a substantial heterogeneity and variation in the selection and combination of allostatic load measures (Mauss et al. 2015). Up to now, this diversity prevented scientific progress due to lack of standardization and comparability of findings. More recently, some measurement convergence was observed. This can be observed in Table 7.1, where, in addition to the original components of the MacArthur network (Seeman et al. 2001), an AL index examined in the English Longitudinal Study on Aging (ELSA) (Coronado et al. 2018) and an AL index developed in the prospective French cohort study CONSTANCES (Wahrendorf et al. 2022) are listed.

Table 7.1 indicates an unequal number of AL components (10, 15, 10), and limited comparability. However, information on BP, body weight, metabolic risk, blood lipids, and some data on HPA axis and immune function are comparable at least across two of the three studies. Importantly, ELSA and CONSTANCES offer biomarker data on the cardiovascular, metabolic, anthropometric, and immune/inflammatory systems, and in addition, MacArthur and ELSA include neuroendocrine data.

What is the relationship between stressful work and allostatic load? In the systematic review mentioned, five studies analysed this association cross-sectionally, mainly based on the DC model. They all reported some significant link, at least with single model components (Mauss et al. 2015). The ELSA study differs from these reports in two important aspects. Firstly, it covers a large sample of older adults in England followed prospectively over eight years. Secondly, exposure was measured several times during follow-up, thus relating a cumulative measure of stressful work in terms of the ERI model to the prospectively assessed AL index (Coronado et al. 2018). This study reported a significantly elevated AL index in the group defined by cumulative work stress. Further support of an association of adverse work with allostatic load came from the UK Household Longitudinal Study. The

Table 7.1 Three examples of an Allostatic Load (AL) Index

Seeman et al., 2001	Coronado et al., 2018	Wahrendorf et al., 2022
Adrenaline	IGF 1	
Noradrenaline	Cortisone	
Cortisol	Cortisol	
DHEA-S	White blood cells count	White blood cells count
	C-reactive protein	
	Fibrinogen	
SBP	SBP	SBP
DBP	DBP	DBP
	Antihypertension medication	FEV_1, FVC
	Pulse rate	
HbA1c	HbA1c	Fasting glucose
Cholesterol	Total chol/HDL ratio	Total chol/HDL ratio
HDL		LDL
	Triglyceride	Triglyceride
		Creatinine clearance rate
Waist to hip ratio	Waist to height ratio	Waist to hip ratio
	% underweight	

DBP, diastolic blood pressure; DHEA-S, de-hydro-epi-androsterone sulfate; FEV_1, FVC, ratio of forced expiratory volume in 1 s to forced vital capacity; HbA1c, glycated haemoglobin level; HDL, high density lipoprotein; IGF-1, insulin growth factor; LDL, low density lipoprotein; SBP, systolic blood pressure.

investigators identified an increased AL score among formerly unemployed people who were re-employed in a disadvantaged, dissatisfying job, compared to scores of those who remained unemployed (Chandola and Zhang 2018). The finding may indicate that exerting unrewarding efforts evokes stronger stress reactions than remaining in a passive state of worklessness.

A different conceptual approach was applied in the CONSTANCES study that analysed retrospectively assessed employment histories (Wahrendorf et al. 2022). Occupational careers were classified according to duration, timing, and sequence of events over time (e.g. job changes).

This enabled the definition of several types of critical employment trajectories, such as precarious careers, discontinuous careers, and careers characterized by cumulative disadvantage (see also Section 3.2). Informed by core stress-theoretical notions of job security, control, fairness, and reward, these critical trajectories are assumed to activate chronically stressful experience among exposed workers. Based on the biomarkers listed in Table 7.1, a composite AL score was constructed, and associations with critical job careers were examined in regression analyses. Results indicated higher AL levels among men and women with employment careers characterized by repeated periods of unemployment or years out of work. Strongest associations were obvious in the group of workers in a continuously disadvantaged occupational position (Wahrendorf et al. 2022).

These latter studies point to promising further developments of life-course occupational health research, by extending exposure assessment over time, and by proposing integrated measures of psychobiological markers reflecting the physiologic burden of chronically stressful experience at work. With improved standardization and improved sets of biomarkers, research along these lines is likely to uncover new insights.

7.3 Future directions

Chapters 6 and 7 demonstrated a substantial extension of the knowledge base in occupational health research in the recent past, with a special focus on health effects of adverse psychosocial work environments. Each study design, the prospective epidemiological cohort study, the naturalistic observational investigation, and the laboratory experiment, contributed to this development. The three complementary sources of evidence offer opportunities of triangulating different research approaches. However, integrating experimental and naturalistic investigations in large epidemiological cohort studies must be considered a challenging task. As documented in one such, successfully accomplished project, dealing with associations of cognitively stimulating work and prevention of dementia (Kivimäki et al. 2021; see Box 6.2), it requires a sustainable transdisciplinary collaboration between several research teams, based on a well-functioning network and solid research funding. Such conditions are still rare in current scientific work arrangements.

Strengthening transdisciplinary research collaboration is one step towards increasing impact in this field of scientific development. Four more steps are briefly mentioned here. Firstly, several further directions of advances in epidemiological research methodology deserve attention. For instance, new sophisticated statistical models need to be applied to the analysis of large datasets with multiple measurement waves, allowing advances in conducting causal analysis, mediation, and moderation analysis, and in disentangling bi-directional associations between work and health in longitudinal research (see also Chapter 5). A second step concerns a conceptual extension of exposure assessment. The dominant theoretical models offer opportunities for extending their meso-level approach by integrating relevant macro-structural conditions. Moreover, exposure dynamics need to be analysed in a life-course perspective (e.g. Wahrendorf and Demakakos 2020). Importantly, available theoretical models are expected to address essential recent changes in the nature of work and employment relationships, with a focus on challenges and threats in the face of increased unpredictability, instability, and discontinuity (see also Chapters 2 and 3). Finally, in view of the planetary challenge of climate change and related global public health crises, a broader assessment of the exposome (the totality environmental factors that an individual is exposed throughout life) will be required, including environmental and socioeconomic adversities that transcend and modify the work context (see Chapters 2 and 11).

As a third step, advances in the explanation of psychobiological pathways are expected by including new stress-related biomarkers from cutting-edge research developments, in particular in the fields of genetics and epigenetics. First pioneering studies applying advances in the analysis of DNA methylation, oxidative stress, and cell regulation in social and occupational epidemiology are already available. One such example concerns the epigenetic modification of distinct inflammatory genes by socioeconomic position (Stringhini et al. 2015) (see also Section 3.3). With discoveries in telomere biology (Rentscher et al. 2020) and in epigenetics of biological ageing (Palma-Gudiel et al. 2020), far-reaching new insights are expected to occur. This latter research identified several DNA methylation-based markers of ageing in different tissues ('epigenetic clocks'). These markers are used to calculate epigenetic age acceleration, a measure that reflects an increase in biological age in comparison to chronological age. For instance, preliminary evidence indicates that cumulative social disadvantage, as indicated by a continued low occupational position over adult life, precipitates the biological aging process. Based on data from three epidemiological cohort studies, mean biological aging in the disadvantaged group was found to be accelerated by about one year if compared to the ageing in the so-cially privileged group (Fiorito et al. 2017). So far, it seems premature to reach conclusions with regard to associations of psychosocial stress at work with markers of accelerating ageing. In a Finnish study, a posi-tive effect of long working hours, and a negative, age-retarding effect of working in an active job was observed, whereas job strain and ERI were not associated with these markers (Freni-Sterrantino et al. 2022b). Yet, in the British 'Understanding Society' study, participants with distinct features of employment-related stress, job insecurity and job loss, were at risk of accelerated aging (Freni-Sterrantino et al. 2022a). This study also documented an association with exposure to night shift, a finding confirmed in an investigation of nurses, where the aging effect was add-itionally associated with experienced work stress, as measured by ERI (Carugno et al. 2021).

Alongside such innovations in epigenetic research, progress in func-tional neuroimaging techniques opened a new window of opportunity, exploring links between stress-induced activation of prefrontal and limbic brain structures and peripheral organ dysfunction. Results from some preliminary longitudinal studies support this assumption (Osborne et al. 2020). In a pioneering investigation with 293 patients who were free from cardiovascular disease and followed over a mean 3.7 years, amygdalar ac-tivation was assessed at baseline. During follow-up, 22 cardiovascular dis-ease events occurred. The hazard ratio of incident cardiovascular disease was 1.59 (1.27; 1.98) among participants with a high level of amygdalar ac-tivation. In addition, this association was in part mediated by arterial in-flammation (Tawakol et al. 2017). The single innovative studies mentioned here will need replication and extension, but they may break the paths of conventional occupational health research.

As a fourth step of future directions of research, more in-depth inves-tigations on interventions of health-promoting work environments are expected (see Chapter 10). This is an era of strongly underdeveloped know-ledge producing findings with relevance to practical application. Despite the many methodological limitations, theory-based programmes pro-moting personnel and organizational developments in diverse work set-tings deserve more attention. Testing multi-mode approaches, extending the duration and monitoring quality of intervention and evaluation pro-jects, and intensifying research on precarious employment groups and novel nonstandard working conditions are some of the priorities in this area. Overall, there is a strong case for investments in innovative developments of occupational psychosocial health research.

7.4 Summary

Readers of this chapter are now in a position to judge the scientific evidence on psychobiological pathways linking stressful work with the development of chronic disorders. They are familiar with basic concepts and their application in epidemiological, naturalistic, and experimental studies. This new knowledge broadens the awareness of how even subtle repression of basic psychosocial and material needs at work can impair people's health and well-being.

7.5 Relevant questions

- Why is it important to study psychobiological processes in research on work-related stress and health?
- Despite available evidence documented in this chapter, there are several discordant findings and open questions. In your view, what is the most pressing open question to be tackled by further research?
- From a practical point of view, how would you prioritize the usefulness of knowledge, comparing the new epidemiological (Chapter 6) and psychobiological (Chapter 7) findings?

Recommended reading

❖ Bellingrath, S., and Kudielka, B. M. (2016), 'Psychobiological pathways from work stress to reduced health: naturalistic and experimental studies on the ERI model'. In J. Siegrist and M. Wahrendorf (eds.), *Work stress and health in a globalized economy*. Cham: Springer, 145–70.

❖ Nakata, A. (2012), 'Psychosocial job stress and immunity: a systematic review'. In Q. Yan (ed.), *Psychoneuroimmunology: methods and protocols*. Totowa, NJ: Humana Press, 39–75.

❖ Osborne, M. T., Shin, L. M., Mehta, N. N., et al. (2020), 'Disentangling the links between psychosocial stress and cardiovascular disease', *Circ Cardiovasc*, 13 (8), e010931.

❖ Steptoe, A., and Kivimaki, M. (2012), 'Stress and cardiovascular disease', *Nat Rev Cardiol*, 9 (6), 360–70.

Useful websites

❖   Psychoneuroendocrinology: https://www.sciencedirect.com/journal/psychoneuroendocrinology
❖   Psychosomatic Medicine: https://journals.lww.com/psychosomaticmedicine/pages/default.aspx
❖   Wikipedia: Stress (biology). https://en.wikipedia.org/wiki/Stress_(biology)

References

Adam, E. K., Quinn, M. E., Tavernier, R., et al. (2017), 'Diurnal cortisol slopes and mental and physical health outcomes: A systematic review and meta-analysis', *Psychoneuroendocrinology*, 83, 25–41.

Babu, G. R., Jotheeswaran, A. T., Mahapatra, T., et al. (2014), 'Is hypertension associated with job strain? A meta-analysis of observational studies', *Occup Environ Med*, 71 (3), 220–7.

Bathman, L. M., Almond, J., Hazi, A., et al. (2013), 'Effort-reward imbalance at work and pre-clinical biological indices of ill-health: the case for salivary immunoglobulin A', *Brain Behav Immun*, 33, 74–9.

Bellingrath, S., and Kudielka, B. M. (2016), 'Psychobiological pathways from work stress to reduced health: naturalistic and experimental studies on the ERI model'. In J. Siegrist and M. Wahrendorf (eds.), *Work stress and health in a globalized economy*. Cham: Springer, 145–70.

Bellingrath, S., Weigl, T., and Kudielka, B. M. (2008), 'Cortisol dysregulation in school teachers in relation to burnout, vital exhaustion, and effort-reward imbalance', *Biol Psychol*, 78 (1), 104–13.

Bellingrath, S., Rohleder, N., and Kudielka, B. M. (2010), 'Healthy working school teachers with high effort-reward-imbalance and overcommitment show increased pro-inflammatory immune activity and a dampened innate immune defence', *Brain Behav Immun*, 24 (8), 1332–9.

Berger, E., Castagne, R., Chadeau-Hyam, M., et al. (2019), 'Multi-cohort study identifies social determinants of systemic inflammation over the life course', *Nat Commun*, 10 (1), 773.

Bierhaus, A., Wolf, J., Andrassy, M., et al. (2003), 'A mechanism converting psychosocial stress into mononuclear cell activation', *Proc Natl Acad Sci USA*, 100 (4), 1920–5.

Carugno, M., Maggioni, C., Ruggiero, V., et al. (2021), 'Can night shift work affect biological age? Hints from a cross-sectional study on hospital female nurses', *Int J Environ Res Public Health*, 18 (20), 10639.

Chandola, T., and Zhang, N. (2018), 'Re-employment, job quality, health and allostatic load biomarkers: prospective evidence from the UK Household Longitudinal Study', *Int J Epidemiol*, 47 (1), 47–57.

Chrousos, G. P., and Gold, P. W. (1992), 'The concepts of stress and stress system disorders. Overview of physical and behavioral homeostasis', *JAMA*, 267 (9), 1244–52.

Collins, S. M., Karasek, R. A., and Costas, K. (2005), 'Job strain and autonomic indices of cardiovascular disease risk', *Am J Ind Med*, 48 (3), 182–93.

Coronado, J. I. C., Chandola, T., and Steptoe, A. (2018), 'Allostatic load and effort-reward imbalance: associations over the working-career', *Int J Environ Res Public Health*, 15 (2), 191.

Dekker, J. M., Crow, R. S., Folsom, A. R., et al. (2000), 'Low heart rate variability in a 2-minute rhythm strip predicts risk of coronary heart disease and mortality from several causes: the ARIC Study. Atherosclerosis Risk In Communities', *Circulation*, 102 (11), 1239–44.

Duchaine, C. S., Brisson, C., Talbot, D., et al. (2021), 'Cumulative exposure to psychosocial stressors at work and global cognitive function: the PROspective Quebec Study on Work and Health', *Occup Environ Med*, 78 (12), 884–92.

Eddy, P., Wertheim, E. H., Kingsley, M., et al. (2017), 'Associations between the effort-reward imbalance model of workplace stress and indices of cardiovascular health: a systematic review and meta-analysis', *Neurosci Biobehav Rev*, 83, 252–66.

Eddy, P., Heckenberg, R., Wertheim, E. H., et al. (2016), 'A systematic review and meta-analysis of the effort-reward imbalance model of workplace stress with indicators of immune function', *J Psychosom Res*, 91, 1–8.

Falk, A., Kosse, F., Menrath, I., et al. (2018), 'Unfair pay and health', *Manag Sci*, 64 (4), 1477–88.

Faruque, M. O., Framke, E., Sorensen, J. K., et al. (2022), 'Psychosocial work factors and blood pressure among 63,800 employees from the Netherlands in the Lifelines Cohort Study', *J Epidemiol Community Health*, 76 (1), 60–66.

Fiorito, G., Polidoro, S., Dugue, P. A., et al. (2017), 'Social adversity and epigenetic aging: a multi-cohort study on socioeconomic differences in peripheral blood DNA methylation', *Sci Rep*, 7 (1), 16266.

Freni-Sterrantino, A., Fiorito, G., d'Errico, A., et al. (2022a), 'Association between work characteristics and epigenetic age acceleration: cross-sectional results from UK – Understanding Society study', *Aging*, 14 (19), 7752–73.

Freni-Sterrantino, A., Fiorito, G., D'Errico, A., et al. (2022b), 'Work-related stress and well-being in association with epigenetic age acceleration: a Northern Finland Birth Cohort 1966 Study', *Aging*, 14 (3), 1128–56.

Fuchs, F. D., and Whelton, P. K. (2020), 'High blood pressure and cardiovascular disease', *Hypertension*, 75 (2), 285–92.

Furman, D., Campisi, J., Verdin, E., et al. (2019), 'Chronic inflammation in the etiology of disease across the life span', *Nat Med*, 25 (12), 1822–32.

Gilbert-Ouimet, M., Trudel, X., Brisson, C., et al. (2014), 'Adverse effects of psychosocial work factors on blood pressure: systematic review of studies on demand-control support and effort-reward imbalance models', *Scand J Work Environ Health*, 40 (2), 109–32.

Gruenewald, T. L., Seeman, T. E., Ryff, C. D., et al. (2006), 'Combinations of bio-markers predictive of later life mortality', *Proc Natl Acad Sci USA*, 103 (38), 14158–63.

Hamer, M., Williams, E., Vuonovirta, R., et al. (2006), 'The effects of effort-reward imbalance on inflammatory and cardiovascular responses to mental stress', *Psychosom Med*, 68 (3), 408–13.

Hintsanen, M., Elovainio, M., Puttonen, S., et al. (2007), 'Effort-reward imbalance, heart rate, and heart rate variability: the Cardiovascular Risk in Young Finns Study', *Int J Behav Med*, 14 (4), 202–12.

Jarczok, M. N., Jarczok, M., and Thayer, J. F. (2020), 'Work stress and autonomic nervous system activity'. In T. Theorell (ed.), *Handbook of socioeconomic determinants of occupational health: from macro-level to micro-level evidence.* Cham: Springer, 625–56.

Jarczok, M. N., Jarczok, M., Mauss, D., et al. (2013), 'Autonomic nervous system activity and workplace stressors—a systematic review', *Neurosci Biobehav Rev*, 37 (8), 1810–23.

Johnston, D., Bell, C., Jones, M., et al. (2015), 'Stressors, appraisal of stressors, experienced stress and cardiac response: a real-time, real-life investigation of work stress in nurses', *Ann Behav Med*, 50 (2), 187–97.

Kim, E., Zhao, Z., Rzasa, J. R., et al. (2021), 'Association of acute psychosocial stress with oxidative stress: evidence from serum analysis', *Redox Biol*, 47, 102138.

Kirschbaum, C., Pirke, K. M., and Hellhammer, D. H. (1993), 'The "Trier Social Stress Test" – a tool for investigating psychobiological stress responses in a laboratory setting', *Neuropsychobiology*, 28 (1-2), 76–81.

Kivimäki, M., Walker, K. A., Pentti, J., et al. (2021), 'Cognitive stimulation in the workplace, plasma proteins, and risk of dementia: three analyses of population cohort studies', *BMJ*, 374, n1804.

Kunz-Ebrecht, S. R., Kirschbaum, C., and Steptoe, A. (2004), 'Work stress, socioeconomic status and neuroendocrine activation over the working day', *Soc Sci Med*, 58 (8), 1523–30.

Landsbergis, P. A., Dobson, M., Koutsouras, G., et al. (2013), 'Job strain and ambulatory blood pressure: a meta-analysis and systematic review', *Am J Public Health*, 103 (3), e61–71.

Lewington, S., Clarke, R., Qizilbash, N., et al. (2002), 'Age-specific relevance of usual blood pressure to vascular mortality: a meta-analysis of individual data for one million adults in 61 prospective studies', *Lancet*, 360 (9349), 1903–13.

Loerbroks, A., Schilling, O., Haxsen, V., et al. (2010), 'The fruits of one's labor: effort-reward imbalance but not job strain is related to heart rate variability across the day in 35-44-year-old workers', *J Psychosom Res*, 69 (2), 151–9.

Magnusson Hanson, L. L., Virtanen, M., Rod, N. H., et al. (2019), 'Does inflammation provide a link between psychosocial work characteristics and diabetes? Analysis of the role of interleukin-6 and C-reactive protein in the Whitehall II cohort study', *Brain Behav Immun*, 78, 153–60.

Magnusson Hanson, L. L., Westerlund, H., Goldberg, M., et al. (2017), 'Work stress, anthropometry, lung function, blood pressure, and blood-based biomarkers: a cross-sectional study of 43,593 French men and women', *Sci Rep*, 7 (1), 9282.

Maina, G., Bovenzi, M., Palmas, A., et al. (2009), 'Associations between two job stress models and measures of salivary cortisol', *Int Arch Occup Environ Health*, 82 (9), 1141–50.

Mauss, D., Li, J., Schmidt, B., et al. (2015), 'Measuring allostatic load in the workforce: a systematic review', *Ind Health*, 53 (1), 5–20.

Nakata, A. (2012), 'Psychosocial job stress and immunity: a systematic review'. In Q. Yan (ed.), *Psychoneuroimmunology: methods and protocols*. Totowa, NJ: Humana Press, 39–75.

Nyberg, S. T., Fransson, E. I., Heikkila, K., et al. (2013), 'Job strain and cardiovascular disease risk factors: meta-analysis of individual-participant data from 47,000 men and women', *PLoS One*, 8 (6), e67323.

Osborne, M. T., Shin, L. M., Mehta, N. N., et al. (2020), 'Disentangling the links between psychosocial stress and cardiovascular disease', *Circ Cardiovasc*, 13 (8), e010931.

Palma-Gudiel, H., Fañanás, L., Horvath, S., et al. (2020), 'Psychosocial stress and epigenetic aging', *Int Rev Neurobiol*, 150, 107–28.

Penz, M., Siegrist, J., Wekenborg, M. K., et al. (2019), 'Effort-reward imbalance at work is associated with hair cortisol concentrations: prospective evidence from the Dresden Burnout Study', *Psychoneuroendocrinology*, 109, 104399.

Pruessner, J. C., Wolf, O. T., Hellhammer, D. H., et al. (1997), 'Free cortisol levels after awakening: a reliable biological marker for the assessment of adrenocortical activity', *Life Sci*, 61 (26), 2539–49.

Rentscher, K. E., Carroll, J. E., and Mitchell, C. (2020), 'Psychosocial stressors and telomere length: a current review of the science', *Annu Rev Public Health*, 41, 223–45.

Romanowska, J., and Theorell, T. (2020), 'Using arts to support leadership development'. In T. Theorell (ed.), *Handbook of socioeconomic determinants of occupational health: from macro-level to micro-level evidence*. Cham: Springer, 489–504.

Romanowska, J., Larsson, G., Eriksson, M., et al. (2011), 'Health effects on leaders and co-workers of an art-based leadership development program', *Psychother Psychosom*, 80 (2), 78–87.

Schnall, P. L., Schwartz, J. E., Landsbergis, P. A., et al. (1998), 'A longitudinal study of job strain and ambulatory blood pressure: results from a three-year follow-up', *Psychosom Med*, 60 (6), 697–706.

Seeman, T. E., McEwen, B. S., Rowe, J. W., et al. (2001), 'Allostatic load as a marker of cumulative biological risk: MacArthur studies of successful aging', *Proc Natl Acad Sci USA*, 98 (8), 4770–75.

Siegrist, J., and Sies, H. (2017), 'Disturbed redox homeostasis in oxidative distress: a molecular link from chronic psychosocial work stress to coronary heart disease?', *Circ Res*, 121 (2), 103–05.

Siegrist, J., and Li, J. (2017), 'Work stress and altered biomarkers: a synthesis of findings based on the effort-reward imbalance model', *Int J Environ Res Public Health*, 14 (11), 1373.

Stalder, T., and Kirschbaum, C. (2012), 'Analysis of cortisol in hair – state of the art and future directions', *Brain Behav Immun*, 26 (7), 1019–29.

Steptoe, A. (2006), 'Psychobiological processes linking socio-economic position with health'. In J. Siegrist and M. Marmot (eds.), *Social inequalities in health: new evidence and policy implications*. Oxford: Oxford University Press, 101–26.

Steptoe, A., and Willemsen, G. (2004), 'The influence of low job control on ambulatory blood pressure and perceived stress over the working day in men and women from the Whitehall II cohort', *J Hypertens*, 22 (5), 915–20.

Steptoe, A., and Kivimaki, M. (2012), 'Stress and cardiovascular disease', *Nat Rev Cardiol*, 9 (6), 360–70.

Steptoe, A., Siegrist, J., Kirschbaum, C., et al. (2004), 'Effort-reward imbalance, overcommitment, and measures of cortisol and blood pressure over the working day', *Psychosom Med*, 66 (3), 323–9.

Steptoe, A., Kunz-Ebrecht, S., Owen, N., et al. (2003), 'Influence of socioeconomic status and job control on plasma fibrinogen responses to acute mental stress', *Psychosom Med*, 65 (1), 137–44.

Stringhini, S., Polidoro, S., Sacerdote, C., et al. (2015), 'Life-course socioeconomic status and DNA methylation of genes regulating inflammation', *Int J Epidemiol*, 44 (4), 1320–30.

Takaki, J. (2013), 'Associations of job stress indicators with oxidative biomarkers in Japanese men and women', *Int J Environ Res Public Health*, 10 (12), 6662–71.

Tawakol, A., Ishai, A., Takx, R. A. P., et al. (2017), 'Relation between resting amygdalar activity and cardiovascular events: a longitudinal and cohort study', *Lancet*, 389 (10071), 834–45.

Theorell, T. (2009), 'Anabolism and catabolism'. In S. Sonnentag, P. L. Perrewé, and D. S. Ganster (eds.), *Occupational stress and wellbeing. Current perspectives on job-stress recovery*, vol. 7. London: Emerald Group Publishing Limited, 249–76.

Theorell, T. (2016), 'Reward, flow and control at work'. In J. Siegrist and M. Wahrendorf (eds.), *Work stress and health in a globalized economy*. Cham: Springer, 315–32.

Theorell, T. (2020), 'Regeneration and anabolism: the good perspective'. In T. Theorell (ed.), *Handbook of socioeconomic determinants of occupational health: from macro-level to micro-level evidence*. Cham: Springer, 1–13.

Thielmann, B., Hartung, J., and Bockelmann, I. (2022), 'Objective assessment of mental stress in individuals with different levels of effort reward imbalance or overcommitment using heart rate variability: a systematic review', *Syst Rev*, 11 (1), 48.

Trudel, X., Brisson, C., Gilbert-Ouimet, M., et al. (2018), 'Psychosocial stressors at work and ambulatory blood pressure', *Curr Cardiol Rep*, 20 (12), 127.

Trudel, X., Brisson, C., Milot, A., et al. (2013), 'Psychosocial work environment and ambulatory blood pressure: independent and combined effect of demand-control and effort-reward imbalance models', *Occup Environ Med*, 70 (11), 815–22.

Trudel, X., Brisson, C., Milot, A., et al. (2016), 'Effort-reward imbalance at work and 5-year changes in blood pressure: the mediating effect of changes in body mass index among 1400 white-collar workers', *Int Arch Occup Environ Health*, 89 (8), 1229–38.

Trudel, X., Milot, A., Gilbert-Ouimet, M., et al. (2017), 'Effort-reward imbalance at work and the prevalence of unsuccessfully treated hypertension among white-collar workers', *Am J Epidemiol*, 186 (4), 456–62.

Vrijkotte, T. G., van Doornen, L. J., and de Geus, E. J. (2000), 'Effects of work stress on ambulatory blood pressure, heart rate, and heart rate variability', *Hypertension*, 35 (4), 880–6.

Wahrendorf, M., and Demakakos, P. (2020), 'Childhood determinants of occupational health at older ages'. In T. Theorell (ed.), *Handbook of socioeconomic determinants of occupational health: from macro-level to micro-level evidence*. Cham: Springer, 1–18.

Wahrendorf, M., Chandola, T., Goldberg, M., et al. (2022), 'Adverse employment histories and allostatic load: associations over the working life', *J Epidemiol Community Health*, 76 (4), 374–81.

PART IV
EFFECTS OF HEALTH ON WORK

8

Working with a disease or disability

8.1 Health and work trajectories

8.1.1 Bi-directional relationships between work and health

Modern societies increasingly face an ageing workforce. Despite a continuous growth of healthy life expectancy, a substantial part of older working people suffers from some degree of health impairment. Prevalent chronic diseases and disabilities often impair people's work ability, increase absenteeism and longer periods of sick leave, and contribute to higher rates of early retirement (OECD 2010). A strong link of disability with reduced employment is of particular concern (see 8.1.2.1). Leaving paid work due to disabling conditions is considered the tip of an iceberg. A substantial part of adults with age-related functional decline or presence of a chronic disease continue to work. They are faced with a recurrent challenge to maintain their functioning and work ability. Medical treatment and supervision, extended periods of sick leave, medical and vocational rehabilitation measures, and a variety of return-to-work programmes are available to this end. In all these instances, to a different extent, reduced health affects people's daily work experience and work ability.

- Whereas the former chapters of this book focused on the pathway leading from adverse working conditions to poor health, this part of the book emphasizes the reverse pathway by demonstrating effects of reduced health on work ability and job continuity (see also Tang 2014).
- Analysing this bi-directional relationship in a life-course perspective is a core task of occupational health research. Although the pathway from health to work may matter more in later stages of occupational careers, both directions deserve attention at each stage of development as they often interact.

Psychosocial Occupational Health. Johannes Siegrist and Jian Li, Oxford University Press.
© Oxford University Press 2024. DOI: 10.1093/oso/9780192887924.003.0008

- When putting the main focus on the pathway from health to work, different steps of an aggravating process can be distinguished in an analytical perspective. Starting from mild impairment with tangible effects on work ability and workload, reduced health may result in periods of sick leave, requiring medical treatment and rehabilitation. Further steps are (a) efforts to return to work and, if not feasible, (b) exit from paid work.

In this chapter, it is not possible to provide an in-depth analysis of each step of this aggravating process. Following a brief description of each step, we focus on two steps with outstanding relevance for individual workers and for social, health and labour policies: (1) voluntary or involuntary early exit from paid work due to disability or chronic disease, and (2) return to work following medical or vocational rehabilitation. These two topics are addressed at different depth. Restricting essential information on determinants and consequences of exit from paid work to the presentation and discussion of selected recently published high-quality studies will result in a relatively short section that appears first (Section 8.1). More space is devoted to the analysis of complex processes of return to work (Section 8.2). Here, we elaborate three different scenarios of return to work. In the first scenario, we identify conditions that enable job continuation following recovery from disease. We chose ischaemic heart disease as a disorder providing some empirical illustration of this trajectory. The second scenario deals with job change following an incident event that disrupts the previous occupational career. Spinal cord injury was chosen to exemplify of how a severe disability affects the option of return to work. In the third scenario, job instability defines the analytical focus. Here, a precarious trajectory characterized by periods of worklessness, recurrent health impairment, and involuntary job change is described, and a highly prevalent mental disorder, depression, was selected to document respective developments. These three scenarios cannot cover the broad spectrum of processes enabling the integration of people with impaired health into work, but they may reveal some general features of strengths and limitations within the practices and outcomes of return to work.

These two steps are best understood as stages of an aggravating process starting with impact of reduced health on people's work ability. Pain, restricted movements, reduced muscle strength, and lack of energy and attention are examples of this impact. To what extent they compromise work ability and result in practical consequences depends on a variety of factors. These factors include the severity of health impairments, the nature and specific requirements of job tasks, the visibility and control of work performance, and the tolerance accorded to workers with reduced job performance by the organization's management. Staying at work with reduced work ability is likely to overstretch available coping resources due to enhanced compensatory energy mobilization. As a result, increased workload is experienced. As more physical energy is required to meet the regular demands at work, less energy is available to tackle subsequent obligations, triggering a state of exhaustion. In consequence, physical exhaustion may worsen the manifestation of symptoms and bodily restrictions, thus initiating a vicious circle of work-related impaired health. This vicious circle is not restricted to physical workload. Longitudinal studies of associations of psychosocial work characteristics with impaired health collecting data over several subsequent measurement waves support a bi-directional relationship between work and health. For instance, in a Swedish study on musculoskeletal pain with four sets of measurements made every two years from 2010 to 2016, stressful work in terms of the effort-reward imbalance (ERI) model was associated with increased risk of onset of neck-shoulder and low back pain during a two-year follow-up-period. Conversely, presence of musculoskeletal pain predicted high levels of stressful work during the respective follow-up period (Halonen et al. 2018; Halonen et al. 2019). Similarly, in a study of older workers, continued stressful work predicted the onset of sleep disturbance over a four-year period, while sleep disturbances at study onset equally increased the risk of subsequent high levels of work stress (Cho and Chen 2020). Earlier on, we pointed to impressive evidence on bi-directional associations between stressful work and symptoms of burnout provided by longitudinal studies, based on the job demands-resources (JD-R) model (Lesener et al. 2019). In a systematic review focusing on the job strain model, effects of work stressors on strain were stronger than those of the reverse pathway (Tang 2014).

The vicious circle may be maintained for a certain time by presenteeism, but it often ends in periods of sick leave. In most modern welfare systems, long-term absenteeism due to continued health impairment is covered for a certain time by sickness benefits paid by employers (often six weeks). Thereafter, sickness funds provide benefits in terms of a reduced amount of employees' previous salary, again for a certain time period (e.g. in Finland up to one year). If chronic health problems cannot be improved by medical and vocational rehabilitation, the aggravating process leads to early exit from paid work as mentioned (see next section).

Rich knowledge is available from officially recorded data on absenteeism and its occupational determinants despite their methodological liniations (Loisel and Anema 2013). A multitude of studies examined associations of a variety of psychosocial work characteristics with absenteeism, including the DC model (e.g. North et al. 1996), the OJ model (e.g. Head et al. 2007), the ERI model (e.g. Duchaine et al. 2020), and the JD-R model. Yet, as the quality of evidence is often limited in these investigations, they are not discussed here.

8.1.2 Chronic disease or disability and exit from work

Labour market policies at the national level play a crucial role in the management of disability and chronic disease at work. While active labour market policies aim at reinforcing and extending participation in paid work through a set of legal, organizational, and individual measures (see below), passive labour market policies are designed to support those who are no longer capable of staying at work, mainly by providing unemployment benefits, access to early retirement, and disability pensions. There are large variations in the development of these policies across countries, and in addition to legal regulations, characteristics of the labour market and trends of economic development exert a powerful impact on the amount and duration of providing benefits and offering supportive programmes (Dahl and van der Wel 2020; see Chapter 9). National labour and social policies are supported by some supranational activities and regulations. The International Labour Organization's (ILO) 'Social Protection Floor Initiative' (International Labour Organization 2013), the United Nations' 'Convention on the Rights of Persons with Disabilities' (UN General Assembly 2007), and the '2021–2030 European Disability Strategy' implemented in the European Community (Eurofound 2021) are examples. The boundaries between measures of active labour market policies and passive labour market policies are increasingly blurred in view of an overarching trend towards safeguarding and augmenting work participation of people with impaired health. Several countries started to reduce the amount of passive payments of benefits and to limit access to early retirement. Criteria of accordance were tightened, and the time frame of granting disability pensions was limited, urging people to return to work whenever possible. In addition to attempts to raise the age of state pension eligibility, these measures were realized as a reaction to rapidly increasing public spending, specifically of national pension systems and health-care organizations. Moreover, the measures reflect a shift towards strengthening active labour market policies, specifically by extending incentives of supported employment (see below).

In OECD countries, a growing number of disability benefit recipients was observed in recent past, where about six per cent of the working age population were covered by this measure of social protection (OECD 2010). Disability pensions are granted if a medically certified diagnosis indicates an inability of a person's continued work participation due to a physical or mental impairment. Accordingly, many people with disabilities have left the labour market. A respective quantification, labelled disability-employment gap, sheds some light on the policy dimension of this problem. For instance, a European report concluded that the employment rate of persons with disability was 50.8 per cent, compared to 75 per cent among persons without disability (Eurofound 2021). The size of this gap was confirmed by another cross-country study (Barr et al. 2020). This latter study identified a further severe problem related to disability: Substantial social inequalities in employment rates became apparent among persons with disability. For instance, among disabled women with low educational level the employment rate was as low as twenty-five per cent whereas it mounted to around seventy per cent among disabled women with high education. Respective differences for men were around thirty-five per cent versus around seventy per cent (Barr et al. 2020; see also Dahl and van der Wel 2020). Therefore, the analysis of links between work, impaired health, and exit from paid work through provision of a disability pension has to tackle with two interrelated questions:

- What is the evidence of a social gradient of health-related exit from paid work? Is this risk substantially higher among people with low educational or occupational position than among those with more privileged socioeconomic positions?
- What is the contribution of adverse working conditions to elevated risks of health-related exit from paid work? Is there evidence of a direct impact of adverse material and psychosocial work characteristics on the frequency of disability pensions? And is this impact particularly strong among socioeconomically deprived people?

Before these questions are answered, it is useful to ask how disability is defined and assessed (see Box 8.1).

Box 8.1 Disability: definition and assessment

- According to WHO's International Classification of Functioning, Disability and Health disability is defined as a dynamic continuum of experiences of bodily impairments and restrictions in activity and participation. In this continuum, personal disability characteristics are modified by enabling or limiting environmental conditions (World Health Organization 2001).
- In a similar way, according to the United Nations, people with disability are characterized by the presence of long-term physical, mental, intellectual, or sensory impairment that interferes with their full participation in their communities (UN General Assembly 2007).
- A variety of assessment methods were introduced to measure disability, such as self-assessed or expert-assessed scales, that is, Activities of Daily Living (ADL), Instrumental Activities of Daily Living (IADL), Global Activity Limitation Indicator (GALI) and tests of cognitive function (e.g. Free and Cued Selective Reminding Test (FCSRT) and of physical function (e.g. standing balance; for references e.g. Wahrendorf et al. 2019). However, most assessments consider physical and mental impairments without documenting their impact on participation.

8.1.2.1 Exit from paid work and socioeconomic position

The first question concerning evidence of a social gradient of health-related exit from paid work has been investigated in a series of influential scientific analyses, using disability pension (DP) as the relevant outcome criterion for exit from paid work. As health status is a powerful determinant of DP, it is important to disentangle three interrelated links, (a) the link between socioeconomic position (SEP) and health, (b) the link between health and DP, and (c) the link between SEP and DP, considering health. The association between SEP and health has received most extensive attention in research on social determinants of health. A strong, consistent social gradient of major chronic diseases according to SEP has been documented. In particular, this holds true for morbidity and mortality from cardiovascular and metabolic diseases, respiratory diseases, distinct cancers, accidents, and affective disorders

(Mackenbach 2019). Relative morbidity risks are around twice as high among working age people with lowest SEP as compared to those with highest SEP (see also, Marmot 2004). Social gradients of similar strength were identified for levels of physical and cognitive functioning from early life to midlife (Hurst et al. 2013). This evidence is even more compelling if the link of SEP with functional impairment is analysed in early old age. Several ageing studies document steep social gradients of physical and cognitive functioning (Makaroun et al. 2017; Wahrendorf et al. 2013). Taken together, this elevated burden of disease and disability accumulating during midlife puts people who live and work in socially disadvantaged conditions at heightened risk of suffering from impaired health at advanced working age, thus urging them to premature, involuntary exit from work.

What is known about the link (b) between impaired health and risk of DP? A systematic literature review of twenty-nine studies concluded that poor self-rated health, prevalence of chronic disease, and mental health problems predict elevated risks of involuntary exit from employment, either in terms of DP or of unemployment (van Rijn et al. 2014). A third way of leaving work, early retirement, that is based on people's voluntary decision, was only weakly related to these indicators of poor health. If low SEP is related to poor health, and if poor health increases the probability of receiving DP, can we conclude that SEP is negatively associated with an elevated risk of health-related exit from work? A robust answer to this question is given by the findings of an investigation that included prospective data of seven large cohort studies from Europe and the US, using education and occupational grade as separate indicators of SEP, and adjusting the effects on a measure of health-related work exit for self-rated health and birth cohort. Results are displayed in Figure 8.1 (Carr et al. 2018).

Findings are indicated as hazard ratios (HR) of the lowest of three occupational groups, compared to the highest occupational group (HR = 1.0), separately for men and women. In all but one case, HRs of health-related work exit were significantly increased in the lowest occupational group, with a slightly stronger significance among men. Within this range, HRs vary considerably between 1.61 and 4.60. Men and women in the second occupational group also experienced higher risks of health-related work exit, but effects were weaker and less consistent. This pattern was replicated with educational degree as stratifying variable, but the results with occupational grade as SEP indicator were most compelling.

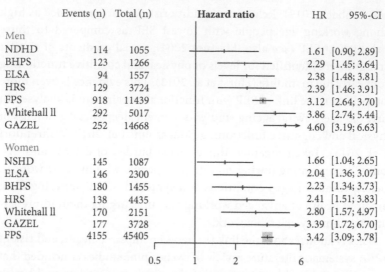

	Events (n)	Total (n)	Hazard ratio	HR	95%-CI
Men					
NDHD	114	1055		1.61	[0.90; 2.89]
BHPS	123	1266		2.29	[1.45; 3.64]
ELSA	94	1557		2.38	[1.48; 3.81]
HRS	129	3724		2.39	[1.46; 3.91]
FPS	918	11439		3.12	[2.64; 3.70]
Whitehall ll	292	5017		3.86	[2.74; 5.44]
GAZEL	252	14668		4.60	[3.19; 6.63]
Women					
NSHD	145	1087		1.66	[1.04; 2.65]
ELSA	146	2300		2.04	[1.36; 3.07]
BHPS	180	1455		2.23	[1.34; 3.73]
HRS	138	4435		2.41	[1.51; 3.83]
Whitehall ll	170	2151		2.80	[1.57; 4.97]
GAZEL	177	3728		3.39	[1.72; 6.70]
FPS	4155	45405		3.42	[3.09; 3.78]

Adjusted for poor self-rated health (all studies) and birth cohort (all studies except NSHD).

Figure 8.1 Association of low occupational grade with risk of health-related work exit (disability pension) in seven cohort studies. BHPS, British Household Panel; ELSA, English Longitudinal Study of Ageing; FPS, Finnish Public Sector Study; GAZEL, Electricité De France-Gaz De France; HRS, Health and Retirement Study; NSHD, National Survey of Health and Development.

Source: Reproduced with permission from Carr, E., Fleischmann, M., Goldberg, M., et al. (2018), 'Occupational and educational inequalities in exit from employment at older ages: evidence from seven prospective cohorts', *Occup Environ Med*, 75 (5), 369–77. [Figure 4, p. 374] (Creative Commons Attribution 4.0 International License, https://crea tivecommons.org/licenses/by/4.0/).

8.1.2.2 Working conditions as determinants of disability pension

With our second question, we were wondering whether adverse working conditions determine risks of receiving a DP. We also asked whether these risks were particularly pronounced among employed people with low oc- cupational positions. A comprehensive systematic review concluded that a variety of psychosocial working conditions are associated with elevated risks of DP, but that moderating factors, such as low occupational position, deserve more attention in future research (Knardahl et al. 2017). This latter shortcoming was extensively analysed in a series of high-quality studies per- formed by a Dutch team led by Alex Burdorf. In a first prospective study of 14,700 employees followed up to ten years, the influence of SEP (measured by education), health, unhealthy behaviour, and work characteristics on involuntary (DP; unemployment) and voluntary (early retirement; economic inactivity) early exit from work was investigated (Robroek et al. 2015). The main findings of interest in this context refer to the two variables, SEP and DP. If compared to the highest of three educational groups, the lowest group had significantly increased risks of poor health, of performing unhealthy behaviour, and of being exposed to heavy physical workload and low job task control. Risks of receiving disability pension or of becoming unemployed were also significantly increased. An additional analysis revealed that elevated DP risks were predicted by low SEP, low job control, high physical workload, and low reward (Robroek et al. 2015). In a longitudinal study from Germany, part of the association of DP with low SEP was explained by a low level of work ability and poor health (Rohrbacher and Hasselhorn 2022). The findings of these studies from the Netherlands and Germany corroborate evidence on social inequalities in involuntary early exit from paid work, and they emphasize the role of distinct mediating factors. As precarious work is more prevalent among employees with low SEP, it may additionally contribute to the burden of DP. In a Finnish study, two indicators of precarious work—previous unemployment and poor employability prospects—were linked to a higher risk of depression-related DP among men, but not among women (Pyöriä et al. 2021).

With the advent of two new metrics—related to early exit from paid work—the working life expectancy (WLE) and working years lost (WYL), a relevant improvement in the standardization of measurement was achieved (see Box 8.2). These measures are instructive for policy reasons. For instance, one Dutch study analysed changes in working careers over a twenty-year period, comparing WLE at the age of 58 years between healthy workers and workers with functional disability. In the former group, a mean increase in WLE of 1.8 years was observed, compared to an increase of 0.7 years in the latter group (Burdorf and Robroek 2020).

To disentangle the effects of chronic disease, SEP, and poor working conditions on WLE and WYL data from a further large longitudinal study in the Netherlands (STREAM) were analysed (Schram et al. 2022). This investigation included 11,808 employed men and women aged 50 to 66 years, with information from annual online questionnaires and linked data from statistical offices. While the previously reported results of a social gradient and an impact of chronic disease on involuntary exit from work were confirmed, new data illustrated the effects of adverse working conditions on WLE as well as their differential strength according to SEP. Five working

Box 8.2 **Working life expectancy and Working years lost**

- Working life expectancy (WLE): Number of years a person is expected to stay at work until leaving for statutory retirement.
- Working years lost (WYL): Number of working years lost due to premature exit from paid employment.
- Information is usually based on employment statistics with data on monthly transitions (employed, involuntary or voluntary exit, mortality) retrieved over time at individual level. Transition rates are calculated for a distinct age period, for example, 50–65 years (Schram et al. 2022).

conditions were measured with standardized questionnaire data, physical workload, job demands, autonomy, emotional demands, and social support at work. For each one of the three SEP categories (educational level), WLE was estimated by applying a multistate model with estimation of transition states between different types of being employed or not, resulting in WLE 'as the number of years in the work state, conditional on being in paid employment at the starting age' (Schram et al. 2022, p. 393). Accordingly, WYL indicated the mean number of working years lost due to premature exit from work for each category. In Table 8.1, a selection of results from respective analyses is displayed, with three adverse working conditions (high physical workload; low autonomy; low social support). Given our focus on involuntary work exit, the results presented in this table are limited to this type of labour market exit (Schram et al. 2022; extract from table 4, p. 395).

To our knowledge, this is the first empirical evidence quantifying work years lost due to distinct adverse material and psychosocial working conditions according to the SEP of employed people. Of interest, effects of adverse work on WYL were stronger among participations with low SEP than among those with high SEP. Among the former group, losses were highest for those exposed to low social support (2.37 years) and low autonomy at work (2.01 years). Within each SEP, differences in loss between those exposed and not exposed were also largest in case of exposure to psychosocial work conditions (Schram et al. 2022).

In conclusion, chronic diseases and disabilities in ageing working populations are main risk factors of involuntary exit from paid employment,

Table 8.1 Working years lost (95 per cent CI) due to involuntary exit from paid employment according to educational level and selected unfavourable working conditions

Educational level	Physical workload		Autonomy		Social support	
Low	Low	1.84 (1.55–2.12)	High	1.80 (1.55–2.08)	High	1.66 (1.41–1.91)
	High	1.93 (1.65–2.20)	Low	2.01 (1.72–2.31)	Low	2.37 (2.04–2.74)
Intermediate	Low	1.60 (1.46–1.76)	High	1.58 (1.44–1.71)	High	1.46 (1.33–1.59)
	High	1.68 (1.51–1.87)	Low	1.74 (1.55–1.94)	Low	2.08 (1.86–2.32)
High	Low	1.40 (1.31–1.48)	High	1.38 (1.29–1.46)	High	1.27 (1.19–1.35)
	High	1.46 (1.31–1.62)	Low	1.51 (1.37–1.66)	Low	1.82 (1.65–1.97)

Source: Adapted with permission from Schram, J. L. D., Schuring, M., Oude Hengel, K. M., et al. (2022), 'The influence of chronic diseases and poor working conditions in working life expectancy across educational levels among older employees in the Netherlands', *Scand J Work Environ Health*, 48 (5), 391–98. [Table 4, p.395]; (Creative Commons Attribution 4.0 International License, https://creativecommons.org/licenses/by/4.0/).

resulting in unemployment, early retirement, or receipt of a disability pension. As poor health is more frequent among employees with low SEP, a social gradient of health-related work exit was expected. This assumption was supported by strong empirical evidence (Figure 8.1). At the same time, adverse material and psychosocial working conditions were shown to increase the probability of involuntary work exit, in addition to their direct effects on the progression of disease and disability. Therefore, due to accumulation of adversities and disadvantages, the toll of lost working years is highest among employees in low SEP (Table 8.1). Leaving work prematurely due to impairment goes along with far-reaching financial restrictions and a disruption of social roles and relationships. These consequences result in people's increased psychological, social, and economic vulnerability. Whereas extensive social protection measures mitigate some of these distressing consequences, a high burden of chronic difficulties remains to be tackled, at the level of individuals and their families, and at the level of society at large. Therefore, increased investments into measures of worksite health promotion and return to work are a high priority policy target.

8.2 Return to work with chronic disease or disability

8.2.1 Basic notions

Work is a key activity in adult life. It offers people a social role within the societal structure, defined by a formal contract with recurrent obligations and a corresponding revenue. It protects people against basic life risks by providing health insurance, unemployment insurance, and pensions. Moreover, under favourable conditions, work and employment meet important human needs, such as the development of capabilities and skills, the promotion of personal growth and career advancement, and the recurrent experience of control, mastery, recognition, and self-esteem. Given these fundamental benefits of work, it is basically unfair that substantial parts of adult populations are excluded from labour market participation, either due to unemployment, lack of training, disease or disability, or social discrimination. In a human rights perspective, the right to work needs to be included in a list of basic human rights. In fact, the United Nations' 'Universal Declaration of Human Rights' had already recognized this obligation in 1948 (United Nations 1948). More recent declarations, including the 'Convention on the Rights of Persons with Disabilities' (CRPD), confirmed and strengthened this responsibility of nations (Bickenbach 2020; UN General Assembly 2007). Specifically, people with disabilities and chronic health impairments are often excluded from opportunities of full participation in paid work, as documented, for instance, in the World Report on Disability (World Health Organization 2011). Therefore, there is a strong need to extend and intensify initiatives and programmes of including these population groups into paid work. This is one aspect to be emphasized in the analysis of return-to-work processes.

A second aspect of this analysis concerns the institutional and organizational features of return-to-work programmes (see Schultz and Gatchel 2016 and Chapter 9). To what extent do legal rules prevent or promote return to work? What is the role of social insurance authorities providing compensations, health-care providers, and employers? In what organizational contexts are workers supported to return to work? For instance, medical rehabilitation may be well developed at the expense of vocational rehabilitation. Or, several countries favour rehabilitation clinics as setting for return-to-work programmes, whereas in other countries, these processes are carried out in ambulatory settings. Analysis of the contribution of organizational aspects to return to work needs to include labour market barriers. Return-to-work programmes may be successfully accomplished for some employable groups with disabilities, but the absence of suitable job opportunities deprives these groups of work participation. For instance, in a European-wide survey on environmental and personal factors limiting access to work, around thirty per cent of respondents reported that lack of suitable job opportunities was a decisive factor (Eurofound 2017). As indicated below, this complaint is of key importance among people with disability who aim at returning to work.

Thirdly, return-to-work programmes require the collaboration of multidisciplinary teams. Distinct from acute medical treatment that is under control of physicians, medical and vocational rehabilitation activities involve professionals from additional disciplines, such as physiotherapy, psychotherapy, nursing, vocational counselling, nutritional sciences, sports sciences, educational sciences, and human resource management. Successful performance requires a problem-oriented division of work and cooperation. Opportunities of offering multi-disciplinary programmes heavily depend on legal, financial, and organizational circumstances. One can argue that specialized rehabilitation clinics are better prepared to offer such programmes as they have recruited diverse professional groups and developed standardized programmes targeting patient groups with specific health problems. On the other hand, ambulatory settings may offer more flexibility, although logistic problems can interfere with treatment efficacy. In several countries where the biomedical model is dominant, interdisciplinary teamwork has not yet been developed, and a lack of training options towards greater professionalization of paramedical disciplines prevents progress.

Finally, in every analysis of return-to-work activities, disease-specific aspects deserve the highest attention. Considering the broad spectrum of disabilities and chronic diseases one recognizes the need to select or weight different programme components according to underlying treatment needs. This does not preclude extending a specific element within a specialized rehabilitation programme to other patient groups. For instance, behavioural psychotherapy may be applied to patient groups with different disorders. Equally so, distinct elements within the Individual Placement and Support (IPS) practice, which was originally developed for people with serious mental illness, were applied to other disability conditions more recently (Bond et al. 2019). Yet, whether the improvement of physical functioning, of emotional and social capabilities, of cognitive and intellectual skills, or of sensory functioning is a predominant target requires different therapeutic approaches. Moreover, treatment success and probability of sustainable reintegration into work varies largely across different types of disabilities and illnesses. Therefore, when discussing new knowledge on psychosocial aspects of return to work in this section, we focus our analysis on three representative disorders that illustrate three different scenarios of return to work, one characterized by job continuation, one necessitating job change, and one defined by job instability and precarious interruptions. As mentioned, despite their diversity, the three scenarios may reveal some general features within the dynamics of return-to-work programmes (see also Bültmann and Siegrist 2020).

8.2.2 Job continuation: The case of ischaemic heart disease

Acute myocardial infarction (AMI) is a dominant manifestation of ischaemic heart disease. Due to atherosclerotic and thrombotic narrowing of coronary arteries oxygen supply to the myocardium is restricted, resulting in ischaemic lesion and cardiac arrhythmias. AMI is a serious health complication with increased risk of sudden cardiac death. However, progress in intense care treatment and success in controlling main cardiovascular risk factors (e.g. hypertension, hyperlipidaemia) reduced mortality risks and improved longer-term survival (Amini et al. 2021). Once released from hospital, cardiac patients are offered cardiac rehabilitation, delivered in rehabilitation centres, clinics, or in ambulatory settings under the control of physicians. Cardiac rehabilitation is additionally offered to patients who underwent coronary artery bypass graft (CABG) surgery or percutaneous coronary intervention (PCI). The main aim of cardiac rehabilitation consists in shaping and reinforcing a lifestyle that protects patients from recurrent cardiac events and contributes to healthy life expectancy. Specifically, adherence to medical therapy, regular physical activity, healthy diet, smoking cessation, as well as improvement of mental health and personal coping ability are expected to enable patients to continue their regular life and to return to work. There are large variations across countries in coverage, intensity, and duration of rehabilitation measures as well as in their organizational contexts (see Chapter 9). As a general trend, a strong emphasis on biomedical and behavioural aspects is observed, whereas psychosocial and occupation-related aspects with relevance to cardiac patients are often neglected (Jelinek et al. 2015; Reibis et al. 2019).

It is evident that the severity of disease, the functional limitations due to ischaemia and angina pectoris, heart failure, and cardiac arrhythmias reduce options for returning to work, and especially of return to physically strenuous work. Yet, even among cardiac patients with successful medical outcomes distinct occupational risk factors can interfere with return to work as they may augment the occurrence of recurrent coronary events. These risk factors include material conditions such as shift work, noise, and exposure to toxic chemical substances (de Rijk 2020; Theorell 2020) as well as psychosocial features (see Chapter 6, Table 6.1; de Rijk 2020; Gragnano et al. 2018). Opportunities of return to work are determined by external conditions (e.g. lower labour market access for low skilled workers (Butt et al. 2018); e.g. disincentives of financially attractive early exit offers), but personal characteristics of AMI patients are relevant as well (e.g. depressive symptoms (de Jonge et al. 2014), older age, female gender (Dreyer et al. 2016), and negative beliefs about their own capability (Reibis et al. 2019; Soderberg et al. 2015)).

We are now interested to learn how successful the rate of return to work is among cardiac patients after discharge from hospital due to AMI, CABG, or PCI, taking these enabling or limiting factors into account. To what extent are these men and women able to return to their previous employment,

Box 8.3 **Estimates of return-to-work rates among cardiac patients**

- After one year, return-to-work rates were reported as 76 per cent in a European survey of cardiac patients (de Cauter et al. 2019), as 80 per cent in a nationwide Danish study of patients with CABG (Butt et al. 2018).
- After two to three years, return-to-work rates were still very high, for example around seventy-nine per cent among AMI patients in a study in Israel (two years; Zack et al. 2022), around seventy per cent among PCI patients in a Norwegian study (three years; Olsen et al. 2020).
- In an intervention study (see Table 8.2), the return-to-work rate to the previous job was ninety-four and ninety-eight per cent respectively after one and two years in the intervention group, but significantly lower in the control group (Zack et al. 2022).
- Overall, the return-to-work rate among cardiac patients is high, and a large majority continues to work in the previous job. However, a strong social gradient of return-to-work according to occupational position is observed. Based on a systematic review and meta-analysis of forty-three prospective studies, the return rate was around eighty-one per cent among white collar workers, compared to sixty-five per cent among blue-collar workers (Kai et al. 2022).

thus experiencing job continuation? Some robust estimates are given in Box 8.3. These data indicate that cardiac patients have a high probability of continuing their job career, and even to return to the job held previously. A large majority of patients is capable of working full-time, and these high rates are rather stable over a couple of years. However, large variations are observed according to socioeconomic, work-related, health-related, and psychological characteristics of patients (Kai et al. 2022). For instance, social support provided by partners and friends was shown to be an important determinant of rehabilitation success. In one study, 85 per cent of cardiac patients who were in employment after one year were married, but this percentage was as low as 56 per cent among those who were not yet returned to work at this time (Zack et al. 2022). Marital support in promoting adaptation to the work role and in reconciling work and family obligations represents a crucial factor in the rehabilitation process from hospital discharge to re-entry to the labour market. These enabling and limiting factors need to be assessed by professional members of the cardiac rehabilitation team, and results should instruct the implementation of specific interventions according to need.

As research evidence on rehabilitation after acute cardiac events has been developed quite extensively in a couple of advanced countries, this knowledge was applied in a series of intervention studies (randomized controlled trials (RCTs)) aiming to strengthen return to work. A meta-analysis of thirty-nine RCTs found little support for person-directed interventions, but some modest support for programmes that combined person- and work-directed elements (Hegewald et al. 2019). A recent intervention trial provided some more encouraging findings (Zack et al. 2022). Importantly, this RCT included 71 cardiac patients in an intensive case management programme and 77 patients in the usual rehabilitation programme. Case managers assessed the patients' own perceptions and expectations regarding their health and their work, explored their occupational background, and referred patients to psychotherapy if needed (e.g. for treating depressive symptoms). Moreover, an occupational physician was recruited for cooperation. Subsequently, a tailored integration plan was discussed between case manager, patient, and employer, and the employer was instructed about the patient's needs and options. Similarly, the patient's family was included in this process. Once patients had returned to work, regular supervision by calls from the case managers was provided. For those patients who had not returned to work after six months, an intensive training programme of twelve sessions was offered. This comprehensive intervention resulted in remarkable achievements, as displayed in Table 8.2.

Return-to-work rates at six, twelve, and twenty-four months were 15 to 17 per cent higher in the intervention group, compared to the control group. Differences in full-time rates amounted to 23 per cent between the two groups. A similar difference was observed with regard to return to the same job as before the cardiac event. Here, rates were 23, 20, and 21 per cent higher after six, twelve, and twenty-four months in the intervention group (Zack et al. 2022).

In conclusion, cardiac patients who experienced an AMI or underwent CABG or PCI have good opportunities to return to work after rehabilitation and to continue their previous job. These opportunities vary according to the presence or absence of reliably identified risk factors. It is therefore a

Table 8.2 Return-to-work rate and employment status at follow-up of the intervention and control groups

Study groups	Employed vs non-employed		Occupational status of employed patients		
	Employed	Non-employed	Full-time job	Part-time job	Same job
Return-to-work within 6 months (N [%])					
Intervention group (N = 74)	66 (89%)	8 (11%)	53 (80%)	13 (20%)	65 (98%)
Controls (N = 77)	57 (74%)	20 (26%)	36 (63%)	21 (37%)	42 (73%)
p-value	0.0105		0.0275		< 0.0001
Employment status at 12 months (N [%])					
Intervention group (N = 74)	68 (92%)	6 (8%)	57 (84%)	11 (16%)	64 (94%)
Control group (N = 77)	58 (75%)	19 (25%)	41 (71%)	17 (29%)	44 (75%)
p-value	0.0053		0.0390		0.0036
Employment status at 24 months (N [%])					
Intervention group (N = 74)	65 (87%)	9 (12%)	57 (87%)	8 (12%)	64 (98%)
Control group (N = 77)	56 (72%)	21 (28%)	36 (64%)	20 (36%)	43 (76%)
p-value	0.0162		0.0022		0.0002

Source: Adapted with courtesy of Zack, O., Melamed, S., Silber, H., et al. (2022), 'The effectiveness of case-management rehabilitation intervention in facilitating return to work and maintenance of employment after myocardial infarction: results of a randomized controlled trial', *Clin Rehabil*, 36 (6), 753–66. [Table 3, p. 760].

priority aim of cardiac rehabilitation to minimize these risk factors, as far as they are modifiable, and to strengthen patients' resources to cope with the challenge of this disease. As was argued, sustained success is best achieved by intense case management targeting work-directed aspects early on, including family members, employers, and occupational professionals.

8.2.3 Job change: The case of spinal cord injury

Although AMI and stroke are severe acute clinical events their adverse long-term effects are often prevented by sudden intense care intervention and subsequently continued medical treatment. In case of spinal cord injury (SCI) this option is less realistic. SCI often results in severe physical disability. In consequence, motor control from the brain to peripheral parts of the body and flow of sensory information from the periphery to the brain are hampered. The severity of injury depends on the level of the affected spinal cord and on the degree of damage (complete or incomplete). If the cervical spinal cord is damaged, functions in all bodily parts are affected (tetraplegia). Damage in lower parts of the spinal cord results in more restricted loss of sensory function or motor control of arms, legs, or other parts (paraplegia). SCI is a disabling condition often requiring people to use a wheelchair for daily activities. Often, secondary health problems, such as decreased pulmonary function, bladder dysfunction, pain, and pressure sores, aggravate the condition. Despite its low incidence, SCI is a highly threatening event disrupting established ways of life, compelling people to undergo far-reaching adaptive changes, and requiring costly long-term treatment and rehabilitation (Bickenbach et al. 2013).

Given these conditions, there is no surprise that employment rates and return-to-work rates are substantially lower than those reported for cardiovascular diseases. A recent estimate of the amount of employment among people with SCI derived from a survey in twenty-two countries reports a mean employment rate of thirty-five per cent, where this rate is defined as the percentage of a working age population engaged in paid work (Post et al. 2020). In Europe, employment rates of people with SCI are mostly above fifty per cent (Leiulfsrud et al. 2020). Switzerland seems to be a special case, given a progressive health, social, and labour market policy for people with disabilities. In a longitudinal study from this country with one of the largest samples of people with SCI, fifty-six per cent of participants were employed at baseline, and sixty-one per cent five years later

(Schwegler et al. 2021). Although the large majority was working part-time, there was a high continuity of labour market participation in this cohort. Return to work was more likely among men and women with higher education and those working in middle-class occupations before injury. This finding was in line with the one derived from a comparative study of four European countries. The probability of returning to the same occupational category as pre-injury was about twice as high among those with middle-class (mostly white-collar) occupations compared to the probability of working-class (mostly blue-collar) occupations. However, a sizeable proportion of working-class occupations experienced occupational mobility due to vocational training, thus improving their opportunity of re-entering the labour market. Social inequalities in access to the labour market were larger among women, where those in pre-injury working-class occupations had very restricted chances of being reemployed (Leiulfsrud et al. 2020).

Due to their functional limitations and reduced health, a majority of people suffering from SCI are forced to change the job, either by being offered other, manageable job tasks, or by entering a new job where new skills acquired during vocational training are applied. Part-time work is highly prevalent under both conditions. Such changes can result in maintaining one's previous socioeconomic status, or in experiencing occupational downward mobility. For manual workers with high skill level, some options of social upward mobility are likely. Overall, job change is experienced as a challenge, requiring sustained efforts of coping with and adapting to new working and living conditions. This process is illustrated by a case history presented in Box 8.4.

The case history illuminates the depth and range of life-changing experiences as well as the resources needed to cope with chronic difficulties and threats. It also emphasizes an important role of labour market options, of skill level in search for work, and of strong support from one's social network. In a qualitative study, the psychosocial costs of these adaptive changes were described in more detail (Marti et al. 2017). For a person forced to disrupt his/her previous professional career and the related social identity, it is hard to develop a new employment identity. In the beginning, there are intense feelings of uncertainty of whether the new demands at work can be met, and of whether one's achievements are recognized by colleagues and superiors. How well has the person been prepared by vocational training for new tasks and obligations? Is there help available, for instance by a job coach, the former employer, or by colleagues? Is the new work environment supportive, providing accommodation, or is the burden

Box 8.4 Case history: Returning to work after traumatic spinal cord injury

Charlotte was 45 years old when she slipped from the ladder while helping her mother cleaning the windows. The fall ended up in a rib fracture and a traumatic injury of the spinal cord at the thoracic level T6. As the emergency team immediately recognized the severity of the accident, she was admitted to the university hospital of the next larger town. Charlotte underwent a spinal surgery the same day and was diagnosed with a complete paraplegia, indicating a complete lesion of motor and sensory functions below the lesion level of the sixth thoracic vertebra (T6). She spent the acute phase in the university hospital and was then transferred to first rehabilitation in a specialized clinic, offering a broad range of therapies to manage the consequences of her spinal cord injury. Besides physiotherapy, bladder and bowel management, occupational therapy and psychological support to adapt to the new life situation, Charlotte had the opportunity to participate in vocational rehabilitation.

Given her wheelchair dependency, returning to the previous job as a real estate broker was hardly possible. The job coach contacted her previous employer and invited him to discuss potential alternatives that would fit her special needs. However, it turned out difficult and the pre-injury employer could not offer her an adequate solution as there were no vacancies and no budget to create new jobs in the company. Charlotte was deeply disappointed but quickly understood that flexibility and openness for new possibilities would be necessary strategies to deal with the new situation. Together with her job coach, she identified a retraining program for accounting in real estate management.

After discharge from 28 weeks of first rehabilitation, Charlotte was optimistic and with the help of her network, she found a wheelchair accessible apartment and soon started the retraining [...]. After two years, she received her diploma and finally found a part-time job nearby. The new colleagues and the employer were supportive and Charlotte received an adapted workplace. The supportive environment and her ability to quickly adapt to new situations helped her keeping the job.

Source: Reproduced with permission from Finger, M. E., and Fekete, C. (2020), 'Shifting the focus from work reintegration to sustainability of employment'. In U. Bültmann and J. Siegrist (eds.), *Handbook of disability, work and health*. Cham: Springer, 633–59. [p. 635f.]; license no.: 5503040089269.

of adaption aggravated by experiences of social distance, social exclusion, and discrimination? A further difficulty mentioned in this study relates to the uncertainty of whether the new employment arrangement can be sustained in view of additional family obligations, given functional limitations, and extended time requirements (Marti et al. 2017). The case history, as well as a substantial amount of research on disability, reveal two main entry points for measures to improve a sustained employment participation of people with SCI.

- Vocational rehabilitation: Here, the availability of professionals working in an established organizational setting with close links to rehabilitation clinics and services is an essential prerequisite. However, even in high-income countries, these services are not as widely provided as needed. Although dealing with, and recovering from the injury takes several months, an early integration of vocational aspects into a comprehensive rehabilitation strategy can improve the chances of later employment (Bickenbach et al. 2013). Vocational rehabilitation as a multi-disciplinary approach includes a detailed assessment of the patients' previous work history, skill level, and occupational goals and expectations, followed by training of new skills and explorations of new job opportunities. Strengthening psychological coping resources, in particular promoting self-efficacy and self-confidence, and reducing anxiety and depression, are very relevant components of this programme. This task goes along with addressing specific ergonomic and technical issues required for new employment options. Job application skills, job search abilities, supported by job placement services and vocational counsellors, define a subsequent step. To this end, the strategy of IPS was shown to improve return to work opportunities and trajectories. This programme offers tailored individual support through different stages of the reemployment process, building on the abilities of job-seeking people. It gives advice on job searching, facilitating contacts with employers, prepares people for their entry into a new job, improves the implementation of job accommodation, and provides continued post-placement help (see below). Beneficial effects of this approach were documented, among others, in an intervention study among working-age persons with SCI, offering supportive employment to the intervention group while providing conventional vocational rehabilitation to the control group. Reemployment after twelve months was twenty-five per cent in the group supported by IPS as compared to ten per cent in the control group. After twenty-four months, the rate in the IPS group reached a level of forty-three per cent (Ottomanelli et al. 2017).

- Removing or reducing barriers to employment: Interventions need to be guided by available research evidence. There is robust knowledge on enabling and obstructive factors in return to work after SCI. These factors can be classified into non-modifiable (e.g. ethnicity, early life educational background, severity of SCI) and modifiable conditions (e.g. work content, workplace accessibility, improved functioning with assistive technology, management of secondary health problems) at the individual or organizational level. Additionally, macro-level determinants matter, for example, labour market opportunities and incentives or disincentives of disability pension and retirement policies. Using an innovative counterfactual prediction model to identify modifiable conditions that increase employment opportunities among persons with SCI, based on longitudinal data, a Swiss research team revealed a strong impact of the following four factors (Schwegler et al. 2021):

  - Improved functional independence, for example by continued physiotherapy, training, and application of assistive technologies;
  - Improved educational skills acquired during the rehabilitation phase;
  - Progress in managing pain and other secondary health conditions related to SCI;
  - Shifting from either low or full-level of disability pension to ½ or ¾ level of disability pension to enable part-time employment.

Indirect support validating main predictions comes from a large survey from Australia, analysing responses from 1,189 working-aged people with SCI. The main complaints of those who returned to work were 'problems with completing work' (where part-time employment could mitigate the problems), and 'unmet needs relating to assistive devices' (whose availability could improve functional independence) (Borg et al. 2022). These two entry points need to be extended to include other policy-related factors. Specifically, facilitating return to work among employees at older age, among women, and among those exposed to precarious work should be a priority aim.

To conclude, although relatively rare in working-age populations, SCI is a severe, life-disrupting condition requiring strong, enduring, and costly adaptive efforts. Return to work chances are reduced, and jobs often need to be changed, based on skills acquired through vocational training. Nevertheless, in high-income countries, health care, and labour and social policies offer opportunities of full social participation to many people with SCI. Moreover, seminal scientific research started to instruct interventions and to implement models of best practice. There is still large room for improvement, specifically to tackle social inequalities of life chances among people with disabilities. In contrast, in low-income countries, SCI remains a huge problem for policy efforts as traumatic injury continues to be a devastating, often terminal condition (Bickenbach et al. 2013). Guided by the principles of the United Nations convention on the rights of persons with disabilities, governments are called to address these adversities by strengthening prevention and rehabilitation.

8.2.4 Job instability

The term 'common mental disorders' was introduced as a summary label of highly prevalent affective disorders (i.e. depression and anxiety disorders), where depression deserves special attention, due to its far-reaching impact on health and quality of life. Depressive episodes have a major negative impact on work ability, productivity, and quality of life across working populations, given their frequent first manifestation in early adulthood and their risk of relapse and chronicity (Vigo et al. 2016). At least two circumstances aggravate the situation. Firstly, recognition and treatment of symptoms of this disorder are often delayed, in part caused by people's efforts to hide the symptoms due to their fear of being stigmatized as mentally ill. In part, the health-care system contributes to delay by physicians' incorrect diagnoses and by a shortage of specialized services. Secondly, up to now there is only limited knowledge on the causes of this disorder, and it is assumed that depressions are caused by a complex interaction of personal, environmental and psychosocial factors. In consequence, sustainable treatment success is restricted, despite proven efficacy of pharmacotherapy and psychotherapy. We already mentioned the bi-directional associations between work and depression. In Chapter 6, we discussed the impact of adverse psychosocial work environments on disease incidence, and Chapter 7 introduced supplementary evidence on psychobiological pathways underlying these relationships. The focus of this chapter is on the ways that the disorder affects the working person's opportunities to fully participate in the labour market.

Compared to the previous two chronic health impairments, this impact is more complex. In case of ischaemic heart disease, we saw high return-to-work rates with a large majority being employed in the previous job. People with SCI went through a critical stage of medical and vocational rehabilitation, and about half of working-age patients were able to return to work, often changing their job in relation to their functional capacity, and often confined to part-time work. Risks of job instability and unemployment were relatively low after extended preparation of return to work. The pattern of reintegration of persons with depression deviates from both trends due to specific features of this disorder and due to extrinsic barriers against reemployment.

Importantly, depression is a chronic disorder with an unpredictable, rather high probability of relapse. Based on longitudinal data, around one third of persons with a first depressive episode suffer from a recurrent event within the first year. After two years, the cumulative probability of recurrence is over forty per cent. Commonly, an episode lasts several months, even under treatment, and for every third episode full recovery is not observed before two years (Keller 1999). Therefore, the occurrence of a depressive episode results in long-term sickness absence, with a variety of options for treatment and for medical and vocational rehabilitation (see below). Severity of disease is a crucial prognostic factor for threatening risks, such as comorbid events, suicide, and exit from paid work. These disease-specific conditions complicate the development and implementation of a unified, standardized vocational rehabilitation approach. They contribute to barriers to rapid reintegration into paid work. In addition to extrinsic barriers (see below), the symptomatology of this disease often aggravates efficient return to and continuation of work.

Loss of energy, increased tiredness, and exhaustion are core symptoms that interfere with the usual level of work performance. Impaired concentration is another critical symptom as it may induce inattentiveness, mistakes during task handling, and erroneous decision making. Due to emotional pain and anxiety, depressed people shift their attention from extrinsic to intrinsic conditions, specifically to their feelings and bodily sensations. Constrained by these concerns, they more easily forget imminent tasks and obligations, or delay appointments. Indifference and lack of empathy during social exchange, increased social isolation, and avoidance of public contact are further symptoms that interfere with a variety of job tasks, mostly so in the service sector. Empirical studies aiming at quantifying the consequences of these symptoms for loss of productivity revealed rather far-reaching effects. For instance, in one analysis, loss of productivity over one month amounted to 2.3 full working days among persons with depression, compared to the productivity of workers without this disorder (Wang et al. 2004). Several other reports support this finding. In a large cross-sectional study from Australia, work productivity was substantially reduced among employees with depression and anxiety symptoms (Deady et al. 2022). With a landmark study, Adler et al. compared the scores of a validated questionnaire measuring job performance deficits in a group of employed depressive patients with the scores of a group of healthy controls, and additionally with a group of patients with a physical impairment (rheumatoid arthritis) (Adler et al. 2006). The depression group recruited from primary care centres included three diagnostic groups of major depressive disorder, dysthymia, and double depression. Importantly, these groups were followed over a period of eighteen months, and in addition to the comparison of job performances scores between the groups over time, changes of disease severity were correlated with changes in job performance. Work limitations were assessed in terms of amount of time experienced during the previous two weeks when one's job performance was reduced due to the presence of emotional or physical symptoms. Items included difficulties with time management, output achievement, and interference with mental and interpersonal tasks. Higher scores indicate more work performance deficits. Figure 8.2 demonstrates the main findings. The scores indicating performance deficits were significantly higher among the three groups of depressive patients compared to the other two groups, and these differences remained significant despite some improvement over time. A further finding, not demonstrated here, confirmed that improved depressive symptomatology was highly correlated with improved job performance (Adler et al. 2006).

Due to tangible interference with job performance, depressive patients often interrupt the job trajectory with periods of extended sickness absence. Therefore, a valid estimate of loss of productivity has to combine the results from work limitations with the indirect costs resulting from sickness absence. These losses were shown to be substantial (e.g. Greenberg et al. 2015).

These difficulties are increased by extrinsic barriers to reintegration into employment. Negative attitudes and behaviours of employers and employees at the worksite play an important role. Insecurity about employability and work capacity, combined with prejudices about mental illness, promote social distance as well as latent or overt signs

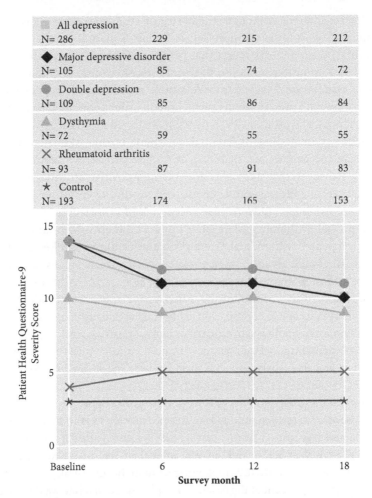

Figure 8.2 Mean scores of the scale measuring job performance deficits between depressive patients (3 groups; N = 286), patients with rheumatoid arthritis (N = 93) and healthy controls (N = 193) over eighteen months; adjusted for age, gender, and number of chronic conditions.

of discrimination. Although a majority of studies exploring discrimination at work focus on more severe forms of mental illness (schizophrenia), some reports reveal that people with depression experience avoidance and discrimination in their work environment (Frank et al. 2022). In a national survey from Australia, around fourteen per cent of employees with mild or moderate mental disorder confirmed respective experiences, and around eleven per cent observed avoidance behaviour. Lack of understanding, differential treatment, change of responsibility, and reduced contact are examples of such experiences (Reavley et al. 2017). However, this study also documented positive attitudes and behaviour from colleagues and superiors in around twenty-four per cent of cases. Among employers, insecurity, lack of knowledge, and scepticism prevail, with potential negative impact on their behaviour towards working people with mental health problems (Follmer and Jones 2017). Yet, distinct policies and campaigns seemed to raise awareness and proactive attitudes among stakeholders (Little et al. 2011). Additional barriers to return to work following a depressive episode were identified in several systematic reviews. Most often, low educational level, older age, female gender, low self-efficacy or lack of positive work expectancy, high job demands, lack of contact with medical specialists and with enterprise, and low worksite social support were mentioned (Fisker et al. 2022; Gragnano et al. 2018; Nigatu et al. 2017).

How do these barriers affect the work trajectories of people with depressive disorder? A few longitudinal studies provide answers to this question. In a large investigation from Norway, 619 patients with depression were observed one year before and one year after their treatment. At the end, a majority was returned to full employment, but in the 'high-risk group' comprising twenty per cent of the baseline sample, the return rate was less than fifty per cent. This group was characterized by low educational level, older age, and low self-efficacy (Sandin et al. 2021). One of two smaller studies reported low job stability one year after return to work in every fourth employee with depression (Ubalde-Lopez et al. 2017), whereas in the second study, forty-two per cent of depressed patients returning to work experienced a slow recovery after twelve months. Their trajectories contained a high amount of work- and health-related difficulties (Arends et al. 2019). In an investigation from the US conducted among 229 employees with depression and two comparison groups (including a healthy control group of 173 employees) followed over six months after baseline, the following results were observed (Lerner et al. 2004):

- Twelve per cent of participants with depression lost their job during this time, compared to two per cent among healthy employees.
- Twenty per cent of participants with depression experienced job turnover during this time, compared to five per cent among healthy participants; job turnover resulted mainly in lower earnings.

These and similar findings (see also Mojtabai et al. 2015) lend some support to the notion that people who are prepared to return to work following a depressive episode face an elevated risk of job instability. Whereas legal regulations in a large number of advanced societies prevent redundancy of employees with chronic disorders after rehabilitation, these groups nevertheless often experience disadvantaged job conditions when returning to work, including forced mobility and job change, reduced working time, and lower earnings.

To conclude, a high burden of psychosocial and material adversity at work among employees returning to work following depression calls for interventive efforts. In fact, impressive efforts to this end were developed in several countries, such as the Netherlands, Germany, Scandinavian countries, and the United Kingdom (see also Chapter 9). There is a consensus among professionals that these interventions should by multidimensional and include early contact with the workplace (Mikkelsen and Rosholm 2018; Nieuwenhuijsen et al. 2020). Ideally, programmes are expected to start during medical rehabilitation and to continue during early stages of the return-to-work process, including experts from medical, psychological, and occupational fields. The current evidence on best practice models is mixed, but the following conclusions deserve attention:

- Interventions focusing on cognitive psychotherapy were shown to produce a small significant beneficial effect, compared to usual care. However, in a majority of cases, they fail to integrate worksite problems into their approach (Finnes et al. 2019).
- Pre-vocational training programmes ('first train, then place') aim at stabilizing work-related competences, while neglecting the real work context. Evidence on sustainable effects is scarce so far (Chuang et al. 2015).
- The supported employment strategy ('first place, then train') helps people to readjust to the work setting by preparing the return process early on, and by offering coaching during the initial employment phase. The IPS model is the most established application with documented efficacy over a period of up to two years (Frederick and

VanderWeele 2019). Yet, according to a careful report, long-term effects after six years are no longer observed (Pichler et al. 2021).

- More specifically, IPS integrates employment services with mental health treatment, giving attention to workers' preferences. Moreover, individualized long-term support at the workplace is offered, and in case of poor job match, professional help in search for a new job is given (Bond et al. 2020).
- A comprehensive strategy termed IGLOO was proposed, addressing five levels of work domains where resources can be improved: Individual (coping strategies), Group (peer support), Leader (supervisor support), Organisation (human resource models; occupational health services), Overarching context (social and health policies) (Nielsen et al. 2018).

Given these models and their documented effects, the main problem at large is not insufficient knowledge on how to intervene, but rather insufficient investments in the application of interventions in a broader context of secondary and tertiary prevention.

8.3 Summary

Job trajectories following the manifestation of chronic disease or disability are multifaceted and diverse. Using concepts and metrics introduced in this chapter, readers are prepared to disentangle these complexities. Moreover, updated scientific knowledge is provided on three scenarios of return to work, illustrated by three different conditions of impaired health, and promising intervention approaches are depicted.

8.4 Relevant questions

- There is strong evidence that involuntary early exit from paid work is particularly high among employees in low socioeconomic positions. According to your view, which one of the following approaches is most promising to reduce this social inequality, and why?
  a) Strengthening employees' health through prevention early on;
  b) Improving quality of work and employment in companies;
  c) Modifying national legislation of disability pension and unemployment.

- Return to work was analysed with regard to three specific diseases. Musculoskeletal disorders are a further frequent diagnosis with high relevance to return to work. If you had to develop a rehabilitation programme for employees with such a disorder which ones of the elements discussed in this chapter would you propose and why?

Recommended reading

❖ Bültmann, U., and Siegrist, J. (eds.) (2020), *Handbook of disability, work and health*. Cham: Springer.

❖ Eurofound (2021), 'Working conditions and sustainable work: An analysis using the job quality framework. ', (Luxembourg: Publications Office of the European Union).

❖ Loisel, P., and Anema, J. R. (eds.) (2013), *Handbook of work disability. Prevention and management*. New York, NY: Springer.

❖ Schultz, I. Z., and Gatchel, R. J. (eds.) (2016), *Handbook of return to work. From research to practice*. New York, NY: Springer.

Useful websites

❖ Journal of Occupational Rehabilitation https://www.springer.com/journal/10926

❖ Centre for Mental Health (UK): IPS centres of Excellence https://www.centreformentalhealth.org.uk/ips-centres-excellence

❖ Disability and Rehabilitation https://www.tandfonline.com/journals/idre20

❖ U.S. Department of Labor, Vocational Rehabilitation FAQs https://www.dol.gov/agencies/owcp/dlhwc/FAQ/RehabFAQs

References

Adler, D. A., McLaughlin, T. J., Rogers, W. H., et al. (2006), 'Job performance deficits due to depression', *Am J Psychiatry*, 163 (9), 1569–76.

Amini, M., Zayeri, F., and Salehi, M. (2021), 'Trend analysis of cardiovascular disease mortality, incidence, and mortality-to-incidence ratio: results from global burden of disease study 2017', *BMC Public Health*, 21 (1), 401.

Arends, I., Almansa, J., Stansfeld, S. A., et al. (2019), 'One-year trajectories of mental health and work outcomes post return to work in patients with common mental disorders', *J Affect Disord*, 257, 263–70.

Barr, B., McHale, P., and Whitehead, M. (2020), 'Reducing inequalities in employment of people with disabilities'. In U. Bültmann and J. Siegrist (eds.), *Handbook of disability, work and health*. Cham: Springer, 309–27.

Bickenbach, J. (2020), 'A human rights perspective on work participation'. In U. Bültmann and J. Siegrist (eds.), *Handbook of disability, work and health*. Cham: Springer, 331–45.

Bickenbach, J., Officer, A., Shakespeare, T., et al. (eds.) (2013), *International perspectives on spinal cord injury*. Geneva: World Health Organization.

Bond, G. R., Drake, R. E., and Pogue, J. A. (2019), 'Expanding individual placement and support to populations with conditions and disorders other than serious mental illness', *Psychiatr Serv*, 70 (6), 488–98.

Bond, G. R., Drake, R. E., and Pogue, J. A. (2020), 'Facilitating competitive employment for people with disabilities'. In U. Bültmann and J. Siegrist (eds.), *Handbook of disability, work and health* Cham: Springer, 571–87.

Borg, S. J., Borg, D. N., Arora, M., et al. (2022), 'Factors related to engagement in employment after spinal cord injury in Australia: a cross-sectional study', *Arch Phys Med Rehabil*, 103 (12), 2345–54.

Bültmann, U., and Siegrist, J. (eds.) (2020), *Handbook of disability, work and health*. Cham: Springer.

Burdorf, A., and Robroek, S. (2020), 'Trajectories from work to early exit from paid employment'. In U. Bültmann and J. Siegrist (eds.), *Handbook of disability, work and health*. Cham: Springer, 71–83.

Butt, J. H., Rorth, R., Kragholm, K., et al. (2018), 'Return to the workforce following coronary artery bypass grafting: a Danish nationwide cohort study', *Int J Cardiol*, 251, 15–21.

Carr, E., Fleischmann, M., Goldberg, M., et al. (2018), 'Occupational and educational inequalities in exit from employment at older ages: evidence from seven prospective cohorts', *Occup Environ Med*, 75 (5), 369–77.

Cho, E., and Chen, T. Y. (2020), 'The bidirectional relationships between effort-reward imbalance and sleep problems among older workers', *Sleep Health*, 6 (3), 299–305.

Chuang, W. F., Hwang, E., Lee, H. L., et al. (2015), 'An in-house prevocational training program for newly discharged psychiatric inpatients: exploring its employment outcomes and the predictive factors', *Occup Ther Int*, 22 (2), 94–103.

Dahl, E., and van der Wel, K. A. (2020), 'Policies of reducing the burden of occupational hazards and disability pensions'. In U. Bültmann and J. Siegrist (eds.), *Handbook of disability, work and health*. Cham: Springer, 85–104.

de Cauter, J. V., Bacquer, D., Clays, E., et al. (2019), 'Return to work and associations with psychosocial well-being and health-related quality of life in coronary heart disease patients: Results from EUROASPIRE IV', *Eur J Prev Cardiol*, 26 (13), 1386–95.

de Jonge, P., Zuidersma, M., and Bültmann, U. (2014), 'The presence of a depressive episode predicts lower return to work rate after myocardial infarction', *Gen Hosp Psychiatry*, 36 (4), 363–7.

de Rijk, A. (2020), 'Coronary heart disease and return to work'. In U. Bültmann and J. Siegrist (eds.), *Handbook of disability, work and health*. Cham: Springer, 431–50.

Deady, M., Collins, D. A. J., Johnston, D. A., et al. (2022), 'The impact of depression, anxiety and comorbidity on occupational outcomes', *Occup Med (Lond)*, 72 (1), 17–24.

Dreyer, R. P., Xu, X., Zhang, W., et al. (2016), 'Return to work after acute myocardial infarction: comparison between young women and men', *Circ Cardiovasc Qual Outcomes*, 9 (2 Suppl 1), S45–52.

Duchaine, C. S., Aube, K., Gilbert-Ouimet, M., et al. (2020), 'Psychosocial stressors at work and the risk of sickness absence due to a diagnosed mental disorder: a systematic review and meta-analysis', *JAMA Psychiatry*, 77 (8), 842–51.

Eurofound (2017), 'Reactivate: employment opportunities for economically inactive people', (Luxembourg: Publications Office of the European Union).

Eurofound (2021), 'Working conditions and sustainable work: An analysis using the job quality framework', (Luxembourg: Publications Office of the European Union).

Finger, M. E., and Fekete, C. (2020), 'Shifting the focus from work reintegration to sustainability of employment'. In U. Bültmann and J. Siegrist (eds.), *Handbook of disability, work and health*. Cham: Springer, 633–59.

Finnes, A., Enebrink, P., Ghaderi, A., et al. (2019), 'Psychological treatments for return to work in individuals on sickness absence due to common mental disorders or musculoskeletal disorders: a systematic review and meta-analysis of randomized-controlled trials', *Int Arch Occup Environ Health*, 92 (3), 273–93.

Fisker, J., Hjorthoj, C., Hellstrom, L., et al. (2022), 'Predictors of return to work for people on sick leave with common mental disorders: a systematic review and meta-analysis', *Int Arch Occup Environ Health*, 95 (7), 1–13.

Follmer, K. B., and Jones, K. S. (2017), 'Stereotype content and social distancing from employees with mental illness: the moderating roles of gender and social dominance orientation', *J Appl Soc Psychol*, 47 (9), 492–504.

Frank, B. P., Theil, C. M., Brill, N., et al. (2022), 'Leave me alone with your symptoms! Social exclusion at the workplace mediates the relationship of employee's mental illness and sick leave', *Front Public Health*, 10, 892174.

Frederick, D. E., and VanderWeele, T. J. (2019), 'Supported employment: metaanalysis and review of randomized controlled trials of individual placement and support', *PLoS One*, 14 (2), e0212208.

Gragnano, A., Negrini, A., Miglioretti, M., et al. (2018), 'Common psychosocial factors predicting return to work after common mental disorders, cardiovascular diseases, and cancers: a review of reviews supporting a cross-disease approach', *J Occup Rehabil*, 28 (2), 215–31.

Greenberg, P. E., Fournier, A. A., Sisitsky, T., et al. (2015), 'The economic burden of adults with major depressive disorder in the United States (2005 and 2010)', *J Clin Psychiatry*, 76 (2), 155–62.

Halonen, J. I., Lallukka, T., Virtanen, M., et al. (2019), 'Bi-directional relation between effort-reward imbalance and risk of neck-shoulder pain: assessment of mediation through depressive symptoms using occupational longitudinal data', *Scand J Work Environ Health*, 45 (2), 126–33.

Halonen, J. I., Virtanen, M., Leineweber, C., et al. (2018), 'Associations between onset of effort-reward imbalance at work and onset of musculoskeletal pain: analyzing observational longitudinal data as pseudo-trials', *Pain*, 159 (8), 1477–83.

Head, J., Kivimaki, M., Siegrist, J., et al. (2007), 'Effort-reward imbalance and relational injustice at work predict sickness absence: the Whitehall II study', *J-Psychosom Res*, 63 (4), 433–40.

Hegewald, J., Wegewitz, U. E., Euler, U., et al. (2019), 'Interventions to support return to work for people with coronary heart disease', *Cochrane Database Syst Rev*, 3 (3), CD010748.

Hurst, L., Stafford, M., Cooper, R., et al. (2013), 'Lifetime socioeconomic inequalities in physical and cognitive aging', *Am J Public Health*, 103 (9), 1641–48.

International Labour Organization (2013), *World of work report*. Geneva: ILO.

Jelinek, M. V., Thompson, D. R., Ski, C., et al. (2015), '40 years of cardiac rehabilitation and secondary prevention in post-cardiac ischaemic patients. Are we still in the wilderness?', *Int J Cardiol*, 179, 153–9.

Kai, S. H. Y., Ferrieres, J., Rossignol, M., et al. (2022), 'Prevalence and determinants of return to work after various coronary events: meta-analysis of prospective studies', *Sci Rep*, 12 (1), 15348.

Keller, M. B. (1999), 'The long-term treatment of depression', *J Clin Psychiatry*, 60 (Suppl. 17), 41–5.

Knardahl, S., Johannessen, H. A., Sterud, T., et al. (2017), 'The contribution from psychological, social, and organizational work factors to risk of disability retirement: a systematic review with meta-analyses', *BMC Public Health*, 17 (1), 176.

Leiulfsrud, A. S., Solheim, E. F., Reinhardt, J. D., et al. (2020), 'Gender, class, employment status and social mobility following spinal cord injury in Denmark, the Netherlands, Norway and Switzerland', *Spinal Cord*, 58 (2), 224–31.

Lerner, D., Adler, D. A., Chang, H., et al. (2004), 'Unemployment, job retention, and productivity loss among employees with depression', *Psychiatr Serv*, 55 (12), 1371–8.

Lesener, T., Gusy, B., and Wolter, C. (2019), 'The job demands-resources model: a meta-analytic review of longitudinal studies', *Work Stress*, 33 (1), 76–103.

Little, K., Henderson, C., Brohan, E., et al. (2011), 'Employers' attitudes to people with mental health problems in the workplace in Britain: changes between 2006 and 2009', *Epidemiol Psychiatr Sci*, 20 (1), 73–81.

Loisel, P., and Anema, J. R. (eds.) (2013), *Handbook of work disability: prevention and management*. New York, NY: Springer.

Mackenbach, J. P. (2019), *Health inequalities*. Oxford: Oxford University Press.

Makaroun, L. K., Brown, R. T., Diaz-Ramirez, L. G., et al. (2017), 'Wealth-associated disparities in death and disability in the United States and England', *JAMA Intern Med*, 177 (12), 1745–53.

Marmot, M. G. (2004), *Status syndrome: how social standing affects our health and longevity*. London: Bloomsbury.

Marti, A., Escorpizo, R., Schwegler, U., et al. (2017), 'Employment pathways of individuals with spinal cord injury living in Switzerland: a qualitative study', *Work*, 58 (2), 99–110.

Mikkelsen, M. B., and Rosholm, M. (2018), 'Systematic review and meta-analysis of interventions aimed at enhancing return to work for sick-listed workers with common mental disorders, stress-related disorders, somatoform disorders and personality disorders', *Occup Environ Med*, 75 (9), 675–86.

Mojtabai, R., Stuart, E. A., Hwang, I., et al. (2015), 'Long-term effects of mental disorders on employment in the National Comorbidity Survey ten-year follow-up', *Soc Psychiatry Psychiatr Epidemiol*, 50 (11), 1657–68.

Nielsen, K., Yarker, J., Munir, F., et al. (2018), 'IGLOO: an integrated framework for sustainable return to work in workers with common mental disorders', *Work Stress*, 32 (4), 400–17.

Nieuwenhuijsen, K., Verbeek, J. H., Neumeyer-Gromen, A., et al. (2020), 'Interventions to improve return to work in depressed people', *Cochrane Database Syst Rev*, 10 (10), CD006237.

Nigatu, Y. T., Liu, Y., Uppal, M., et al. (2017), 'Prognostic factors for return to work of employees with common mental disorders: a meta-analysis of cohort studies', *Soc Psychiatry Psychiatr Epidemiol*, 52 (10), 1205–15.

North, F. M., Syme, S. L., Feeney, A., et al. (1996), 'Psychosocial work environment and sickness absence among British civil servants: the Whitehall II study', *Am J Public Health*, 86 (3), 332–40.

OECD (2010), *Sickness, disability and work: breaking the barriers. A synthesis of findings across OECD countries*. Paris: OECD.

Olsen, S. J., Schirmer, H., Wilsgaard, T., et al. (2020), 'Employment status three years after percutaneous coronary intervention and predictors for being employed: a nationwide prospective cohort study', *Eur J Cardiovasc Nurs*, 19 (5), 433–39.

Ottomanelli, L., Goetz, L. L., Barnett, S. D., et al. (2017), 'Individual placement and support in spinal cord injury: a longitudinal observational study of employment outcomes', *Arch Phys Med Rehabil*, 98 (8), 1567–75 e1.

Pichler, E. M., Stulz, N., Wyder, L., et al. (2021), 'Long-term effects of the individual placement and support intervention on employment status: 6-year follow-up of a randomized controlled trial', *Front Psychiatry*, 12, 709732.

Post, M. W., Reinhardt, J. D., Avellanet, M., et al. (2020), 'Employment among people with spinal cord injury in 22 countries across the world: results from the International Spinal Cord Injury Community Survey', *Arch Phys Med Rehabil*, 101 (12), 2157–66.

Pyöriä, P., Ojala, S., and Nätti, J. (2021), 'Precarious work increases depression-based disability among male employees', *Eur J Public Health*, 31 (6), 1223–30.

Reavley, N. J., Jorm, A. F., and Morgan, A. J. (2017), 'Discrimination and positive treatment toward people with mental health problems in workplace and education settings: findings from an Australian National Survey', *Stigma Health*, 2 (4), 254.

Reibis, R., Salzwedel, A., Abreu, A., et al. (2019), 'The importance of return to work: how to achieve optimal reintegration in ACS patients', *Eur J Prev Cardiol*, 26 (13), 1358–69.

Robroek, S. J., Rongen, A., Arts, C. H., et al. (2015), 'Educational inequalities in exit from paid employment among Dutch workers: the influence of health, lifestyle and work', *PLoS One*, 10 (8), e0134867.

Rohrbacher, M., and Hasselhorn, H. M. (2022), 'Social inequalities in early exit from employment in Germany: a causal mediation analysis on the role of work, health, and work ability', *Scand J Work Environ Health*, 48 (7), 569–78.

Sandin, K., Anyan, F., Osnes, K., et al. (2021), 'Sick leave and return to work for patients with anxiety and depression: a longitudinal study of trajectories before, during and after work-focused treatment', *BMJ Open*, 11 (9), e046336.

Schram, J. L. D., Schuring, M., Oude Hengel, K. M., et al. (2022), 'The influence of chronic diseases and poor working conditions in working life expectancy across educational levels among older employees in the Netherlands', *Scand J Work Environ Health*, 48 (5), 391–98.

Schultz, I. Z., and Gatchel, R. J. (eds.) (2016), *Handbook of return to work. From research to practice*. New York, NY: Springer.

Schwegler, U., Fekete, C., Finger, M., et al. (2021), 'Labor market participation of individuals with spinal cord injury living in Switzerland: determinants of between-person differences and counterfactual evaluation of their instrumental value for policy', *Spinal Cord*, 59 (4), 429–40.

Soderberg, M., Rosengren, A., Gustavsson, S., et al. (2015), 'Psychosocial job conditions, fear avoidance beliefs and expected return to work following acute coronary syndrome: a cross-sectional study of fear-avoidance as a potential mediator', *BMC Public Health*, 15, 1263.

Tang, K. (2014), 'A reciprocal interplay between psychosocial job stressors and worker well-being? A systematic review of the "reversed" effect', *Scand J Work Environ Health*, 40 (5), 441–56.

Theorell, T. (2020), 'Occupational determinants of cardiovascular disorders including stroke'. In U. Bültmann and J. Siegrist (eds.), *Handbook of disability, work and health*. Cham: Springer, 189–206.

Ubalde-Lopez, M., Arends, I., Almansa, J., et al. (2017), 'Beyond return to work: the effect of multimorbidity on work functioning trajectories after sick leave due to common mental disorders', *J Occup Rehabil*, 27 (2), 210–17.

UN General Assembly (2007), 'Convention on the Rights of Persons with Disabilities: resolution / adopted by the General Assembly, 24 January 2007, A/RES/61/106', https://www.refworld.org/docid/45f973632.html, accessed 20 March 2023.

United Nations (1948), 'Universal declaration of human rights. 217 (III) A', https://www.un.org/en/about-us/universal-declaration-of-human-rights, accessed 20 March 2023.

van Rijn, R. M., Robroek, S. J., Brouwer, S., et al. (2014), 'Influence of poor health on exit from paid employment: a systematic review', *Occup Environ Med*, 71 (4), 295–301.

Vigo, D., Thornicroft, G., and Atun, R. (2016), 'Estimating the true global burden of mental illness', *Lancet Psychiatry*, 3 (2), 171–8.

Wahrendorf, M., Reinhardt, J. D., and Siegrist, J. (2013), 'Relationships of disability with age among adults aged 50 to 85: evidence from the United States, England and continental Europe', *PLoS One*, 8 (8), e71893.

Wahrendorf, M., Hoven, H., Goldberg, M., et al. (2019), 'Adverse employment histories and health functioning: the CONSTANCES study', *Int J Epidemiol*, 48 (2), 402–14.

Wang, P. S., Beck, A. L., Berglund, P., et al. (2004), 'Effects of major depression on moment-in-time work performance', *Am J Psychiatry*, 161 (10), 1885–91.

World Health Organization (2001), *International Classification of Functioning, Disability and Health (ICF)*. Geneva: WHO.

World Health Organization (2011), 'World report on disability', (Geneva: WHO).

Zack, O., Melamed, S., Silber, H., et al. (2022), 'The effectiveness of case-management rehabilitation intervention in facilitating return to work and maintenance of employment after myocardial infarction: results of a randomized controlled trial', *Clin Rehabil*, 36 (6), 753–66.

9
Organizational contexts and social change in rehabilitation

9.1 Legal and structural conditions

The decisions on providing disability pensions and the processes of return to work discussed in Chapter 8 are embedded in a set of legal regulations and structures of medical and vocational rehabilitation services that vary widely across countries. Importantly, these regulations and structures are largely determined by labour and social policies as well as by health-care policies at national level. In many cases, regulations and organizational settings also vary at regional levels within countries. Focusing on legislation offers a useful approach towards analysing national variations in these policies. Three kinds of legislation are of particular interest in this chapter: (1) laws regulating access to regular pensions during retirement, (2) laws setting criteria for granting health-related disability pensions, thus enabling early exit from paid work, and (3) laws with impact on the return-to-work process.

To illustrate the close links between these three regulatory systems, a simple example may be useful. Think of a low-skilled white-collar male employee in a medium-size enterprise who suffered from a stroke at the age of fifty-eight. Thanks to rapid medical intervention, the disablement of this man was limited, enabling him to move, to speak, and to act without cognitive impairment, but with substantial retardation in all activities. What would be an appropriate decision for his future? First of all, he did not fear losing his job as the enterprise was located in a European country with a binding law prohibiting the dismissal of employees immediately after onset of a major disease or disability. As a first option, he could retire as the retirement policy in his country allowed retirement after forty years of employed activity. However, premature retirement would considerably reduce the level of pension. The second option consisted in applying for a disability pension. This option was contingent on a medical certificate. Moreover, depending on the specific regulations, financial compensation

Psychosocial Occupational Health. Johannes Siegrist and Jian Li, Oxford University Press.
© Oxford University Press 2024. DOI: 10.1093/oso/9780192887924.003.0009

would probably result in a tangible income loss. Return to work was the third option, specifically so as the employee's work motivation was high and as he was given the opportunity of reducing his working time. The example sheds light on the intertwined legal regulations and the complexity of related decision-making.

As mentioned, variations of these legal regulations across countries are substantial. The next section underlines these variations with some examples, and it documents the far-reaching influence of policies on practices and outcomes of return to, or exit from, work at all three levels, those concerning regular pensions, those dealing with disability pensions, and those directed towards return to work.

9.1.1 National policies

Pension systems are a crucial pillar of a nation's welfare policy, providing income in old age. Payments largely depend on the duration of employment of recipients, and more specifically on contributions during their occupational career. In addition, basic income in old age is provided to those who were not economically active during major parts of their adult life. Pension systems vary widely across countries, embedded in different socio-political, economic, and cultural backgrounds. Level of generosity, conditions and modalities of financing, and criteria of access to regular pension payments are the main sources of variation (OECD 2010). Describing them is far beyond the aims of this book, requiring a detailed exploration of national specifications. Readers interested in a comparative review of pension systems in Europe and beyond are referred to excellent documentation prepared by the Max Planck Institute for Social Law and Social Policy (Schneider et al. 2021). Here, we only illustrate some of these variations with brief examples. For instance, while the standard age of pension access is sixty-five years in many countries, it varies from age sixty (e.g. Poland) to age sixty-seven (e.g. USA, Sweden). The mean level of pension, compared to previous earning, may sum up to fifty-two per cent (e.g. Germany), or it may be as high as eighty-nine per cent (Austria). Large differences are observed in the ways of how old age security is financed. As an example from northern Europe, Norway has introduced a tax-based basic old age pension for all citizens, where the formerly employed people are granted an income-based pension. In addition, employers and employees are obliged to contribute to an occupational pension system. In southern European countries, such as

Greece, a mix of statutory pension and benefits based on private insurance is more common. The old age security system in France is of special interest as its regulations privilege distinct occupational groups. In this system, the statutory old age pension is supplemented by private insurance plans that are partly shared by employees and employers. Additional benefits are provided for raising children and caring for sick persons. Compared with other North and West European systems the French regime seems rather privileged.

Similar country differences are given with regard to disability pensions, where two distinct types of policies are observed. One type, labelled passive spending, favours the provision of supply in terms of income compensation. This measure prevents, or at least reduces, poverty among people with disability. The other type, labelled active spending, focuses on ways of supporting people with health impairment by integrating them into the labour market, thus prioritizing investments in rehabilitation over accordance of pension. In recent decades, a shift from passive to active labour market policies has been documented, most obviously in Scandinavian countries and in countries with a liberal welfare system (Dahl and van der Wel 2020). Other countries, including some southern European nations, continue to focus on supply-oriented approaches. Nevertheless, given a high proportion of claimants in times of restricted public spending, all welfare systems are faced with the problem of reducing generosity in distributing disability pensions by sharpening criteria of admission, by introducing part-time pensions, and by limiting level and duration of benefits received. Overall, in high-income countries, and specifically in Europe, employment-oriented active policies prevail, supported by regulations that provide an appropriate level of social protection.

It is important to mention that labour market policies for people with disability cover three different dimensions: social protection, labour market integration, and civil rights (Diderichsen 2020). These policies are composed of a variety of elements including, but not restricted to, legislation. For instance, ensuring civil rights to a large extent depends on anti-discrimination laws, whereas in the case of strengthening labour market integration a mix of legal measures and non-governmental programmes initiated by professional groups, employer organizations, trade unions, and others contribute to its advancement. In an instructive review of active labour market interventions to support employment of sick and disabled people, Barr et al. (2020) identified four different types of measures directed at the work environment:

- Tackling discrimination;
- Improving workplace accessibility;
- Offering financial incentives to employers;
- Enhancing return to work.

The first measure prohibits employers from excluding disabled and chronically ill persons from labour market participation, according to national legislative acts. The second measure is realized by legal or financial regulations that reduce barriers to accessibility to work for these groups. Thirdly, job creation incentives are expected to increase employment opportunities for people with disability or chronic disease. Finally, return-to-work procedures are strengthened by measures of integrating services and agencies involved in this process. These interventions directed at a supportive work environment are complemented by a set of measures focusing on the disabled people themselves in order to increase their employability through skill development. More specifically, these measures are:

- Providing individual case management;
- Promoting training and education;
- Managing health conditions;
- Easing transition from benefits to work.

The first type of initiative is most important as it offers individual counselling, advice, and support during a critical stage of transition from passiveness to work. Several approaches are available to this end, following two different strategies, either 'first train, then place' or 'first place, then train' (see Chapter 8). Both strategies rely on programmes that promote training and skill development. Managing health conditions is a core activity of medical rehabilitation services before return to work, and of occupational health agencies after inclusion into paid work. Again, coordination of services and continuity of care are essential obligations. The fourth type of measure includes disincentives to rely on disability benefits and financial incentives to return to work.

This typology reflects the extension of initiatives of active labour market policies beyond the entitlement of laws. National differences in comprehensiveness and rigour of these types of measures are significant. In a cross-country perspective, it is probably accurate to conclude that Scandinavian countries, the United Kingdom, and some Western European countries like Germany and the Netherlands, developed the broadest spectrum of active labour market initiatives addressing disability and covering the three dimensions mentioned (Diderichsen 2020). Denmark with its 'flexicurity' approach is considered an exception to this pattern as the core measure of social protection, job security, has a low priority, whereas labour market integration and civil rights are highly prioritized. This system enables dismissals and lay-offs of employees, but it compensates elevated risks of unemployment by a generous unemployment insurance. At the same time, by rendering employment more flexible and by supporting return to work, reintegration rates are rather high (Dahl and van der Wel 2020; Diderichsen 2020). It is still a matter of debate, and further scientific inquiry is needed to identify the most successful mix of integrative labour market programmes in attempts to reduce the disability-employment gap.

Legislation directed at the return-to-work-process has been less extensively developed so far, if compared to the regulation of disability pensions and of general retirement policies. However, Canada, Scandinavian countries, and Germany are places with corresponding legal innovations. In Canada, at the level of provinces, coordinated programmes between workers compensation boards, employers, and occupational health-care services promote return to work in systematic ways. With its 'rehabilitation chain' legislation, Sweden obliges employers to take an active role in rehabilitation by developing return-to-work plans with employees, and by implementing the plan in coordination with stakeholders of social insurance and health-care organizations (Barr et al. 2020). In Germany, a law enacted in 2004 requires distinct engagements from all enterprises towards reintegrating sick and disabled employees into work. The process is initiated by the employer's interview with the employee exploring options and preferences for future work. As a result, a detailed plan of practical measures is set up. Measures include the continuation of medical and vocational rehabilitation, the recruitment of job coaching services, and the design of a graded return-to-work-process. In this latter case, reduced income is supplemented by sick-leave benefits, and employers receive some compensation for productivity loss.

Taken together, legislation proves to be an indispensable determinant of successful measures of reintegration of workers with chronic disease or disability into paid work. Gains are particularly prominent in the case of active labour market policies. Despite these merits, several future challenges deserve continued attention. One such challenge concerns measures to counteract disincentives to work inherent in some disability and retirement policies. While tangible reductions in generosity of welfare benefits have occurred in recent years, it is still difficult to tailor support according to need, based on justified eligibility criteria. For instance, in countries like Switzerland, Canada, and the United Kingdom, it was observed that in a number of cases, the level of disability benefit was very close to the level of earnings achieved through employment, thus deterring people from returning to work. The introduction of part-time work supplemented by sickness pay can offer a way to meet this challenge. Another disincentive is given by generous legislation related to early retirement. For instance, in France and in Austria, thresholds of exit from paid work in case of disability are very low. Under these conditions, integrating sick and disabled workers aged in their fifties seems rather unlikely (Barr et al. 2020).

Reducing social inequalities in return to work by appropriate legal regulations is a further, more serious challenge. Despite the universal orientation of several legal declarations, susceptibility to discrimination at work continues to be pronounced among disadvantaged groups in the labour market. Legal attempts towards reducing the employment gap in case of disability are less successful among people with low socioeconomic status. Similarly, poverty risks remain substantially higher in these groups. While legal regulations, in general, were developed with the intention of supporting all population groups in need, their implementation was sometimes restricted to more educated populations or those working in more privileged employment conditions. For instance, flexicurity measures in Denmark were less accessible to low-skilled workers (Diderichsen 2020), or access-to-work programmes were less often available to socially deprived groups (Barr et al. 2020). In a register-based study on some 219,000 insured persons in Germany, social inequalities in three outcomes of medical rehabilitation were documented: (1) the patient's work ability, as assessed by physicians at the end of medical rehabilitation; (2) the probability of return to work in subsequent years; and (3) early exit from work due to receipt of a disability pension during follow-up (seven years) (Götz et al. 2020). Relative risks of these outcomes according to three indicators of socioeconomic position (education, occupational class, income) were analysed with multiple adjustments. For all three outcomes and all three socio-economic indicators, significantly elevated risks were observed among more disadvantaged groups. Figure 9.1 displays the predicted frequencies of the three outcomes, based on predicted proportions for the three socioeconomic indicators, adjusted for age: gender, medical diagnosis, repeated rehabilitation and sickness absence before rehabilitation (Götz et al. 2020). These findings are challenging as Germany has

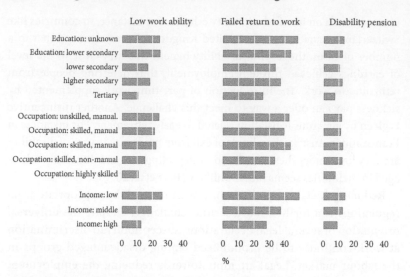

Figure 9.1 Predicted frequencies of three rehabilitation outcomes (predicted proportions adjusted for age, sex, diagnosis, repeated rehabilitation, sickness absence).

Source: Reproduced with permission from Götz, S., Wahrendorf, M., Siegrist, J., et al. (2020), 'Social inequalities in medical rehabilitation outcomes—a registry-based study on 219,584 insured persons in Germany', *Eur J Public Health*, 30 (3), 498–503. [Figure 1, p. 501]; license no.: 5503040691215.

developed a comprehensive medical rehabilitation system accessible to all socio-economic population groups, a system supported by elaborated legal regulations and by substantial public spending.

Legal regulations as crucial elements of national labour and social policies define one dimension of macro-level determinants of return-to-work processes. Health-care policies structuring the organizational settings of medical and vocational rehabilitation and their transfer into occupational life define a further dimension of determinants of these processes. Again, as illustrated in the next section, these policies and the related organizational settings vary widely across countries.

9.1.2 Organizational settings

Ideally, health-care systems are organized along three different principles of providing health care:

- State-dependent, centralized, taxation-funded provision of health care, with an important role of general practitioners as gatekeepers in primary health care ('Beveridge' model);
- Social insurance-based provision of health care contingent on mandatory payments of employees and employers, with strong impact of medical professions and sickness funds ('Bismarckian' model);
- Market-based provision of health care by private insurers who reimburse (at least partially) patients' payments, committed to cost containment (e.g. Health Maintenance Organization).

Although the United Kingdom represents the Beveridge model, Germany the Bismarckian model, and the US the free market model, each country has incorporated distinct elements from these models, thus representing a variety of organizational structures. In essence, these variations concern the interaction between five principal actors: consumers, first-line providers (office-based general practitioners or specialized physicians), second-line providers (hospitals), governments, and insurers (Stevens 2001). Despite these variations, there is a growing tendency towards convergence, due to economic constraints in face of rising health-care expenses.

Health care provided by services of medical rehabilitation is organized in different forms across countries. Even within Europe, rehabilitation services are provided at least in three organizational settings, as evident from a comparative review (Mittag and Welti 2017). Outpatient care is the most common setting, either organized in community centres or in collaboration with physicians located in residential areas. The close link to everyday life, including workplaces, is considered a clear advantage of this approach. It is well established in Finland and in the United Kingdom, where nurses have an important role. In other countries, including Switzerland and the Netherlands, referrals are mainly initiated by acute clinics after dismissal or by occupational physicians who monitor employees on long-term sick leave. For severe diseases (e.g. neurological injuries, strokes) these countries provide specialized clinics. Acute hospitals with affiliated departments of rehabilitation represent a second form that is prevalent in France. Close links with acute treatment represent an advantage, but at the same time the gap to everyday life and work settings of patients is huge. Germany is the country that represents most convincingly a third organizational form, specialized rehabilitation clinics that provide a comprehensive three-week programme on site for targeted patient groups (mainly cardiovascular, orthopaedic, cancer, or mental health diseases). Based on contracts between social security (pension) funds and private or public providers, patients are referred to these clinics after dismissal from hospitals although they are free to initiate the application. While these clinics are located rather far away from patients' residence, they confront patients with an intense intervention performed by an interdisciplinary team of professionals.

Across countries, one often observes a mix between elements of these three types. For instance, in countries like Austria, Switzerland, and Germany, rehabilitation clinics and outpatient programmes act as alternatives in a competitive market. It is important to mention that rehabilitation services are provided independent of the specific funding mechanism (state-dependent, social insurance-driven, or market-driven system). Moreover, so far there is no convincing evidence of superiority of outcome efficiency between these different settings. However, the integration of medical and vocational rehabilitation varies widely. Advantages of a close collaboration and problems of a more distant collaboration are briefly illustrated with the three diseases that were discussed with regard to return to work.

How relevant an optimal coordination of medical and vocational rehabilitation is can be studied in case of spinal cord injury. In countries like Switzerland, Germany, and Australia, specialized rehabilitation clinics address vocational aspects in an early stage of treatment. Once the patient has coped with the shock of a profound life-changing event, prospects of future life are carefully explored with the help of professional experts, where work and employment play a significant role. To this end, the patient's expectations, interests, and abilities are discussed, and rehabilitation needs are specified. Validated assessment tools that cover relevant biopsychosocial aspects are used to document (and later evaluate) the rehabilitation process (Escorpizio et al. 2015). As a next step, an intervention programme is developed and implemented, guided by an expert in vocational rehabilitation who collaborates closely with the clinical team on site, being involved in case conferences and discharge planning. Tasks include training in job-seeking skills, counselling activities, workplace visits, contacts with employers, and preparation for continued job coaching during the return to work. The evaluation of early access to vocational rehabilitation programme conducted in Australia revealed that more than half of participants with spinal cord injury were in paid employment or in vocational training several months after discharge (Middleton et al. 2015).

Coordination of medical and vocational rehabilitation proved to be more difficult in the case of cardiovascular disease treated in rehabilitation clinics, as for those widely established in Germany. These intense, comprehensive three-week interventions are unique in that an interdisciplinary team collaborates with patients on site, applying validated programmes and transmitting the competences of different disciplines. The majority of patients are recovering from acute myocardial infarction. The teams working with these patients regularly include physiotherapists, psychologists, social workers, and experts in sports, nutrition, and health education. Yet, teams are working under the dominance of cardiologists who still mainly adhere to a biomedical model of disease. In addition, the treatment occurs at distance from the everyday life of patients, and the transfer of newly acquired health behaviour to the future living and working environment remains an unmet challenge. It is no surprise to learn that sustainable long-term effects of this type of in-patient cardiac rehabilitation are quite modest (Mittag et al. 2011). Although courses on successful coping with stress are regularly included in these programmes, their individual-centred design does not address the extrinsic constraints of future work environments. More recently, the need to prioritize work reintegration was recognized by professional bodies in cardiac rehabilitation (De Sutter et al. 2020; Kai et al. 2022).

This tension between medical and vocational rehabilitation is probably most worrying in the case of common mental disorders, and in particular depression. Several reasons account for this. Unlike somatic disorders where reduced physical functioning and fitness have direct impact on work ability, thus requiring some coordinated action from medical and vocational rehabilitation, reduced mental health does not seem to necessitate vocational training. Moreover, the treatment of depression during medical rehabilitation includes psychotherapy, but main psychotherapeutic approaches, similar to those applied in cardiac rehabilitation, focus on individual coping and problem solving, with little relationship to future work. While these interventions promote the patient's recovery process, their impact on return was shown to be modest (Martin et al. 2009). However, more recent approaches including contact with management and workplaces and offering multicomponent interventions resulted in positive and sustainable effects on workers' health (Mikkelsen and Rosholm 2018; Nazarov et al. 2019; Nieuwenhuijsen et al. 2020).

Fear of being stigmatized and hesitation to disclose one's diagnosis are conditions that contribute to a delay of coping with return to work during rehabilitation. What can be done at the level of companies and enterprises to promote work integration following a depressive episode? Several companies developed their own strategy of support. An approach initiated in some businesses in Germany in collaboration with university-based professionals in psychosomatics and psychiatry illustrates this activity (Rothermund et al. 2016; see Box 9.1). Implementing a psychosomatic or psychotherapeutic consultation in collaboration with a company's occupational health service has several advantages. For sick employees it is easier to disclose their disease in a medically protected environment. For employees suffering from mental strain without accessing the health-care system, it provides an opportunity of early detection and treatment. For occupational physicians, it enriches their professional impact and range of activities. For

---

Box 9.1 Company-supported mental health care

- The company agrees on a treatment contract with the sickness fund that includes the majority of employees as insured members. The company's occupational health service acts as a coordinating centre. As a third partner, an out-patient psychiatric consultation team or a specialized centre of psychotherapy offers treatment for patients referred by the coordination centre.
- Given the professional discretion of occupational physicians, employees are confident to attend the consultation offered by the coordination centre. Fees for the first two consultation sessions are paid by the company. Subsequent treatment sessions following referral are paid by the sickness fund.
- Consultation is not restricted to patients who return to work, but it is open to all employees suffering from mental strain, thus combining primary and secondary prevention. In most cases, treatments are provided as a series of sessions of brief psychotherapy, but they include stay in a clinic in more severe cases. Occupational physicians are gatekeepers and contribute to the reintegration by their involvement in work accommodation.
- As the programme is open to all insured employees, support is also provided to low educated or migrant groups who otherwise encounter difficulties in accessing psychiatric health care (for details, see Rothermund et al. 2016).

Source: Data from Rothermund, E., Gundel, H., Rottler, E., et al. (2016), 'Effectiveness of psychotherapeutic consultation in the workplace: a controlled observational trial', *BMC Public Health,* 16 (1), 891.

companies, it is cost-saving as sickness absence was shown to be reduced as a result of psychotherapeutic intervention (Kant et al. 2008). Moreover, employers are given a pro-active role in joint efforts of improving workers' mental health (Jansen et al. 2021).

In view of the high prevalence of mental disorders, the contribution of these company-based approaches to pertinent problem-solving is still modest. Preventive programmes at large scale are required to improve the adaptation of employees with mental health problems to the demands of their work and to increase early recognition and treatment of these disorders. As regulatory frameworks, responsible stakeholders, models of good practice, and assessment tools are available in the field of occupational health in a variety of countries, the main problem is no longer a lack of knowledge, but a lack of implementation. This is even more worrying as several evaluations documented the cost-effectiveness of such programmes (Vlasveld et al. 2012; Wang et al. 2007).

In conclusion, different organizational settings are available for integration of medical and vocational rehabilitation of persons with chronic disease or disability. These settings seem to work independently of the specific principle of health-care system functioning (state-dependent, social-security-driven, or market-driven), and they are generally supported by legal policies endorsed at national level. Overall, there are obvious gaps in integrating medical and vocational tasks in professional attempts towards increasing return-to-work rates. Several entry points to a reduction of these gaps are obvious. One such entry point concerns the approximation of rehabilitation services to the lived environments of employees, that is, to their workplaces, strengthening the role of occupational health services, and mobilizing the engagement of the company's stakeholders. Furthering interdisciplinary collaboration within organizational settings is a second entry point. Importantly, professionalization and specialization of paramedical disciplines is a promising development towards this aim as transdisciplinary exchange enriches the collaboration and increases the quality of service. Moreover, gendered team composition weakens the traditional male dominance in medicine, giving more weight to openness, tolerance, and empathy as essential prerequisites of sustainable collaboration. The fact that more women have entered medicine in recent times, combined with the observation that women working as nurses transformed their status from a subordinated caring position into a role as collaborative professional expert, supports this process (Davies 1996; Gutenbrunner et al. 2022). Patients with a chronic disease or disability can contribute quite strongly to efficient cooperation of medical and vocational rehabilitation and its successful outcome. Rather than being passive, subordinate subjects of medical decisions, they can actively use their autonomy, motivation, and competences, thus providing a third entry point for change. Given the significance of a major societal change, often interpreted in terms of increased empowerment, this third step is discussed in some more depth in the next section.

9.2 Empowering people with chronic disease or disability

9.2.1 Conceptual clarification

Women and men with a chronic disease or disability have to cope with this experience for a long time, and often over their lifetime. With this flow of experience, they accumulate particular knowledge, and they develop skills and ways of adapting to, and managing the restrictions imposed by their health condition. Moreover, they are prepared to improve their health and well-being by mobilizing available resources. This source of coping with disease and disability has been largely ignored by the profession of medicine in an era of rapid scientific and technological progress of modern medicine, where physicians exerted extensive control over diagnostic procedures and treatment decisions on chronic diseases, most explicitly in clinical settings of acute care. Numerous scientific investigations on patient-physician relationships in clinical settings documented the structural inequalities in communication, information, and decision-making, as well as their adverse consequences for patients' well-being and health outcomes related to this 'paternalistic' regime of providing health care (Cockerham 1998; Freidson 1970). During the second half of the twentieth century, a new social movement emerged, initiated by particular minority groups in Western societies who suffered from restricted civil rights, thus rising their voice, and asking for more influence, autonomy, and power. People with a disability were one such disadvantaged minority group claiming their right to full social participation. This group was particularly influential in extending opportunities for social participation and in removing barriers and negative attitudes towards people with disability. At the international level, the endorsement of the Convention on the Rights of Persons with Disabilities by the United Nations is the most visible and sustainable proof of success of collective empowerment achieved by a socially disadvantaged group (United Nations

2006). Within this process of social change by extending rights and actions of formerly deprived population groups, self-help movements of citizens played an important role, strengthening solidarity and mutual help, and striving for public impact. Early on, distinct groups of patients with chronic disease (e.g. type 2 diabetes, rheumatic diseases, mental disorders) joined these movements in order to demonstrate and mitigate their concerns. Strengthening their marginal role within the health-care system, and specifically extending their influence against the dominance of medical experts were important aims. The introduction of legislative regulations strengthening patient rights supported these movements, and in recent times, patients as consumers and evaluators of health-care services were given extended opportunities of exerting some control (White 2000). Beyond the level of national regulations and policies, the World Health Organization promoted this social movement of empowering people with chronic disease and disability through its Ottawa Charta for Health Promotion. Although this document stressed primary prevention and health promotion in different societal settings, strengthening competences, knowledge, and autonomous actions of people with disease and disability was a relevant component within this programme (World Health Organization 1986).

Before continuing our argument, it is important to clarify the meaning of the notion of empowerment as applied to people with chronic disease and disability. In a masterly review analysing the use of the concept of patient empowerment in research literature, a Belgian and Dutch team of social and behavioural scientists proposed several crucial distinctions (Castro et al. 2016). Firstly, they argue that applying this concept is particularly useful at the micro-level of analysis, dealing with relationships between patients and health-care professionals. To be enacted, empowerment of patients requires a certain opportunity structure, specifically a health-care system that offers patients some possibilities of participation, and it requires that patients are equipped with basic competences and knowledge about their own disease. Secondly, when discussing the core notion of patient empowerment, these authors propose to focus on personal agency, that is, a motivation to be in control of tangible aspects of one's own condition (the disease), and of strengthening self-motivation in order to improve one's condition. Thirdly, concerning the consequences of empowerment, the authors suggest that shared decision-making between professionals and patients as a means of improving coping with the disease is considered the most important outcome (Castro et al. 2016). Conceptualizing patient empowerment as activity of an agentic self, aiming at improving self-regulation and control, and considering shared decision-making in a patient-centred health-care system the crucial outcome has the advantage of being based on a solid theoretical ground, the self-determination theory (Ryan and Deci 2018). This theory claims that human motivation is determined by extrinsic and intrinsic incentives, and that the need for positive self-regulation, including personal growth, provides a strong intrinsic motivation. This need is satisfied if opportunities for experiencing autonomy, competence, and interpersonal relatedness are given. Translated to the field of patient empowerment this theory posits that patients who share a common goal, supporting each other (relatedness), who are well informed about their disease (competence), and who are given the opportunity to act and to be involved in shared decision-making (autonomy) develop a strong intrinsic motivation to strengthen their self-efficacy and self-management, thus fostering personal growth and well-being (see also Coulter and Fitzpatrick 2000).

Viewed from this theoretical perspective, patient empowerment acts as a personal resource of successful coping with the challenges of a chronic disease or disability. Activating this resource in patient-centred clinical work may have unexpected positive effects on collaboration and adherence, on health-promoting behaviour, on patients' well-being and quality of life, and on reintegration into paid work. In addition, from a stress-theoretical point of view, strong positive emotions emanating from experienced empowerment may protect the individual from a deterioration in the course of disease. It is therefore of interest to explore to what extent empirical evidence supports these assumptions. Yet, reviewing this field of research is rather difficult as it includes a variety of concepts and methods, applies different research designs, and is often based on small samples. This heterogeneity, together with a lack of replication studies, complicates the search for cumulative knowledge. Rather than presenting selected findings we illustrate the promise of this approach with reference to one specific category of disorders, cardiometabolic diseases.

9.2.2 The case of empowering people with cardiometabolic diseases

Why is empowerment important for people with cardiometabolic disease who are prepared to return to work or to remain engaged in work? Firstly, controlling the main cardiovascular risk factors is an important daily task, and improved self-management skills facilitate this task. Secondly, having acquired improved coping skills increases successful management of critical transition periods, such as the time after discharge from hospital. A further reason concerns longer-term outcomes of this disease. People who are capable of experiencing autonomy and control in their daily environments are somehow protected against the risks of aggravation of their chronic disease. Glycaemic control in patients with type 2 diabetes mellitus (T2DM) is an essential goal of self-help programmes, given the fact that only around one third of patients with T2DM are able to effectively manage their disease. Around half of these patients had poor control of their glycaemic level, and lack of risk factor control increases the occurrence of serious complications, such as visual loss, amputation, neuropathy, and end-stage renal disease (Lambrinou et al. 2019). Empowerment of T2DM patients requires knowledge, self-motivation, and distinct skills of handling therapy and improving health behaviour. Different approaches were developed to enable empowerment. They include face-to-face communication with professionals, group sessions, support from trained peers, guidance through telemonitoring, websites or social media, distribution of booklets and guidelines, and application of smartphone devices (Lambrinou et al. 2019).

So far, few and mixed findings are available on the effectiveness of these methods (Chan et al. 2014; Deakin et al. 2005). The promotion of shared decision-making by the team seemed to be particularly important (McGill et al. 2017). Moreover, improved knowledge on the disease and its treatment strengthened self-efficacy (Y.-J. Lee et al. 2016; E.-H. Lee et al. 2021).

Whether patient empowerment results in a reduction of adverse clinical events was examined in a prospective cohort study in China (Wong et al. 2015). A large sample of 13,639 T2DM patients who were offered a structured patient empowerment programme by trained professional educators was matched with a sample of the same size of T2DM patients receiving usual care. All participants were free from cardiovascular disease (CVD) at baseline. In this publication, the details of the patient empowerment programme were not explained, but it obviously contained elements of improved knowledge and skill training. After a mean observation period of 21.5 months, the incidence rates of CVD and of all-cause mortality were compared between the two samples, applying Kaplan–Meier survival curves. Figure 9.2 displays respective results for all-cause mortality and incident cardiovascular events (Wong et al. 2015). The statistical significance of hazard ratios between the two groups was examined by multivariable Cox proportional hazards regression analysis. Findings indicated significantly reduced hazard ratios for all-cause mortality, incident CVD, and incident stroke in the treatment group. In a sensitivity analysis of the sub-sample that completed the full programme over time, the significant effects of the first two outcomes were confirmed. However, it should be noted that these findings are not based on a randomized controlled trial and that residual confounding cannot be excluded.

Cardiometabolic diseases include different clinical manifestations. Heart failure is one such manifestation. Some studies explored associations

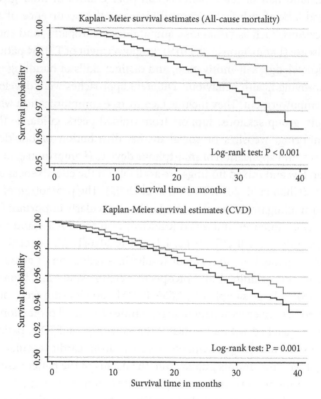

Figure 9.2 All-cause mortality and incident cardiovascular events in two groups of patients with type 2 diabetes mellitus (RCT). Intervention group: patient empowerment program (top line); control group: usual care (bottom line).

Source: Reproduced with permission from Wong, C. K., Wong, W. C., Wan, Y. F., et al. (2015), 'Patient empowerment programme in primary care reduced all-cause mortality and cardiovascular diseases in patients with type 2 diabetes mellitus: a population-based propensity-matched cohort study', *Diabetes Obes Metab,* 17 (2), 128–35. [Figure 1, p. 5]; license no.: 5503041161170.

of patient empowerment with outcomes of this clinical manifestation. To some extent, hospital readmission rates could be reduced (Jovicic et al. 2006; Liu et al. 2022). Acute myocardial infarction is another relevant clinical manifestation already mentioned. Empowerment is part of cardiac rehabilitation programmes with a focus on physical exercise (Dibben et al. 2021). However, in general, longer-term adherence to behavioural change and compliance with treatment guidelines were shown to be rather poor (Ruano-Ravina et al. 2016). There is some promise in applying new information and communication technologies in cardiac rehabilitation (Vahedian-Azimi et al. 2016), specifically if empowerment instructions are based on social cognition theory (Bandura 2004), as evidenced in a 12-week multi-media interactive nurse-led intervention programme (Su and Yu 2021). Despite preliminary advances, sustainable longer-term effects are difficult to reach as they require a more intense, more radical reorientation and reorganization of people's life habits following the survival of a cardiac event. One famous trial based on a joint retreat of an interdisciplinary professional team and a group of motivated cardiac patients consisted in an intensive lifestyle modification through a radical vegetarian diet, regular aerobic exercise, smoking cessation, and stress management (Ornish et al. 1998). Favourable outcomes included a small, but significant regression of coronary artery atherosclerosis and a reduction of recurrent cardiac events. Clearly, such far-reaching investments required from patients and from health-care providers are not realistic at larger scale, and barriers against their implementation are particularly high among working-age populations.

Taken together, empowerment of patients with cardiometabolic risk and disease offers an important, largely underused resource in secondary prevention. Supported by distinct social movements, such as self-help organizations, by improved legislation of patient rights, and by patient-centred approaches of clinical care, the autonomy and responsibility of patients as pro-active partners in rehabilitation programmes was strengthened, resulting in remarkable improvements of health and well-being.

9.3 Some suggestions for further development

In Chapters 8 and 9, we addressed the challenge of an increased burden of chronic disease and disability in aging workforces, causing a high prevalence of sick leaves and productivity losses. Substantial efforts to bring sick people back to work were, and continue to be, developed to mitigate this impact, applying measures of active labour market policies and programmes of medical and vocational rehabilitation. These policies and the organizational structures of rehabilitation services provided to people with chronic disease or disability vary widely across countries. Moreover, success rates of return to work depend on type and severity of disease, on the comprehensiveness of the programme, its translation into action by an interdisciplinary professional team, and on a proactive role given to patients in terms of empowerment. Despite strong efforts to reintegrate people with impaired health into paid work, early exit from work is the only option for many employees with disease or disability. Whether being exposed to unemployment, being granted a disability pension, or getting access to early retirement depends on a variety of institutional, organizational, and personal factors. Overall, early exit from work under these conditions represents a threatening life event with negative financial, mental, and social consequences. Importantly, we argued that in all critical instances, whether returning to work or being excluded from the labour market (mainly due to receiving disability pension or becoming unemployed), pronounced social inequalities are evident, leaving workers with lower socioeconomic positions at higher risk of accumulated disadvantage (Grammenos 2021).

These disturbing facts give rise to some reflections and suggestions on how the health of an aging workforce can be improved, how the success of return to work among employees with chronic disease or disability can be extended, and how pathways to job loss and disability pensions can be modified, specifically with the aim of reducing social inequalities. Among the many measures, organizations, and levels of action the following propositions may deserve particular attention.

To extend the success rate of return to work among employees with chronic disease or disability:

- Develop and implement active labour market policies in countries that lag behind modern welfare states, and enforce anti-discrimination legislation;
- Increase investments in occupational health services in order to extend their capacity for screening risk populations and of providing programmes of primary and secondary prevention;
- Promote the implementation and coordinated action of medical and vocational rehabilitation, with special recognition of different needs according to type and severity of disease or disability;

- Provide evidence-based in-patient and/or out-patient programmes of medical and vocational rehabilitation, led by an interdisciplinary professional team, enabling patient empowerment, and increasing sustainability of effects (e.g. by using innovative health communication technology);
- Offer financial incentives for employers to create/modify jobs and provide training for employees who returned to work, enhancing individual placement and support initiatives;
- Improve the quality of work and employment among those who return to work, in order to prevent relapse and to sustain work ability and well-being.

To modify pathways to job loss and disability pensions, specifically to reduce social inequalities:

- Monitor physically and psychosocially adverse working conditions at early stages within companies and develop preventive measures to mitigate adversity;
- Offer training and qualification opportunities for job change among employees with impaired health;
- Protect employees with disability or chronic disease from job loss by enforcing respective legislation;
- Ensure that disability pensions are fairly granted to employees according to severity of disease or disability, and according to adversity of previous job exposure;
- Implement evidence-based access to early retirement for distinct occupational groups with long-term exposure to physically or psychosocially adverse working conditions.

To improve the health of an aging workforce:

- Make sure that employees are covered by adequate health insurance and that companies enable them to seek medical consultations according to need;
- Ask employers to offer arrangements for physical activity, relaxation and recreation, and promote the delivery of healthy diet;
- Ensure the implementation of regulations that preserve employees from health-adverse working time arrangements and that promote family-friendly working conditions;

- Develop pro-active occupational health and safety programmes at the level of national policies and at the level of corporations, companies, and organizations, with the aim of reducing unhealthy and promoting healthy work;
- Protect workers in precarious, disadvantaged nonstandard employment from poverty and loss by enforcing legal norms and by fostering voluntary agreements at the level of branches or companies.

This last dimension of further development is fundamental as the provision of decent work early on reduces risks of work-induced health impairments at later stages of work trajectories. Given the primacy of preventive efforts, the last two chapters of this book provide an extensive analysis of this topic.

9.4 Summary

With the content of this chapter, we aimed at sensitizing readers to appreciate the important role of legal frameworks, national labour and social policies, and diverse organizational settings in the processes of return to or exit from paid work among people with chronic disease or disability. Furthermore, we emphasized the need of strengthening the empowerment of patients, and we suggested a number of future measures of how to successfully cope with the burden of chronic disease and disability in working populations.

9.5 Relevant questions

- What are the main arguments to strengthen active rather than passive labour market policies in order to reduce the disability employment gap?
- Limited sustainability of improved health behaviour was identified as a weakness in medical rehabilitation programmes. How can innovative health communication technology contribute to strengthen sustainability?
- Why is it important to strengthen empowerment of people with chronic disease or disability, and what are the best strategies to this end?

Recommended reading

❖ Escorpizo, R., Brage, S., Homa, D., et al. (eds.) (2015), *Handbook of vocational rehabilitation and disability evaluation. Application and implementation of the ICF*. Cham: Springer.

❖ Castro, E. M., Van Regenmortel, T., Vanhaecht, K., et al. (2016), 'Patient empowerment, patient participation and patient-centeredness in hospital care: a concept analysis based on a literature review', *Patient Educ Couns*, 99 (12), 1923–39.

❖ OECD (2010), *Sickness, disability and work: breaking the barriers. A synthesis of findings across OECD countries*. Paris: OECD.

Useful websites

❖ Pension maps project website https://www.mpisoc.mpg.de/en/social-law/research/research-projects/pension-maps/project-website/

❖ Journal of Vocational Rehabilitation https://www.iospress.com/catalog/journals/journal-of-vocational-rehabilitation

❖ U.S. Department of Labor, Office of Disability Employment Policy https://www.dol.gov/agencies/odep

References

Bandura, A. (2004), 'Health promotion by social cognitive means', *Health Educ Behav*, 31 (2), 143–64.

Barr, B., McHale, P., and Whitehead, M. (2020), 'Reducing inequalities in employment of people with disabilities'. In U. Bültmann and J. Siegrist (eds.), *Handbook of disability, work and health*. Cham: Springer, 309–27.

Castro, E. M., Van Regenmortel, T., Vanhaecht, K., et al. (2016), 'Patient empowerment, patient participation and patient-centeredness in hospital care: a concept analysis based on a literature review', *Patient Educ Couns*, 99 (12), 1923–39.

Chan, J. C., Sui, Y., Oldenburg, B., et al. (2014), 'Effects of telephone-based peer support in patients with type 2 diabetes mellitus receiving integrated care: a randomized clinical trial', *JAMA Intern Med*, 174 (6), 972–81.

Cockerham, W. C. (1998), *Medical sociology* 4th ed. London: Prentice Hall.

Coulter, A., and Fitzpatrick, R. (2000), 'The patient's perspective regarding appropriate health care'. *The handbook of social studies in health and medicine*. Thousand Oaks, CA: Sage Publications Ltd, 454–64.

Dahl, E., and van der Wel, K. A. (2020), 'Policies of reducing the burden of occupational hazards and disability pensions'. In U. Bültmann and J. Siegrist (eds.), *Handbook of disability, work and health*. Cham: Springer, 85–104.

Davies, C. (1996), 'The sociology of professions and the profession of gender', *Sociology*, 30 (4), 661–78.

De Sutter, J., Kacenelenbogen, R., Pardaens, S., et al. (2020), 'The role of cardiac rehabilitation in vocational reintegration Belgian working group of cardiovascular prevention and rehabilitation position paper', *Acta cardiologica*, 75 (5), 388–97.

Deakin, T., McShane, C. E., Cade, J. E., et al. (2005), 'Group based training for self-management strategies in people with type 2 diabetes mellitus', *Cochrane Database Syst Rev*, (2), CD003417.

Dibben, G., Faulkner, J., Oldridge, N., et al. (2021), 'Exercise-based cardiac rehabilitation for coronary heart disease', *Cochrane Database Syst Rev*, 11 (11), CD001800.

Diderichsen, F. (2020), 'Investing in integrative active labour market policies'. In U. Bültmann and J. Siegrist (eds.), *Handbook of disability, work and health*. Cham: Springer, 661–74.

Escorpizo, R., Brage, S., Homa, D., et al. (eds.) (2015), *Handbook of vocational rehabilitation and disability evaluation: application and implementation of the ICF*. Cham: Springer.

Freidson, E. (1970), *Profession of medicine: a study of the sociology of applied knowledge*. New York, NY: Harper & Row.

Götz, S., Wahrendorf, M., Siegrist, J., et al. (2020), 'Social inequalities in medical rehabilitation outcomes – a registry-based study on 219,584 insured persons in Germany', *Eur J Public Health*, 30 (3), 498–503.

Grammenos, S. (2021), *European comparative data on Europe 2020 and persons with disabilities: labour market, education, poverty and health analysis and trends*. Brussels: Publications Office of the European Union.

Gutenbrunner, C., Stievano, A., Nugraha, B., et al. (2022), 'Nursing–a core element of rehabilitation', *Int Nurs Rev*, 69 (1), 13–19.

Jansen, J., van Ooijen, R., Koning, P. W. C., et al. (2021), 'The role of the employer in supporting work participation of workers with disabilities: a systematic literature review using an interdisciplinary approach', *J Occup Rehabil*, 31 (4), 916–49.

Jovicic, A., Holroyd-Leduc, J. M., and Straus, S. E. (2006), 'Effects of self-management intervention on health outcomes of patients with heart failure: a systematic review of randomized controlled trials', *BMC Cardiovasc Disord*, 6, 43.

Kai, S. H. Y., Ferrieres, J., Rossignol, M., et al. (2022), 'Prevalence and determinants of return to work after various coronary events: meta-analysis of prospective studies', *Sci Rep*, 12 (1), 15348.

Kant, I., Jansen, N. W., van Amelsvoort, L. G., et al. (2008), 'Structured early consultation with the occupational physician reduces sickness absence among office workers at high risk for long-term sickness absence: a randomized controlled trial', *J Occup Rehabil*, 18 (1), 79–86.

Lambrinou, E., Hansen, T. B., and Beulens, J. W. (2019), 'Lifestyle factors, self-management and patient empowerment in diabetes care', *Eur J Prev Cardiol*, 26 (2_suppl), 55–63.

Lee, E.-H., Lee, Y. W., Chae, D., et al. (2021), 'Pathways linking health literacy to self-management in people with type 2 diabetes', *Healthcare (Basel)*, 9 (12), 1734.

Lee, Y.-J., Shin, S.-J., Wang, R.-H., et al. (2016), 'Pathways of empowerment perceptions, health literacy, self-efficacy, and self-care behaviors to glycemic control in patients with type 2 diabetes mellitus', *Patient Educ Couns*, 99 (2), 287–94.

Liu, S., Li, J., Wan, D. Y., et al. (2022), 'Effectiveness of eHealth self-management interventions in patients with heart failure: systematic review and meta-analysis', *J Med Internet Res*, 24 (9), e38697.

Martin, A., Sanderson, K., and Cocker, F. (2009), 'Meta-analysis of the effects of health promotion intervention in the workplace on depression and anxiety symptoms', *Scand J Work Environ Health*, 35 (1), 7–18.

McGill, M., Blonde, L., Chan, J. C. N., et al. (2017), 'The interdisciplinary team in type 2 diabetes management: challenges and best practice solutions from real-world scenarios', *J Clin Transl Endocrinol*, 7, 21–27.

Middleton, J. W., Johnston, D., Murphy, G., et al. (2015), 'Early access to vocational rehabilitation for spinal cord injury inpatients', *J Rehabil Med*, 47 (7), 626–31.

Mikkelsen, M. B., and Rosholm, M. (2018), 'Systematic review and meta-analysis of interventions aimed at enhancing return to work for sick-listed workers with common mental disorders, stress-related disorders, somatoform disorders and personality disorders', *Occup Environ Med*, 75 (9), 675–86.

Mittag, O., and Welti, F. (2017), 'Medizinische Rehabilitation in Deutschland und im restlichen Europa [Comparing medical rehabiltation across Europe and effects of European legislation]', *Bundesgesundheitsbl*, 60 (4), 378–85.

Mittag, O., Schramm, S., Bohmen, S., et al. (2011), 'Medium-term effects of cardiac rehabilitation in Germany: systematic review and meta-analysis of results from national and international trials', *Eur J Cardiovasc Prev Rehabil*, 18 (4), 587–93.

Nazarov, S., Manuwald, U., Leonardi, M., et al. (2019), 'Chronic diseases and employment: which interventions support the maintenance of work and return to work among workers with chronic illnesses? A systematic review', *Int J Environ Res Public Health*, 16 (10), 1864.

Nieuwenhuijsen, K., Verbeek, J. H., Neumeyer-Gromen, A., et al. (2020), 'Interventions to improve return to work in depressed people', *Cochrane Database Syst Rev*, 10 (10), CD006237.

OECD (2010), *Sickness, disability and work: breaking the barriers: a synthesis of findings across OECD countries*. Paris: OECD.

Ornish, D., Scherwitz, L. W., Billings, J. H., et al. (1998), 'Intensive lifestyle changes for reversal of coronary heart disease', *JAMA*, 280 (23), 2001–07.

Rothermund, E., Gundel, H., Rottler, E., et al. (2016), 'Effectiveness of psychotherapeutic consultation in the workplace: a controlled observational trial', *BMC Public Health*, 16 (1), 891.

Ruano-Ravina, A., Pena-Gil, C., Abu-Assi, E., et al. (2016), 'Participation and adherence to cardiac rehabilitation programs: a systematic review', *Int J Cardiol*, 223, 436–43.

Ryan, M. R., and Deci, E. L. (2018), *Self-determination theory: basic psychological needs in motivation, development, and wellness*. New York, NY: Guilford Press.

Schneider, S. M., Petrova, T., and Becker, U. (eds.) (2021), *Pension maps: visualising the institutional structures of old age security in Europe and beyond* 2nd edn. Munich: Max Planck Institute for Social Law and Social Policy.

Stevens, F. (2001), 'The convergence and divergence of modern health care systems'. In W. C. Cockerham (ed.), *The blackwell companion to medical sociology*. Oxford: Blackwell, 159–76.

Su, J. J., and Yu, D. S. (2021), 'Effects of a nurse-led eHealth cardiac rehabilitation programme on health outcomes of patients with coronary heart disease: a randomised controlled trial', *Int J Nurs Stud*, 122, 104040.

United Nations (2006), *Convention of the rights of persons with disabilities*. New York, NY: United Nations.

Vahedian-Azimi, A., Miller, A. C., Hajiesmaieli, M., et al. (2016), 'Cardiac rehabilitation using the Family-Centered Empowerment Model versus home-based cardiac rehabilitation in patients with myocardial infarction: a randomised controlled trial', *Open Heart*, 3 (1), e000349.

Vlasveld, M. C., van der Feltz-Cornelis, C. M., Ader, H. J., et al. (2012), 'Collaborative care for major depressive disorder in an occupational healthcare setting', *Br J Psychiatry*, 200 (6), 510–1.

Wang, P. S., Simon, G. E., Avorn, J., et al. (2007), 'Telephone screening, outreach, and care management for depressed workers and impact on clinical and work productivity outcomes: a randomized controlled trial', *JAMA*, 298 (12), 1401–11.

White, D. (2000), 'Consumer and community participation: a reassessment of process, impact, and value'. In G. L. Albrecht and S. C. Scrimshaw (eds.), *The handbook of social studies in health and medicine*. London: Sage, 465–80.

Wong, C. K., Wong, W. C., Wan, Y. F., et al. (2015), 'Patient empowerment programme in primary care reduced all-cause mortality and cardiovascular diseases in patients with type 2 diabetes mellitus: a population-based propensity-matched cohort study', *Diabetes Obes Metab*, 17 (2), 128–35.

World Health Organization (1986), *Ottawa charter for health promotion*. Copenhagen: WHO Regional Office for Europe.

PART V
PREVENTION
The policy dimension

10

Prevention and health promotion at work

The organizational level

10.1 From risk assessment to workplace health promotion

10.1.1 Basic notions

The previous chapters demonstrated a tangible impact of adverse psycho-social working conditions on health and well-being. Evidence on these associations was shown to be rather strong for cardiovascular disease, type-2 diabetes and metabolic syndrome, and depression. Partial support was obvious for musculoskeletal disorders, addictive disorders, sleep disturbances, and cognitive decline (Chapter 6). Taken together, these manifestations of ill health amount to a considerable burden of work-related diseases. Psychobiological pathways underlying these relationships trigger dysregulation and disturbance of basic autonomic nervous system, cardiovascular, endocrine, immune, and inflammatory processes, resulting in a state of allostatic load (Chapter 7). In consequence, allostatic load increases the organism's vulnerability to pre-clinical stages of disease development and adaptive breakdown. Furthermore, we argued that the associations between adverse working conditions and health are bi-directional, with a main pathway leading from adverse work and employment to reduced health (Chapters 6 and 7), and an additional pathway leading from reduced health to adverse work and employment (Chapters 8 and 9). In this latter case, workers suffering from manifest disorders are exposed to higher levels of stressful work, which in turn aggravate their impaired health. Preventing, or at least reducing the burden of disease attributable to stressful psycho-social working conditions, in addition to chemical, physical, and biological

Psychosocial Occupational Health. Johannes Siegrist and Jian Li, Oxford University Press.
© Oxford University Press 2024. DOI: 10.1093/oso/9780192887924.003.0010

hazards, is one of primary goals of occupational health professionals, health-care systems, occupational health, and social policies. Substantial additional direct and indirect economic costs result from these developments. Reduced productivity in terms of sickness absence, presenteeism, impaired work ability, decrements in performance and motivation, and heightened turnover rates sum up to huge economic losses (Goetzel et al. 2004; World Health Organization 2019). These health-related and business-related losses call for extended activities of prevention and health promotion at work, both at the level of organizations and businesses, and at the level of national and transnational labour, social, and health policies. This chapter deals with the organizational level, whereas Chapter 11 addresses the policy level. The discussion of what types of measures were developed and what effects resulted from the implementation of workplace prevention programmes are the main aims of this chapter.

Workplace prevention and health promotion activities are usually classified according to three different types of practices, and within these practices, different targets are addressed (Daniels et al. 2021; see Box 10.1).

As mentioned in Box 10.1, it is sometimes difficult to draw a clear line between primary and secondary prevention programmes. For instance, a primary prevention programme targeting all members of a company may include persons at risk (e.g. with hypertension, depression, hyperglycaemia etc.) as well as those without risk. Reducing work stress is expected to have beneficial effects on both groups. For instance, in a Canadian primary prevention project, large intervention and control groups were recruited from public organizations with white-collar employees in order to reduce blood pressure and prevalence of hypertension by a theory-based organizational change approach (Trudel et al. 2021). Participants in both groups were either normotensive or hypertensive at entry. Six months and three years after the midpoint of the intervention, a significant reduction in systolic blood pressure was observed in the intervention group, but not in the control group, and the prevalence of hypertension was also significantly reduced in the intervention vs control group (Trudel et al. 2021; see Section 10.2 and Figure 10.1). With regard to mental health, company-based mental health programmes, such as the one described in Chapter 9 (Box 9.1), are another example of blurred boundaries between primary and secondary prevention. Whereas they put their main focus on workers with reduced mental health, some of their actions are open to all members of the organization.

Box 10.1 **Classification and targets of workplace prevention and health promotion activities**

- Primary prevention aims at preventing health risks and promoting health resources among working populations at early stages of exposure to adverse work.
- Secondary prevention is concerned with the strengthening of health resources and prevention of disease development among working populations who are already affected by signs of reduced health or increased vulnerability.
- Tertiary prevention sets out to strengthen adaption to, and coping with adverse work among those who developed chronic disease or disability, and to promote sustainable return to work.
- Rehabilitation is a synonymous term for tertiary prevention (Daniels et al. 2021).

As it is sometimes difficult to clearly distinguish between target populations for primary and secondary prevention (see main text), these two categories are often combined into one category.

Importantly, preventive practices can focus on different aspects. Firstly, and most often, they are directed to individual workers or groups of workers, targeting their personal behaviours, and more specifically their resources for coping with adverse work. Secondly, they address leaders, supervisors, line managers, and other persons with responsibility for subordinates within organizations. Here, indirect effects on workers' health are expected to result from improved leadership behaviour. Finally, distinct features of work organization, work environment, and employment contracts are targeted as far as their improvement is expected to favour employees' health.

In practice, these aspects have been combined in a comprehensive way to define a multi-component prevention. Moreover, the weight attributed to these different aspects varies between primary, secondary, and tertiary prevention. For instance, individual workers are more often targeted in tertiary as compared to primary prevention, and effects of organizational changes are particularly promising at the level of primary prevention.

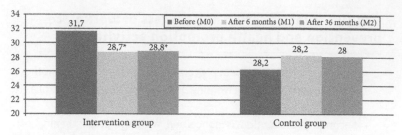

Figure 10.1 Prevalence of hypertension in the intervention group (N = 1,088) and the control group (N = 1,068) in the Canadian White-Collar Workplace Intervention study.

* Group differences are statistically significant at p < 0.05 level.

Source: Reproduced with permission from Trudel, X., Gilbert-Ouimet, M., Vezina, M., et al. (2021), 'Effectiveness of a workplace intervention reducing psychosocial stressors at work on blood pressure and hypertension', *Occup Environ Med,* 78 (10), 738–44. [Figure 2, p. 742]; license no.: 5506981387453.

From an occupational public health perspective, it seems promising to apply a preventive approach to all (or a majority of) members of an organization, despite the challenges of restricted resources and logistical problems (see 10.2). The crucial aspect of any type of preventive activity within organizations concerns the preconditions for its initiation. Given the costs involved in these activities and given widespread resistance from employers and managers against any kind of extrinsic intervention implementing preventive practices at large scale is obviously difficult. To date, external pressures help in reducing these difficulties. Two types of administrative approaches are particularly important: regulatory approaches and voluntary approaches. The first type includes national laws as well as international conventions or directives with relevance to health and safety. Distinct conventions inaugurated by the International Labour Organization (ILO) and a series of directives established by the European Commission illustrate one way that national laws towards strengthening occupational health are extended and coordinated. In addition, national occupational health authorities and institutions support this regulatory approach. Soft laws, such as recommendations/guidelines released by professional bodies, and agreements between social partners (mainly employer organizations and trade unions) are ways of implementing a voluntary approach. These measures include the release of checklists and standards of risk management. Given their flexibility and bottom-up procedures, soft laws often accelerate preventive developments as they are released at different (international,

national, sectoral, enterprise) levels. As mentioned in a recent review (Leka and Jain 2022), promising examples include the global campaign to reduce occupational injuries and diseases ('Vision Zero') initiated by the International Social Security Association (Zwetsloot et al. 2020), and efforts of strengthening occupational well-being through measures of corporate social responsibility, as declared by the leading European business network Corporate Sustainability and Responsibility. A blueprint for integrating the United Nation's Sustainable Development Goal 8 of promoting decent work (United Nations 2015) into training programmes for responsible future business leaders points to the strategic nature of some of these corporate social responsibility initiatives (Wersun et al. 2020). Transnational activities, such as 'Vision Zero' and approaches towards implementing Sustainable Development Goal 8are discussed more extensively in Chapter 11.

What are the main obligations evolving from these regulatory or voluntary approaches? Importantly, a major obligation consists of assessing the occupational risks through monitoring and surveillance. Based on this assessment, intervention programmes need to be developed, either as primary, secondary, tertiary, or multi-component approaches. This is a most critical, relevant step of activity requiring an evidence-based input (e.g. from theoretical and empirical research or from models of good practice). Equally important, once a preventive programme has been prepared, it must be ready for implementation into the everyday world of work and employment. Stakeholders involved in this step of transduction from design to application will experience substantial challenges, considering the difficulties of accomplishing sustainable long-term effects. These core tasks of prevention, risk assessment, and of programme development as well as programme implementation, are discussed in the rest of the present section. In the second part of the chapter, we consider effects of preventive measures in terms of health outcomes, relying mainly on information derived from systematic reviews (Section 10.2).

10.1.2 Risk assessment and surveillance

Systematic data collection of occupational exposures is a fundamental prerequisite of assessing needs for prevention and developing measures of change. In occupational medicine, a number of physical, chemical, and biological hazards at work are objectively assessed, with fixed thresholds of pathological development, as defined by scientific evidence underlying established legal regulations or recommendations from professional bodies. The extent to which occupational health risks are regulated by laws, and are routinely monitored, varies widely across countries. At least with regard to some major, well-established occupational risks, binding conventions were developed by ILO, and countries were expected to ratify these conventions by incorporating them into their national law. For instance, an ILO convention on radiation protection came into force in 1960, ratified by fifty countries, and another convention on banning asbestos was released in 1986 and was ratified by thirty-five countries (Leka and Jain 2020). While the causality of a noxious agent and the definition of noxious thresholds are rather well defined in several cases, such as heavy noise, or exposure to the chemical compound of benzene or to distinct asbestos fibre types, the evidence is less convincing for many other substances. In view of these uncertainties, professional bodies, such as the International Agency for Research on Cancer (IARC), developed a classification of grades of evidence and related guidelines, assisting regulatory organizations in developing recommendations or legal prescriptions to countries that are committed to improving occupational health and safety (Siemiatycki and Xu 2020).

It is much more difficult to establish systematic data collection and definition of noxious thresholds of exposure in case of health-adverse psychosocial work environments than in the case of established physical, chemical, or biological hazards. In consequence, fewer conventions, legal regulations, and recommendations were developed and implemented so far. At the transnational level, an ILO convention on a 'Promotional framework for occupational safety and health' (Convention 187, adopted in 2006 and ratified by forty-two countries) can be interpreted as a general declaration supporting all types of measures promoting healthy work but is lacking specificity and is not obligatory with regard to psychosocial work environments (Leka and Jain 2020). Another transnational declaration, released to its member states as a directive by the European Union, aimed at strengthening employers' obligations to ensure employee health, specifically through systematic risk assessment and inauguration of related preventive activities (Framework Directive 89/391/EEC). Accordingly, several member states of the European Union extended their legal regulations, implemented systematic occupational risk assessments, and reinforced their occupational health and safety institutions (Leka and Jain 2020).

For several reasons, assessing health-adverse psychosocial work environments proves to be a challenging task:

- No agreed-upon objective (e.g. physiological) measure quantifying stressful experience at work is currently available;
- Objective job exposure matrices based on leading theoretical concepts of stressful work are available for a small number of countries and may be too crude to identify detailed occupational risk conditions and to direct the development of preventive measures;
- Standardized, psychometrically validated questionnaires collecting self-reported data on stressful psychosocial work environments, based on leading theoretical concepts, are available (see Chapter 4), and related guidelines for their use were proposed to national statistical offices (OECD 2017). Yet, implementation so far is restricted, given a lack of resources for collecting and analysing data, and a rather low commitment from stakeholders to develop preventive measures in this domain.

Up to now, various forms of assessing psychosocial risks at work were developed, and this variety may have practical and theoretical advantages. At the same time, there are also justifications for prioritizing one specific

Table 10.1 Major psychometrically validated scales measuring psychosocial work environments

Scale	Approach	Author
Job Content Questionnaire (JCQ)	(S)	Karasek et al. 1998
Effort-Reward Imbalance Questionnaire (ERI)	(S)	Siegrist et al. 2004
Job Demand-Resources Questionnaire (JD-R)	(S)	Demerouti et al. 2001
Organizational Justice Scales	(S)	Colquitt 2001; Moorman 1991
Psychosocial Safety Climate Scale (PSC-12)	(S)	Dollard et al. 2019
Employment Precariousness Scale (EPRES)	(S)	Vives et al. 2010
Copenhagen Psychosocial Questionnaire (COPSOQ)	(C)	Kristensen et al. 2005
Job Characteristics Approach	(C)	OECD 2017

(S) = selective; (C) = comprehensive

approach. In Table 10.1 some major psychometrically validated scales proposed and applied for monitoring activities are listed (see also Chapter 4).
They can be divided into selective (S) and comprehensive (C) approaches,
the former measuring a distinct theoretical model and the latter assessing
multiple components derived from several concepts. These scales are available in different versions (long vs short) and languages, and they differ in
the way that thresholds or scores of critical exposure are defined. Moreover,
the robustness of their criterion validity, based on prospective investigations, varies widely.

Despite the difficulties mentioned, several countries developed systematic, routinely implemented risk assessments of adverse psychosocial work
environments and used this information to extend their preventive efforts
at work. Denmark is one such country whose approach is considered a
model of good practice. Essential features are described in Box 10.2.

Box 10.2 Assessing and improving the psychosocial work environment: the case of Denmark

- Companies must perform a regular health and safety assessment that includes critical aspects of the psychosocial work
  environment.
- Employers are responsible for this task, are expected to involve
  employees in the procedure, and to jointly identify targets for
  workplace health promotion.
- Moreover, steps for implementing these targets need to be described, and responsibilities are assigned; to this end, a company-
  based Health & Safety Organization is established.
- The Danish Working Environment Authority elaborates guidelines on assessing and managing psychosocial risks, such as high
  workload, violence, emotionally demanding work. It offers sector-
  specific assessment tools, and it supports training opportunities
  for dealing with these tasks at the company level.
- Labour inspectors of this authority carry out regular checks according to statutory requirements, they advise and control
  companies, and they conduct evaluations as a basis for further
  policy development (European Agency for Safety and Health at
  Work 2022).

In a survey on new and emerging risks at work conducted among member states of the European Union, the implementation of psychosocial risk assessment and preventive activities was one of several topics. Results from Denmark confirmed that this country had the highest coverage of psychosocial risk monitoring and external data inspection through the Working Environment Authority. Moreover, in about two thirds of companies included in the survey, action plans for reducing stressful work were developed, where priorities concerned 'widening employees' decision on how to do the job', 'reorganizing work tasks and structures', and 'reducing long or irregular working hours' (European Agency for Safety and Health at Work 2022).

Similar developments were reported from other parts of the world. For instance, in Japan, legislation on health and safety at work emphasizes the responsibility of employers for health protection of employees, reinforced by distinct guidelines. One such guideline focuses on the promotion and maintenance of mental health of workers, requiring companies to develop participatory approaches and action plans. Furthermore, measures of suicide prevention were implemented, and employers were obliged to refer workers suffering from long working hours and signs of fatigue and exhaustion for professional help. More recently, a stress check programme with regular screening of adverse psychosocial work environments was introduced as a mandatory measure in enterprises with fifty or more employees (Kawakami and Tsutsumi 2016). In Australia, systematic occupational risk management in organizations was inaugurated by the Model Work Health and Safety Act in 2011, where employers' resistance against monitoring carried the risk of financial sanctions. Accordingly, an Australian Workplace Barometer was applied as a tool of benchmarking working conditions (Owen et al. 2016). In this approach, the psychosocial safety climate turned out to be a major indicator of organizational performance, instructing preventive activities (Dollard et al. 2019). Other countries with promising developments of occupational risk assessment can be mentioned, such as Canada, and some of their more specific practical achievements will be discussed in conjunction with research findings derived from intervention studies (Section 10.2).

To conclude, several promising approaches for regular assessment of psychosocial occupational risks were developed, providing a basis for designing and implementing preventive programmes within companies. Despite being anchored in national laws, their translation into action was hampered by constraints at different levels. There is still a long way to go before they are ready to be applied as internationally established standards of surveillance, as is the case for major adverse physical and chemical occupational exposures.

10.1.3 Programme development and implementation

An ideal vision of psychosocial risk assessment might offer individual profiling of stress susceptibility at work, enabling the identification of situational (extrinsic) and personal (intrinsic) targets of intervention. This vision is probably more important for secondary and tertiary prevention, whereas primary prevention mainly addresses employed population groups. Here, information is based on probability statistics derived from epidemiological investigations that identify relative disease risks of exposed populations. One can argue that this epidemiology-based preventive approach does not do justice to individual differences, disregarding relevant interindividual variations in appraisal, coping, and physiological responses to occupational threats. However, it is justified whenever a risk factor to be prevented is highly prevalent in a working population. In this case, even relatively low levels of risk manifestation within a large number of individuals contribute to an increased burden of disease. Reducing a risk factor at the level of total populations is likely to be as efficient as an approach targeting high-risk individuals, or it may even be more efficient (Rose 1992). Different types of primary prevention programmes are described in Box 10.3.

Comparable to the prevalence of health-adverse behaviours, the frequency of health-adverse psychosocial environments is rather high. For instance, several investigations applying measures of the demand-control (DC) or the effort-reward imbalance (ERI) models report a prevalence of stressful work ranging from twenty to thirty per cent of the workforce under study (see Chapters 3 and 6). Under these conditions, measures of primary prevention targeting collectives of individuals rather than single persons seem justified. Accordingly, this section discusses prevention programmes at the company level that address the workforce, either in its totality or focused on distinct subgroups within organizations.

Numerous preventive programmes of behavioural modification were developed, applied, and evaluated over the past few decades, as documented by a huge, rapidly growing number of publications worldwide. Dealing

Box 10.3 Types of primary prevention

There exist several typologies of activities directed at primary prevention. In general, it is convenient to distinguish three types of activities:

- those directed at modifying employees' behaviours, attitudes, and skills;
- those dealing with leadership and collaboration;
- those addressing work organization, work environment, and employment conditions.

Although they might be combined, the first type, behaviour modification, represents by far the most widely applied approach. Internationally leading targets of preventive actions at the workplace are:

- improving physical activity;
- promoting healthy nutrition;
- controlling one's body weight;
- reducing substance use;
- strengthening resilience, coping with stress, and relaxation.

As these actions reach large parts of working-age populations, and as their targets contribute to a reduction of several widely prevalent chronic diseases, they are important in a public health perspective.

with this research is one of the key areas of interest for occupational health psychologists. As excellent textbooks and handbooks inform readers about these developments, our book does not provide a description and discussion of these multiple strategies of workplace behavioural modification (see e.g. Cooper and Quick 2017; Cunningham and Black 2021). This limitation is justified by the fact that the authors' primary expertise, being in sociology (Johannes Siegrist) and an occupational epidemiology (Jian Li), is related to the study of health effects of exposure to adverse psychosocial work environments and its practical implications. Accordingly, we prioritize preventive approaches that address modifiable features of these environments. One major aspect of such approaches concerns leadership behaviour of managers/superiors in organizations, and efforts to improve collaboration and participation among employees. As a another aspect, changes of work organization, work environments, and employment conditions are salient points of structural prevention. The next two sections address these two aspects.

10.1.3.1 Leadership, collaboration, and participation

In any organization requiring some complexity of interpersonal collaboration, leadership is an essential feature of successful performance. It provides guidance, coordination, support, control, and feedback to team members. Leaders are located at different levels of organizational hierarchies, from top operative managers to line managers, the latter being particularly important due to their proximity to collaborating—and formally subordinated—employees. Positive and efficient leadership exerts beneficial effects on employees' commitment and performance, motivation, positive affect, and well-being. Conversely, conflicting, negative leadership behaviour results in decreased motivation and commitment, performance decrement, negative emotions, and reduced well-being. It is no surprise that the analysis of leadership behaviour, its determinants and outcomes, represents a key topic of social and behavioural science research on organizations. Knowledge derived from this research can be successfully applied in interventions that aim at improving organizational performance and employee well-being.

This field of research offers a variety of concepts of leadership and its core features. Given a dynamic research development, several partly overlapping concepts were proposed, and the evidence on determinants and outcomes so far seems inconsistent and incomplete. According to two comprehensive reviews, the following concepts of leadership styles and competencies deserve a short description (Hawkes and Spedding 2022; Yarker et al. 2022):

- Task-oriented vs relationship-oriented leadership: These styles focus on task completion and performance vs consideration of employees' functioning. To achieve successful outcomes a balance between these two styles is needed.
- Transformational leadership: Its main features include inspirational motivation and stimulation, individual consideration, and provision of contingent reward.
- Authentic leadership: Behaviour characterized by inclusive and transparent decision-making, incorporation of ethical values, and unbiased

sharing of information. The concept exhibits strong overlap with the notion of 'ethical leadership'.

- Servant leadership: This style is defined by an altruistic attitude of caring for followers, provision of support, and empowerment.
- Abusive/destructive leadership: In contrast to the former styles and competencies this type is characterized by lack of consideration of followers, egoistic performance, and negative interactions, including hostility and bullying.

To learn how these features of leadership behaviour affect the health and well-being of follower employees it may be helpful to consider those core competencies that were shown to matter for a reduction of stress among subordinates. They can be described by the following terms: (1) respectful and responsible treatment of other members; (2) proactive and problem-solving, supportive action; (3) compassion and individualized concern, including advice seeking (Yarker et al. 2022). Yet, to evaluate the associations between leadership behaviour and employee well-being in more depth, information derived from systematic reviews and meta-analyses is required. To our knowledge, one such meta-analysis offers the most up-to-date and comprehensive information (Montano et al. 2017). In this contribution, studies were classified in five main categories: transformational leadership; task-oriented leadership; relationship-oriented leadership, leader-follower exchange, and destructive leadership. Their associations with indicators of employees' mental health are briefly considered below (see Section 10.2). To teach health-conducive leadership behaviour turned out to be difficult (Kuehnl et al. 2019) and to require innovative approaches (Romanowska and Theorell 2020). Moreover, there are good reasons to extend the frame of analysis beyond leadership behaviour by including the whole staff of a department or its units, the teams composed of leaders and followers. In this perspective, ways of improving collaboration and team climate and opportunities for extending participation of staff members are becoming core topics of interest.

A comprehensive systematic review of organizational- and group-level workplace interventions corroborates this claim (Fox et al. 2021). In one component of this analysis, studies that improved team dynamics were reviewed. Strengthening organizational culture and citizenship, team climate and communication were main aims. A further component of this review concerned interventions that promoted participation among team members in organizations. These programmes were designed either to initiate measures of organizational and personnel development through a structured participatory process, or to increase the engagement of team members by giving them a stronger voice. Encouraging team members to express their views and overcoming behavioural inhibition by pro-active participatory engagement was shown to exert beneficial effects on self-esteem, self-efficacy and related psychobiological responses (Brooks and Wilkinson 2022).

Thus, there are strong arguments in favour of including employee participation in primary workplace prevention programmes, and the different dimensions and modalities of participation were elaborated in some instructive documents (Abildgaard et al. 2020; Aust and Ducki 2004). Taken together, distinct leadership styles and competencies, leader-follower-relationships improving team climate and collaboration, and participation of employees in the design and implementation of preventive programmes can contribute to mental health and well-being at work. Yet, these interpersonal determinants are embedded in structural constraints of the organization. As these organizational constraints matter directly for workers' health and well-being, they deserve further consideration.

10.1.3.2 Work Organization

Preventive measures at the level of organizations are expected to produce more pervasive effects than those attributable to individual- or interpersonal-level interventions as they directly target some of the main determinants of stressful psychosocial work environments. Whether this holds true is an empirical question that is still debated (Section 10.2). Yet, these approaches provide opportunities for reducing organizational constraints and strengthening organizational resources with potential impact on workers' health. Organizational interventions were defined as 'planned, behavioural, and theory-based actions that aim to improve employees' health and well-being by changing the way work is designed, organized, and managed' (Nielsen 2013, p. 1030).

- Organizational interventions include the design, distribution, and division of job tasks, the environmental and temporal conditions of performing work, the contractual features of employees' work, and the vertical and horizontal dimensions of cooperation among staff members.
- It is important to note that organizations are not isolated autonomous entities, but are affected by macrostructural economic, political, and societal conditions, such as legal regulations, economic competition, changing social norms, and technological innovations.

In today's world of work, these latter conditions are even threatening the primacy of organizations as the leading institution of where paid work is performed. With the advances of telecommunication and internet-based production techniques, with increased flexibility of work arrangements, and the expansion of work from home—boosted as a consequence of the COVID-19 pandemic—the boundaries between employees and the employers' firms, enterprises, and other types of organization were weakened. At least, fewer employees are working regularly—and on a daily basis—in a fixed location, the employers' premises or offices as places where work is performed in predefined structural and infrastructural frames. This shift has far-reaching implications, not least for the design and implementation of preventive measures. For instance, it is becoming more difficult for occupational health and safety professionals to monitor and reach employees working at distant places. At the same time, new occupational hazards may evolve in distant unprotected, unregulated workplaces. This shift equally complicates the conduct of research as it reduces opportunities for establishing and continuing longitudinal investigations and controlled trials within stable organizational contexts. In the long run, these difficulties may even challenge established practices of producing scientific knowledge, such as the hierarchy of scientific evidence (see Fig. 5.2, Chapter 5; see also Pfaff and Schmitt 2021).

Readers may become aware that, in view of this growing distance between employees' actual workplaces and employers' organizational settings, some concepts and practices of organizational interventions may no longer be directly applicable. In the near future, it is likely that, in several employment sectors, firms, offices, and factories will no longer be the place frequented by a majority of working individuals on a regular daily basis. Nevertheless, insights on organizational interventions put together in this section still remain relevant for a substantial part of the world's current workforce.

Table 10.2 gives an overview of major targets addressed by organizational interventions with relevance to psychosocial work environments and their impact on workers' health and well-being. The list of targets is not exhaustive, but it reflects main domains of activities. In addition, the salience of each target is indicated by a reference to a publication dealing with the target. As the list is restricted to single targets, more complex intervention approaches applying multi-component programmes are not included (see Section 10.2). Thus, the analytic scheme only partially mirrors the richness of this field of inquiry and evidence.

Table 10.2 Major targets of organizational interventions to improve psychosocial work environments

Target	Main theoretical dimensions	Study author
Shift work scheduling	Demand/Effort—Control	Costa 2020
Reduced working time	Demand/Effort	Voglino et al. 2022
Flexible work arrangement	Control—Reward	Fox et al. 2021
Work-life balance	Control—Support—Resource	Brough et al. 2020
Breaks, reduced pressure	Demand/Effort	Kawakami et al. 1997
Job task enrichment	Control—Resource	Bambra et al. 2007
Job task decision latitude	Control—Resource	Egan et al. 2007
Job rotation	Demand/Effort—Justice	Padula et al. 2017
Skill development	Control—Resource	Trudel et al. 2021
Promotion prospects	Reward—Control—Justice	Bourbonnais et al. 2011
Providing recognition	Reward—Justice	Brisson et al. 2016
Increasing staff	Demand/Effort—Resource	Barck-Holst et al. 2017
Improving pay	Reward—Resource—Justice	Falk et al. 2018
Preventing downsizing	Control—Reward	Cooper et al. 2012

The targets listed in Table 10.2 vary according to opportunity and frequency of implementation and according to the population under study. For instance, changes focusing on working time, including work-life balance, are more frequently addressed than interventions improving pay, or preventing downsizing. Some interventions are directed to specific occupational groups (e.g. job rotation to occupations with strenuous physical work; shift work scheduling to shift workers), whereas their majority of changes apply to a wide range of occupations.

How are the targets transformed into feasible workplace interventions? Depending on available knowledge, models of good practice can be derived from previously conducted interventions, where distinct features of success were identified. For instance, multiple experience with changing shift systems resulted in a series of recommendations and guidelines for optimal ways of implementing shift work cycles and conditions (Costa 2020). As an alternative, workplace interventions can be informed by theoretical models. In this case, psychosocial risk assessment data and extensive preliminary exploratory information are required to apply a general concept to a specific context. One such approach is briefly mentioned here, given its high quality and originality. It concerns an intervention study among white-collar employees working in three semi-public organizations offering insurance services in Canada. Its essential features are described as follows (Brisson et al. 2016):

- The intervention was conceptualized as a quasi-experimental before-after design, with an intervention group and a control group. The findings of an a priori psychosocial risk assessment conducted in the intervention group revealed main problems of concern.
- These problems were identified at the organizational level by measuring the frequency of stressful psychosocial work factors, as defined by leading theoretical models. These problems of concern were prioritized as intervention targets.
- Focus groups composed by representatives of workers, managers, and researchers detailed the intervention targets by developing a list of concrete organizational changes to be considered for implementation ('multi-component' approach).
- The proposed changes were presented to managers in written reports. Based on agreement, they were subsequently implemented in the intervention departments. Detailed records of these changes were documented in a logbook, to help inform the intervention process.
- As the intervention content of organizational changes had to be consistent with the prioritized targets, these changes were classified according to theoretical dimensions (e.g. skill development and training activity as indicators of increased job control).
- Using data from two measurement waves in the intervention and control group (baseline and end of intervention after twelve months), changes in the frequency of stressful psychosocial work factors and effects on health outcomes were analysed in the two groups (intervention effectiveness) (see Section 10.2).

Obviously, developing high-quality interventions along these principles requires substantial research investment that is not easily available. It is therefore a task of occupational health and safety institutions, professional associations, scientists, and other stakeholders to provide manuals, guidelines, tools, and to offer consultation and support to this end. Consultation and support are even more important in view of additional challenges faced during the process of implementation of organizational changes.

10.1.3.3 Programme implementation

Even a well-developed, theoretically grounded organizational change may fail, if the conditions enabling or hindering its implementation are not sufficiently recognized. In recent years, researchers dealing with structural intervention at work became aware of the importance of analysing the process of implementation in a systematic way. Using the so-called Sigtuna principles (von Thiele Schwarz et al. 2021), they aim to produce maximum impact through prioritization of activities according to an optimal balance between investments and anticipated outcomes. Moreover, organizational change needs to be adapted to existing practices and processes within the organization, and continued monitoring, reflection, and organizational learning is required to safely implement the intervention. Another proposal points to the importance of theoretical guidance during the implementation, supporting a realist evaluation and proposing specific hypotheses on core process mechanisms (Roodbari et al. 2021). Yet, few reviews analysed the effectiveness of primary, secondary, or tertiary preventions in a systematic way. One such systematic review identified a number of negative and positive factors to be addressed during the implementation phase of organizational change (Daniels et al. 2021).

Main negative factors include:

- Economic pressure due to competition
- Failure to continuously involve key stakeholders
- Weak participation of professionals
- Limited support from middle-managers
- Lack of clarity in planning the intervention steps.

Main positive factors include:

- Continuity of communication through regular meetings
- Problem-solving capability and organizational learning
- Support from professionals and senior managers
- Functional governance and stepwise development
- Adequate financial resources.

To conclude, implementing organizational change is usually a lengthy and risky process. It occurs in a dynamic environment with unanticipated events, and it can produce unintended, undesired side effects (Semmer 2006). Given these uncertainties, improved process evaluation and best practice models of intervention methods are desirable, and several such models were developed, particularly in some European countries (for review, see Nielsen et al. 2010). In the next section, we consider the main findings from research dealing with effect evaluation, and specifically with health outcomes of organization-level psychosocial workplace interventions. These results play a critical role in terms of scientific credibility of this field of research and in terms of justifying and motivating extended investments in worksite health promotion programmes.

10.2 Health-related intervention effects

Scientific findings derived from classical experiments and randomized controlled trials (RCTs) are recognized as the most reliable and valid sources of scientific proof. This was indicated in Figure 5.2, where a hierarchy of scientific evidence was depicted (Chapter 5). As a standard requirement, randomization occurs at the individual level. In some cases where this is not feasible, randomization is performed at the aggregate level by providing the treatment to all members of a unit A, while all members of a unit B serve as a control group (cluster randomized trials). However, there are additional methodological attempts to meet a high level of scientific credibility. In Chapter 5, we mentioned new statistical models of causal analysis, and we pointed to a relevant intersection between experimental and non-experimental study designs: quasi-experimental, non-randomized studies. In fact, many workplace intervention studies are based on quasi-experimental designs, given the practical difficulties of applying an RCT in a dynamic social environment (Cox et al. 2007). Here, non-equivalent control group designs represent a frequently applied approach. In these studies, participants are not assigned at random to the conditions under study, but outcomes of interest are compared between a treatment group and a control group in a pre-post intervention analysis.

In this section, we demonstrate findings on health effects derived from three types of interventions, (1) those dealing with coping behaviour in organizational contexts, (2) those addressing leadership behaviour, team climate and participation, and (3) those concerned with organizational changes of work and employment conditions. As the selected studies are mainly derived from published systematic reviews, they do not represent an exhaustive, updated account of available evidence. Rather, they enable readers to identify promising examples of intervention and to be informed about major trends of research in this field of inquiry. As was mentioned, our main interest is directed to interventions that target modifiable working and employment conditions at the structural level. The section ends with a short account of economic benefits of psychosocial workplace interventions.

10.2.1 Coping behaviour

Leading literature reviews in this field conclude that a large majority of intervention studies on occupational health address the behaviour of employees, either their health habits and attitudes or their coping capabilities of preventing or reducing stressful experience at work and of strengthening their resilience (Daniels et al. 2021; Fox et al. 2021; Martin et al. 2020; Richardson and Rothstein 2008). This preference resulted in a neglect of organizational-level activities but more recently, this imbalance has been reduced. As a particular strength, evaluations of behavioural modification trials often applied an individual-level randomized design, thereby accumulating solid knowledge about intervention effectiveness. This is documented by several systematic reviews of a selected number of well-studied behavioural modifications aiming to improve working people's mental health. These modifications use psychological and psychotherapeutic approaches, such as cognitive behaviour therapy, mindfulness, resilience, relaxation, and related forms of stress management.

In a rapid review of recently published research dealing with these interventions, Martin et al. (2020) noted that a particularly large number of evaluated programmes used cognitive behaviour therapy, often among health professionals, and that its efficacy to improve mental health was fairly well established (see also Tan et al. 2014). A similar conclusion was drawn from publications reviewing mindfulness. Whereas the diversity of ways of delivering the treatment reduced the generalizability of findings, this evidence was judged to be more robust than that obtained from studies on resilience (Martin et al. 2020). However, for several promising psychological techniques, the empirical basis is still too small to derive firm conclusions.

Examples are programmes that strengthen recovery (Ebert et al. 2015) or those promoting psychological capital (Martin et al. 2020).

A different type of individual-focused interventions concerns health behaviour and related attitudes, the most frequent approach of workplace health promotion programmes (Cunningham and Black 2021). The public health value of these activities is undisputed, and systematic reviews of RCTs addressing weight reduction, physical activity, and healthy nutrition document small positive effects (for review, e.g. Montano et al. 2014b). Yet, the delivery of these activities often suffers from reduced quality and intensity, thus minimizing the sustainability of behavioural changes. In a cluster randomized trial in the US, effects of a workplace wellness programme were analysed in twenty intervention and twenty control departments of a large enterprise. Several modules including weight control, healthy diet, and physical activity were offered over a period of four to eight weeks to the treatment group composed of several thousand participants (Song and Baicker 2019). Compared to the control group, the treatment group reported a modest increase in physical activity and in weight control, but neither clinical data (e.g. blood pressure, BMI, cholesterol) nor administrative employment data (absenteeism) documented any significant group difference.

On balance, behavioural modification initiated by occupational health promotion programmes can exert modest- to moderate beneficial effects on mental health by improving coping behaviour, and they can strengthen health-related behaviour, specifically weight control, physical activity, and healthy nutrition. However, there is weak evidence on longer-term effects of sustainability, and these interventions fail to influence detrimental effects on health due to exposure to adverse psychosocial work environments. Despite some high-quality trials, this line of research is faced with several methodological and conceptual challenges (Burgess et al. 2020).

10.2.2 Leadership, collaboration, and participation

Two systematic reviews provide empirical data on links between these constructs of interpersonal relationships at work and well-being. In the first paper, a meta-analysis of 144 articles exploring associations of different leadership styles with workers' mental health was conducted (Montano et al. 2017). Transformational leadership, relationship-oriented leadership, and positive leader-follower exchange demonstrated rather consistent positive associations with workers' mental health, whereas an opposite effect was observed for destructive leadership. Overall, statistically significant correlations indicated a moderate effect size of leadership behaviour on mental health, thus justifying the conclusion that 'leadership most likely is an important occupational health factor in its own right' (Montano et al. 2017, p. 344). Of interest, while most studies were interested in the well-being of followers, one review focused on leaders' own well-being. Not surprisingly, positive associations with transformational and relationship-focused behaviour, and negative associations with destructive leadership were apparent (Kaluza et al. 2020). A second systematic review, dealing with team dynamics and participation, supplements this knowledge although it does not contain a meta-analysis of findings (Fox et al. 2021). In general, the quality of intervention studies was found to be limited, but high-quality studies pointed to positive effects of team dynamics, collaboration, and organizational culture on job satisfaction, exhaustion, and additional indicators of well-being (Glisson et al. 2006; Glisson et al. 2012). A somewhat larger number of appropriate studies evaluating interventions increasing the effects of organizational participation on well-being was identified. For instance, main results confirmed beneficial effects of improved workflow, communication, and participation in a primary care organizational context (Linzer et al. 2017). In a well-designed intervention on hospital wards, improved participation among health-care professionals contributed to a significant longer-term reduction of work-related burnout (Bourbonnais et al. 2011). On balance, comparing the consistency of favourable mental health effects, intervention studies dealing with leadership behaviour demonstrate stronger links than studies focusing on team climate and participation. Yet, more high-quality studies in this field are required.

10.2.3 Work organization

A variety of systematic reviews aimed to assess the research evidence on health effects of organization-level interventions to improve psychosocial work environments (Bambra et al. 2009; Daniels et al. 2017; Fox et al. 2021; Lamontagne et al. 2007; Tetrick and Winslow 2015). These important contributions reveal an impressive richness of approaches and findings, but they also point to difficulties of harmonizing and generalizing available knowledge. A major difficulty results from the heterogeneity of intervention targets. According to one tradition, intervention targets focus on one specific component within the complexity of psychosocial work environments. Job rotation, flexible work, job enrichment, or skill development are examples. Modifying one distinct component by a preventive programme enables researchers to quantify the effects that are attributable to the intervention. Moreover, replication and standardization of a specific programme seem to be quite feasible. For these reasons, this tradition represents mainstream intervention research. However, another tradition claims that comprehensive, multi-component interventions are likely to result in stronger and more sustainable outcomes, as they simultaneously target different critical drivers of adverse health. For instance, as the main theoretical models of psychosocial work environments predicting adverse health include several components, all components need to be integrated in a preventive programme to produce the intended effect. Another version of the multi-component approach combines material and psychosocial components of work environments, or it integrates traditional safety and health services with the promotion of health behaviour and well-being (the US 'Total Worker Health' approach (see below)). The co-existence of these two traditions of organization-level intervention research and practice enlarges and enriches the scope of available interventions, but it may also delay advancement to a generalized, universally applied approach.

Table 10.3A displays summary information derived from systematic reviews of some workplace health programmes that focus on one specific organizational intervention target. As a selection criterion, at least five independent studies had to be included in a systematic review to provide a minimum level of empirical evidence. In studies evaluating health benefits of work time reduction without reduction of salary, some positive effects were observed, but two studies included a physical activity intervention, and three studies were of poor quality. Therefore, only a tentative conclusion can be drawn (Voglino et al. 2022). Evidence is more robust on positive effects of flexible work schedules on several indicators of well-being, as nine out of eleven studies were of high quality, and as a majority reported positive effects on a spectrum of well-being measures (Fox et al. 2021). This finding is even more important, as this extensive systematic review included additional studies evaluating associations of self-scheduling of working time and of beneficial shift change with well-being. Although of lower methodological quality, a majority of results of these two additional targets supported a health-enhancing effect (Fox et al. 2021). Modifying schedules among shift workers is a particularly relevant time-related

Table 10.3A Health outcomes derived from systematic reviews of some intervention studies targeting a specific organizational component

Author(s) year	Target	Number of studies	Main content	Health outcomes
Voglino et al. 2022	Reduced working time	7	Daily or weekly reduction of work hours by some 25 per cent sleep quality with retained salary	Fatigue ↓, stress ↓
Fox et al. 2021	Flexible work arrangement	11	Flexible schedules of work hours or work location	Burnout ↓, perceived stress ↓, exhaustion ↓, somatic symptoms ↓, sleep quality ↑
Bambra et al. 2007	Task variety	8	Increased responsibility; introduction of new tasks	Exhaustion, somatic symptoms: small or inconclusive effects
Egan et al. 2007	Job control	8	Increased employee participation and / or job autonomy; multi-skilling	Absenteeism ↓, burnout ↓, job stress ↓, mental health ↑

↓, reduction, ↑ improvement.

intervention target, as indicated by a critical review of night shift work interventions and their health effects (Neil-Sztramko et al. 2014). This review was not included in Table 10.3A, as the review included additional types of intervention and as the evidence on health effects was inconsistent. The systematic review of Bambra et al. (2007) analysed three partly overlapping targets—job variety, teamwork, and autonomous groups. Job variety was the category with the closest link to organizational-level change. Half of the eight studies concerned nurses who were trained for new tasks, and no conclusive health effects were observed. Only one study, dealing with manual workers in a postal office, reported reduced musculoskeletal complaints. Similarly, the review by Egan et al. (2007) combined findings from several types of preventive programmes, with job control demonstrating the closest link to organizational change. More than half of programmes with increased job autonomy including multi-skilling pointed to modest improvements in mental health and reduced absenteeism. These latter two

Table 10.3B Health outcomes derived from systematic reviews or original studies of multi-component interventions

Author(s) year	Target	Number of studies	Main content	Health outcomes
Daniels et al. 2017	Job redesign and skills-training	15	Improvement of job tasks and quality of employment in combination with training on the job	Subjective well-being ↑, physical health ↑
Montano et al. 2014b	Material and psychosocial targets	12	Reduced physical workload combined with organizational improvement	↓Back pain, injury, sick leave, eczema
Brisson et al. 2016	Main components of the DC and ERI models as targets	3	Reduced demands, increased support and control; improved esteem/respect	↓ Burnout, distress, blood pressure
Anger et al. 2019	Total worker health (TWH) approach	38	Safety and health measures plus either health promotion or improved psychosocial work	↑ Health behaviour; ↓ weight, pain, injury, absenteeism, exhaustion, blood pressure

↓, reduction, ↑ improvement.

reviews interpreted main findings in terms of the DC model of stressful work, although this model was not explicitly tested in these programmes, in contrast to some multi-component interventions (Table 10.3B).

In Table 10.3B, results from systematic reviews or original studies examining multi-component organization-level programmes are shown. A highly detailed review evaluated the combined effects of job redesign and skills training (Daniels et al. 2017). In a majority of the fifteen investigations analysing this change, some beneficial effects on health and well-being were observed, independent of whether skilling was closely related to redesigning activity or was provided as a general commitment to employees' qualification. The authors concluded that embedding job redesign in wider employment practices of the organization yields positive effects on workers' performance and well-being. A second systematic review was not only interested in comparing material and psychosocial targets of organizational changes, but also in the health effect evolving from multi-component compared to single-component interventions. Twelve out of thirty-three interventions offered combined programmes. Of these, nine found a positive association with the health outcome (Montano et al. 2014a, supplement tables S1 sand S2). The authors tended to support the hypothesis that 'interventions addressing different types of working conditions simultaneously may increase the chances of producing a beneficial effect on the outcome' (Montano et al. 2014a, p. 6). Distinct from systematic reviews, a narrative review summarized health effects of three multi-component organizational interventions that aimed to reduce work-related stress due to high demand/high effort and low control/low reward (Brisson et al. 2016). All three organizations were located in Québec, Canada: a group of long-term care centres, two acute care hospitals, and three large semi-public services with white-collar employees. Significant improvements in mental health were documented in the second and third study. Moreover, small, but significant reductions in systolic and diastolic blood pressure after one year were obvious in the intervention group (Brisson et al. 2016). The programme 'Total Worker Health' (TWH), promoted by the National Institute of Occupational Safety and Health (NIOSH) in the US, represents a further important multi-component intervention approach. It aims to integrate traditional safety and health services with programmes improving workers' health, by strengthening health behaviour and reducing stress at work (Guerin et al. 2021; Punnett 2022; see also Landsbergis et al. 2018). A detailed systematic review of 38 studies with good methodological quality confirms rather consistent beneficial effects of this programme on well-being (mostly improved health behaviour, but also reduced pain, injury, absenteeism, exhaustion, blood pressure) (Anger et al. 2019). Only five studies explicitly addressed the psychosocial work environment as a target.

So far, most organization-level changes reported effects on mental health. Very few documented changes in physical health, such as risk factors for major chronic diseases. The Canadian white-collar workplace change study, described above (Brisson et al. 2016), is an exception. Figure 10.1 displays a reduced prevalence of hypertension in the intervention group after six months and after three years. In addition, a significant difference in mean systolic blood pressure of 2 mmHg between intervention and control group was observed (Trudel et al. 2021).

In the context of measures mitigating climate change a reduction of weekly working days received increased attention. Effects of this measure on limiting the extent of commuting traffic and on widening remote work on working people's well-being and on economic outcomes were analysed in the world's largest four-day working week trial conducted by a team at the University of Cambridge (Lewis et al. 2023). This trial revealed convincing positive effects for employees' well-being as well as for companies' productivity (see Box 10.4). Thus, it represents a promising organizational intervention with beneficial impact on workers' well-being, companies' performances, and environmental protection.

In summary, among the interventions focusing on one target, beneficial effects on health and well-being result from flexible work arrangements and

Box 10.4 The United Kingdom's four-day week pilot

The trial:

- Sixty-one companies from diverse sectors and of different sizes participated in a trial that involved 2,900 employees.
- They agreed to introduce a meaningful reduction in working time, mainly in terms of a four-day week, with pay maintained at 100 per cent.

Main findings:

- Fifty-six companies continued the new working time approach after termination of the trial.
- On average, companies' revenue increased by thirty-five per cent.
- Seventy-one per cent of employees reported a lower level of burnout during the trial, and forty per cent indicated a reduction in sleep difficulties.
- Sixty per cent of employees increased their ability to combine work with core responsibilities, thus improving work-life balance.
- The number of staff leaving the company dropped by fifty-seven per cent over the trial period (Lewis et al. 2023).

from reduced working time. Effects of job variety and increased job control are less well documented. It seems that positive health effects are more likely to result from multi-component approaches as all four types of programmes document some improvement of workers' health and well-being (Table 10.3 B). These results underline a promising role of organization-level interventions that modify psychosocial work environments by structural measures.

10.2.4 Economic evaluation

With our exclusive focus on employees' health and well-being, we did not cover other important benefits. Several publications emphasize that the implementation of organization-level workplace programmes can produce important spill-over effects on the whole organization, strengthening collaboration, motivation, readiness for further change, and productivity gain (Daniels et al. 2017; Lamontagne et al. 2007; Nielsen et al. 2010). For employers and managers, the economic benefits of interventions are of primary interest, and return on investment is a main criterion to decide on further implementation of organizational change. In fact, economic evaluations of workplace prevention programmes were mainly performed from the perspective of employers, calculating cost-effectiveness or via cost-benefit analysis (Johanson and Aboagye 2020). In these cases, intervention costs are compared with costs saved due to reduction of absenteeism or other proxy measures of productivity loss. Although successful workplace interventions are likely to result in some productivity gain, there is an inherent tension between the increase of costs due to the development and implementation of a programme and the delay of return on investment due to longer-term outcomes of employees' presence and performance. This tension eventually prevents employers and managers from making timely decisions to invest in measures of workers' health promotion.

Despite the undisputed relevance of high costs of productivity loss due to work-related ill health, the development of health economic research in this area has been hindered by methodological challenges. Obviously, it is difficult to measure productivity changes and related intervention benefits in a standardized, quantified way. A systematic review of economic evaluations of conventional occupational safety and health interventions concluded that the current state of knowledge is characterized by a low level of standardization and a variety of assessment approaches, aggravating a comparable estimation of costs (Steel et al. 2018). For the more specific field of organization-level workplace interventions the evidence base is even less developed, both in quantitative and qualitative terms. Here, the challenge of enriching the measurement of programme benefit by integrating non-monetary indicators (such as well-being or quality-adjusted life years (QALYs) provides an additional difficulty (Nasamu et al. 2022). A recent systematic review of economic evaluations of mental health interventions with components focusing on the work environment concluded that the paucity of studies dealing with primary and secondary prevention was too small to allow any comparative analysis (Gaillard et al. 2020). Solid evidence of significant return on investment in this review was restricted to studies on tertiary prevention programmes. This gap in knowledge seems critical in view of the large amount of preventive needs due to the tangible impact of adverse psychosocial work environments on workers' mental health (see Chapter 6).

Evidently, more substantial research findings based on standardized assessments are required before solid estimates of economic benefits of organizational changes of adverse psychosocial work environments will be available.

10.3 Summary

The content of this chapter has offered useful information on principles and procedures of workplace health promotion programmes at the level of companies/businesses, their development and implementation, and on the evaluation of health effects attributable to interventions. Several programmes documented beneficial health effects, including cognitive behavioural interventions (individual level), positive leadership styles and enhanced employee participation (group level), flexible work schedules, and multi-component changes of work environments (structural level).

10.4 Relevant questions

- Assume that you organize a well-grounded intervention programme to promote a healthy psychosocial work environment. What are the main obstacles you are likely to face when implementing the programme?

Which ones of these obstacles can be successfully removed, and how?

- Can you briefly describe main strengths and weaknesses of a multi-component workplace health promotion approach, compared to a single-component approach?

In conclusion, if you had a choice, which approach would you prefer?

- Managers usually look for economic efficacy when deciding about a workplace occupational health intervention. Why is it equally important to inform them, based on solid evidence, about the expected health benefits to their employees?

Recommended reading

❖ Brough, P., Gardiner, E., and Daniels, K. (eds.) (2022), *Handbook on management and employment policies*. Cham: Springer.
❖ Cunningham, C. J. L., and Black, K. J. (2021), *Essentials of occupational health psychology*. New York, NY: Routledge.
❖ Landsbergis, P. A., Dobson, M., LaMontagne, A. D., et al. (2018), 'Occupational stress'. In B. S. Levy, D. H. Wegman, S. L. Baron, and R. K. Sokas (eds.), *Occupational and environmental health* 7th edn. Oxford: Oxford University Press, 325–44.
❖ Tetrick, L. E., and Winslow, C. J. (2015), 'Workplace stress management interventions and health promotion', *Annu Rev Organ Psychol Organ Behav*, 2 (1), 583–603.
❖ von Thiele Schwarz, U., Nielsen, K., Edwards, K., et al. (2021), 'How to design, implement and evaluate organizational interventions for maximum impact: the Sigtuna Principles', *Eur J Work Organ Psychol*, 30 (3), 415–27.

Useful websites

- International Labour Organization (ILO), Workplace health promotion and well-being https://www.ilo.org/global/topics/safety-and-health-at-work/areasofwork/workplace-health-promotion-and-well-being/lang--en/index.htm
- World Health Organization (WHO), Mental health at work https://www.who.int/news-room/fact-sheets/detail/mental-health-at-work
- European Agency for Safety and Health at Work (EU-OSHA), Healthy Workplaces Campaign https://healthy-workplaces.eu/
- U.S. National Institute for Occupational Safety and Health (NIOSH), Total Worker Health® Program https://www.cdc.gov/NIOSH/twh/
- Center for Social Epidemiology, Healthy Work Campaign: https://www.healthywork.org/

References

Abildgaard, J. S., Hasson, H., von Thiele Schwarz, U., et al. (2020), 'Forms of participation: The development and application of a conceptual model of participation in work environment interventions', *Econ Ind Democr,* 41 (3), 746–69.

Anger, W. K., Rameshbabu, A., Olson, R., et al. (2019), 'Effectiveness of Total Worker Health® interventions'. In H. L. Hudson, J. A. S. Nigam, S. L. Sauter, L. C. Chosewood, A. L. Schill, and J. Howard (eds.), *Total worker health.* Washington: American Psychological Association, 61–89.

Aust, B., and Ducki, A. (2004), 'Comprehensive health promotion interventions at the workplace: experiences with health circles in Germany', *J Occup Health Psychol,* 9 (3), 258–70.

Bambra, C., Egan, M., Thomas, S., et al. (2007), 'The psychosocial and health effects of workplace reorganisation. 2. A systematic review of task restructuring interventions', *J Epidemiol Community Health,* 61 (12), 1028–37.

Bambra, C., Gibson, M., Sowden, A. J., et al. (2009), 'Working for health? Evidence from systematic reviews on the effects on health and health inequalities of organisational changes to the psychosocial work environment', *Prev Med,* 48 (5), 454–61.

Barck-Holst, P., Nilsonne, Å., Åkerstedt, T., et al. (2017), 'Reduced working hours and stress in the Swedish social services: a longitudinal study', *Int Soc Work,* 60 (4), 897–913.

Bourbonnais, R., Brisson, C., and Vezina, M. (2011), 'Long-term effects of an intervention on psychosocial work factors among healthcare professionals in a hospital setting', *Occup Environ Med,* 68 (7), 479–86.

Brisson, C., Gilbert-Ouimet, M. D., C., Trudel, X., et al. (2016), 'Workplace interventions aiming to improve psychosocial work factors and related health'. In J. Siegrist and M. Wahrendorf (eds.), *Work stress and health in a globalized economy.* Cham: Springer, 333–63.

Brooks, S., and Wilkinson, A. (2022), 'Employee voice as a route to wellbeing'. In P. Brough, E. Gardiner, and K. Daniels (eds.), *Handbook on management and employment practices.* Cham: Springer, 351–68.

Brough, P., Timms, C., Chan, X. W., et al. (2020), 'Work-life balance: definitions, causes, and consequences'. In T. Theorell (ed.), *Handbook of socioeconomic determinants of occupational health: from macro-level to micro-level evidence.* Cham: Springer, 473–87.

Burgess, M. G., Brough, P., Biggs, A., et al. (2020), 'Why interventions fail: a systematic review of occupational health psychology interventions', *Int J Stress Manag,* 27 (2), 195.

Colquitt, J. A. (2001), 'On the dimensionality of organizational justice: a construct validation of a measure', *J Appl Psychol,* 86 (3), 386–400.

Cooper, C. L., Pandey, A., and Quick, J. C. (2012), *Downsizing: is less still more?* Cambridge: Cambridge University Press.

Cooper, C. L., and Quick, J. C. (eds.) (2017), *The handbook of stress and health.* Chichester: Wiley Blackwell.

Costa, G. (2020), 'Shift work and occupational hazards'. In T. Theorell (ed.), *Handbook of socioeconomic determinants of occupational health: from macro-level to micro-level evidence*. Cham: Springer, 207–24.

Cox, T., Karanika, M., Griffiths, A., et al. (2007), 'Evaluating organizational-level work stress interventions: beyond traditional methods', *Work Stress*, 21 (4), 348–62.

Cunningham, C. J. L., and Black, K. J. (2021), *Essentials of occupational health psychology*. New York, NY: Routledge.

Daniels, K., Gedikli, C., Watson, D., et al. (2017), 'Job design, employment practices and well-being: a systematic review of intervention studies', *Ergonomics*, 60 (9), 1177–96.

Daniels, K., Watson, D., Nayani, R., et al. (2021), 'Implementing practices focused on workplace health and psychological wellbeing: a systematic review', *Soc Sci Med*, 277, 113888.

Demerouti, E., Bakker, A. B., Nachreiner, F., et al. (2001), 'The job demands-resources model of burnout', *J Appl Psychol*, 86 (3), 499–512.

Dollard, M. F., Dormann, C., and Idris, M. A. (2019), *Psychosocial safety climate: a new work stress theory*. Cham: Springer.

Ebert, D. D., Berking, M., Thiart, H., et al. (2015), 'Restoring depleted resources: efficacy and mechanisms of change of an internet-based unguided recovery training for better sleep and psychological detachment from work', *Health Psychol*, 34S, 1240–51.

Egan, M., Bambra, C., Thomas, S., et al. (2007), 'The psychosocial and health effects of workplace reorganisation. 1. A systematic review of organisational-level interventions that aim to increase employee control', *J Epidemiol Community Health*, 61 (11), 945–54.

European Agency for Safety and Health at Work (2022), 'Managing psychosocial risks in European micro and small enterprises: Denmark country report', (Bilbao: EU-OSHA).

Falk, A., Kosse, F., Menrath, I., et al. (2018), 'Unfair pay and health', *Manag Sci*, 64 (4), 1477–88.

Fox, K. E., Johnson, S. T., Berkman, L. F., et al. (2021), 'Organisational-and group-level workplace interventions and their effect on multiple domains of worker well-being: a systematic review', *Work Stress*, 36 (1), 30–59.

Gaillard, A., Sultan-Taïeb, H., Sylvain, C., et al. (2020), 'Economic evaluations of mental health interventions: a systematic review of interventions with work-focused components', *Saf Sci*, 132, 104982.

Glisson, C., Dukes, D., and Green, P. (2006), 'The effects of the ARC organizational intervention on caseworker turnover, climate, and culture in children's service systems', *Child Abuse Negl*, 30 (8), 855–80; discussion 49-54.

Glisson, C., Hemmelgarn, A., Green, P., et al. (2012), 'Randomized trial of the Availability, Responsiveness, and Continuity (ARC) organizational intervention with community-based mental health programs and clinicians serving youth', *J Am Acad Child Adolesc Psychiatry*, 51 (8), 780–7.

Goetzel, R. Z., Long, S. R., Ozminkowski, R. J., et al. (2004), 'Health, absence, disability, and presenteeism cost estimates of certain physical and mental health conditions affecting US employers', *J Occup Environ Med*, 46 (4), 398–412.

Guerin, R. J., Harden, S. M., Rabin, B. A., et al. (2021), 'Dissemination and implementation science approaches for occupational safety and health research: implications for advancing total worker health', *Int J Environ Res Public Health*, 18 (21), 11050.

Hawkes, A. J., and Spedding, J. (2022), 'Successful leadership'. In P. Brough, E. Gardiner, and K. Daniels (eds.), *Handbook on management and employment practices*. Cham: Springer, 15–42.

Johanson, U., and Aboagye, E. (2020), 'Financial gains, possibilities, and limitations of improving occupational health at the company level'. In T. Theorell (ed.), *Handbook of socioeconomic determinants of occupational health: from macro-level to micro-level evidence*. Cham: Springer, 537–53.

Kaluza, A. J., Boer, D., Buengeler, C., et al. (2020), 'Leadership behaviour and leader self-reported well-being: a review, integration and meta-analytic examination', *Work Stress*, 34 (1), 34–56.

Karasek, R. A., Brisson, C., Kawakami, N., et al. (1998), 'The Job Content Questionnaire (JCQ): an instrument for internationally comparative assessments of psychosocial job characteristics', *J Occup Health Psychol*, 3 (4), 322–55.

Kawakami, N., and Tsutsumi, A. (2016), 'The Stress Check Program: a new national policy for monitoring and screening psychosocial stress in the workplace in Japan', *J Occup Health*, 58 (1), 1–6.

Kawakami, N., Araki, S., Kawashima, M., et al. (1997), 'Effects of work-related stress reduction on depressive symptoms among Japanese blue-collar workers', *Scand J Work Environ Health*, 23 (1), 54–9.

Kristensen, T. S., Hannerz, H., Hogh, A., et al. (2005), 'The Copenhagen Psychosocial Questionnaire – a tool for the assessment and improvement of the psychosocial work environment', *Scand J Work Environ Health*, 31 (6), 438–49.

Kuehnl, A., Seubert, C., Rehfuess, E., et al. (2019), 'Human resource management training of supervisors for improving health and well-being of employees', *Cochrane Database Syst Rev*, 9 (9), CD010905.

Lamontagne, A. D., Keegel, T., Louie, A. M., et al. (2007), 'A systematic review of the job-stress intervention evaluation literature, 1990–2005', *Int J Occup Environ Health*, 13 (3), 268–80.

Landsbergis, P. A., Dobson, M., LaMontagne, A. D., et al. (2018), 'Occupational stress'. In B. S. Levy, D. H. Wegman, S. L. Baron, and R. K. Sokas (eds.), *Occupational and environmental health* 7th edn. Oxford: Oxford University Press, 325–44.

Leka, S., and Jain, A. (2020), 'Surveillance, monitoring, and evaluation'. In U. Bültmann and J. Siegrist (eds.), *Handbook of disability, work and health*. Cham: Springer, 273–88.

Leka, S., and Jain, A. (2022), 'Managing health, safety, and well-being at work within changing legal and policy frameworks'. In P. Brough, E. Gardiner, and K. Daniels (eds.), *Handbook on management and employment practices*. Cham: Springer, 809 25.

Lewis, K., Schor, J., and Frayne, D. (2023), 'UK's 4 day week pilot results report 2023', https://policycommons.net/artifacts/3450620/uk-4-day-week-pilot-results-report-2023/4250877/, accessed 20 March 2023.

Linzer, M., Poplau, S., Brown, R., et al. (2017), 'Do work condition interventions affect quality and errors in primary care? Results from the Healthy Work Place Study', *J Gen Intern Med*, 32 (1), 56–61.

Martin, A., Shann, C., and LaMontagne, A. D. (2020), 'Promoting workplace mental wellbeing: a rapid review of recent intervention research'. In U. Bültmann and J. Siegrist (eds.), *Handbook of disability, work and health*. Cham: Springer, 289–308.

Montano, D., Hoven, H., and Siegrist, J. (2014a), 'Effects of organisational-level interventions at work on employees' health: a systematic review', *BMC Public Health*, 14, 135.

Montano, D., Hoven, H., and Siegrist, J. (2014b), 'A meta-analysis of health effects of randomized controlled worksite interventions: does social stratification matter?', *Scand J Work Environ Health*, 40 (3), 230–34.

Montano, D., Reeske, A., Franke, F., et al. (2017), 'Leadership, followers' mental health and job performance in organizations: a comprehensive meta-analysis from an occupational health perspective', *J Organ Behav*, 38 (3), 327–50.

Moorman, R. H. (1991), 'Relationship between organizational justice and organizational citizenship behaviors: do fairness perceptions influence employee citizenship?', *J Applied Psychol*, 76 (6), 845–55.

Nasamu, E., Connolly, S., Bryan, M., et al. (2022), 'Workplace well-being initiatives'. In P. Brough, E. Gardiner, and K. Daniels (eds.), *Handbook on management and employment practices*. Cham: Springer, 749–66.

Neil-Sztramko, S. E., Pahwa, M., Demers, P. A., et al. (2014), 'Health-related interventions among night shift workers: a critical review of the literature', *Scand J Work Environ Health*, 40 (6), 543–56.

Nielsen, K. (2013), 'Review article: how can we make organizational interventions work? Employees and line managers as actively crafting interventions', *Hum Relat*, 66 (8), 1029–50.

Nielsen, K., Randall, R., Holten, A.-L., et al. (2010), 'Conducting organizational-level occupational health interventions: what works?', *Work Stress*, 24 (3), 234–59.

OECD (2017), *OECD guidelines on measuring the quality of the working environment*. Paris: OECD.

Owen, M. S., Bailey, T. S., and Dollard, M. F. (2016), 'Psychosocial safety climate as a multilevel extension of ERI theory: evidence from Australia'. In J. Siegrist and M. Wahrendorf (eds.), *Work stress and health in a globalized economy*. Cham: Springer, 189–217.

Padula, R. S., Comper, M. L. C., Sparer, E. H., et al. (2017), 'Job rotation designed to prevent musculoskeletal disorders and control risk in manufacturing industries: a systematic review', *Appl Ergon*, 58, 386–97.

Pfaff, H., and Schmitt, J. (2021), 'The organic turn: coping with pandemic and non-pandemic challenges by integrating evidence-, theory-, experience-, and context-based knowledge in advising health policy', *Front Public Health*, 9, 727427.

Punnett, L. (2022), 'Response to NIOSH request for information on interventions to prevent work-related stress and support health worker mental health', *New Solut*, 32 (3), 223–29.

Richardson, K. M., and Rothstein, H. R. (2008), 'Effects of occupational stress management intervention programs: a meta-analysis', *J Occup Health Psychol*, 13 (1), 69–93.

Romanowska, J., and Theorell, T. (2020), 'Using arts to support leadership development'. In T. Theorell (ed.), *Handbook of socioeconomic determinants of occupational health: from macro-level to micro-level evidence*. Cham: Springer, 489–504.

Roodbari, H., Nielsen, K., Axtell, C., et al. (2021), 'Developing initial middle range theories in realist evaluation: a case of an organisational intervention', *Int J Environ Res Public Health*, 18 (16), 8360.

Rose, G. (1992), *The strategy of preventive medicine*. Oxford: Oxford University Press.

Semmer, N. K. (2006), 'Job stress interventions and the organization of work', *Scand J Work Environ Health*, 32 (6), 515–27.

Siegrist, J., Starke, D., Chandola, T., et al. (2004), 'The measurement of effort-reward imbalance at work: European comparisons', *Soc Sci Med*, 58 (8), 1483–99.

Siemiatycki, J., and Xu, M. (2020), 'Occupational causes of cancer'. In U. Bültmann and J. Siegrist (eds.), *Handbook of disability, work and health*. Cham: Springer, 127–51.

Song, Z., and Baicker, K. (2019), 'Effect of a workplace wellness program on employee health and economic outcomes: a randomized clinical trial', *JAMA*, 321 (15), 1491–501.

Steel, J., Godderis, L., and Luyten, J. (2018), 'Productivity estimation in economic evaluations of occupational health and safety interventions: a systematic review', *Scand J Work Environ Health*, 44 (5), 458–74.

Tan, L., Wang, M. J., Modini, M., et al. (2014), 'Preventing the development of depression at work: a systematic review and meta-analysis of universal interventions in the workplace', *BMC Med*, 12, 74.

Tetrick, L. E., and Winslow, C. J. (2015), 'Workplace stress management interventions and health promotion', *Annu Rev Organ Psychol Organ Behav*, 2 (1), 583–603.

Trudel, X., Gilbert-Ouimet, M., Vezina, M., et al. (2021), 'Effectiveness of a workplace intervention reducing psychosocial stressors at work on blood pressure and hypertension', *Occup Environ Med*, 78 (10), 738–44.

United Nations (2015), 'Transforming our world: the 2030 Agenda for Sustainable Development', https://sdgs.un.org/2030agenda, accessed 27 Feb 2023.

Vives, A., Amable, M., Ferrer, M., et al. (2010), 'The Employment Precariousness Scale (EPRES): psychometric properties of a new tool for epidemiological studies among waged and salaried workers', *Occup Environ Med*, 67 (8), 548–55.

Voglino, G., Savatteri, A., Gualano, M. R., et al. (2022), 'How the reduction of working hours could influence health outcomes: a systematic review of published studies', *BMJ Open*, 12 (4), e051131.

von Thiele Schwarz, U., Nielsen, K., Edwards, K., et al. (2021), 'How to design, implement and evaluate organizational interventions for maximum impact: the Sigtuna Principles', *Eur J Work Organ Psychol*, 30 (3), 415–27.

Wersun, A., Klatt, J., Azmat, F., et al. (2020), *Blueprint for SDG integration into curricula, research and partnership*. New York, NY: Principles for Responsible Management Education (PRME).

World Health Organization (2019), *The WHO special initiative for mental health (2019–2023): universal health coverage for mental health*. Geneva: WHO.

Yarker, J., Donaldson-Feilder, E., and Lewis, R. (2022), 'Management competencies for health and wellbeing'. In P. Brough, E. Gardiner, and K. Daniels (eds.), *Handbook on management and employment practices*. Cham: Springer, 91–115.

Zwetsloot, G., Leka, S., Kines, P., et al. (2020), 'Vision zero: developing proactive leading indicators for safety, health and wellbeing at work', *Saf Sci*, 130, 104890.

11
Healthy work in a national and international perspective

11.1 Impact of labour and social policies on occupational health

11.1.1 Basic notions

In a world of growing globalization, transnational collaboration, and world-wide connectivity one may ask why national states continue to play a decisive role for their inhabitants. Apart from protection of a legalized territory against all kinds of external threats, national states provide substantial frameworks for the political, economic, social, and cultural functioning of their population. As welfare states, they offer resources to their citizens to meet basic social and economic needs. These resources are transmitted to the public by distinct policies. Policies can be defined as regulatory programmes providing services and benefits to inhabitants according to legally predefined conditions. Labour and social policies are of extraordinary significance in this regard. Important areas of concerns for these policies include the prevention of poverty due to unemployment, access to the labour market and its relevant prerequisites (such as training, reskilling, upskilling), support in case of disease and disability, provision of pensions in old age, good quality and safety at work, reconciliation of work and family life, and welfare measures for children and vulnerable population groups. The provision of some form of labour and social policy is a basic requirement for every national government, and economically advanced, modern societies promoted welfare state policies most markedly during the twentieth century.

The programmes of these policies can be distinguished according to their main target populations. Of central importance is the distinction between protective (or passive) and integrative (or active) labour market policies.

Psychosocial Occupational Health. Johannes Siegrist and Jian Li, Oxford University Press.
© Oxford University Press 2024. DOI: 10.1093/oso/9780192887924.003.0011

The former approach is designed to support working-age people who for different reasons are not employed in paid work. Unemployment benefits and disability pensions are provided via contributory schemes to secure a decent living standard. As a special part of protective programmes, disability policies additionally include measures to reduce the occurrence and severity of disability and to enable return to work, as well as measures that protect against discrimination and social exclusion (Dahl and van der Wel 2020). However, these latter measures also include elements of integrative or active labour market policies that can be defined as efforts to increase supply and demand of labour and as attempts to adapt people's capabilities to the demands of the job market. Within disability programmes, so-called support-side policies are a prominent component of active labour market measures as they proactively integrate people with disability into workplaces by training and professional support in close collaboration with employers (Dahl and van der Wel 2020). The 'Individual Placement and Support' model of supported employment is a widely established approach to this end (see Chapters 8 and 9).

Active (or integrative) labour market policies targeting the supply side address people who are ready to enter or re-enter the labour market and people who need skills and competences to be ready for integration into paid work. Training opportunities, counselling services, and employment projects are the main tools to increase employment participation. Reducing the level and shortening the length of provision of protective benefits are ways of motivating and incentivizing non-working people to re-enter the labour market. These measures need to be supplemented by efforts to improve employability and work ability, and by developing skills and competencies. In addition, demand-side actions are directed towards employers by stimulating the creation of new jobs, by increasing work participation through flexible work schedules and family-friendly working conditions, and by imposing legislation against discrimination (Diderichsen 2020). Evidently, several components of active and passive national labour policies are advanced and extended by supranational regulations and prescriptions. The UN convention on the rights of persons with disabilities (UN General Assembly 2007) and the convention on fundamental rights of workers declared by the International Labour Organization (International Labour Organization 2013) are relevant examples (see below).

In order to bridge gaps between labour and social policies distinct 'reconciliation' programmes were developed to better integrate work and family life obligations (Lunau et al. 2020a). They regulate options of leaving paid work for a limited time (e.g. maternity leave), provide access to child-care services for employed parents, and enable enhanced labour market participation by offering flexible work and employment schemes. The generosity of these measures varies considerably across countries. Up to now, Scandinavian countries have pioneered these developments. In this context, the advantages of flexible work and employment regulations have to be balanced against the risks of reduced security. Income insecurity and job insecurity are potential threats of enhanced flexibilization, specifically among socially less protected, more precarious employment groups.

Other links between labour and social policies, and additional areas of social programmes within national welfare states are not described here as the focus of analysis is on employment opportunities and their impact on quality of life and health. As a core message of these basic notions, it seems evident that active, integrative labour policies provide a promising strategy towards enhancing labour market participation and towards strengthening quality of work and employment. It is therefore of interest to analyse these associations more closely by focusing on countries with strongly developed welfare programmes. While several such countries may serve as models, such as Australia, Canada, or Japan, our emphasis, for two reasons, is on European countries. Firstly, new findings from a number of recent comparative studies across European countries are available that document links between the level of labour policies implemented and the quality of psychosocial work environments. Demonstrating such links offers an important argument in favour of extending the perspective of occupational health promoting activities beyond the meso-structural level of workplace interventions within companies and enterprises (see Chapter 10). Secondly, in addition to advanced developments in single countries, Europe—by establishing the European Union—has developed a comprehensive supranational framework of labour and social policies that strengthen and extend national achievements.

11.1.2 National policies, working conditions, and health—the European experience

Europe is a small continent composed by some fifty countries. It has a long and ambivalent history. On one side, the two world wars during the twentieth century were initiated by European countries, and, in earlier times, Europe was actively involved in many wars and in economic and political expansion, giving rise to colonialism with its unjustified exploitation. On the other side, Western civilization originates from European countries, most markedly from ancient Greek, Roman, and Jewish traditions. Later on, some five or six centuries ago, Europe advanced the global process of modernization, characterized by an unprecedented growth in economic, socio-cultural, technological, and scientific developments. Two advances during the second half of the eighteenth century were decisive forces shaping the new world, the industrial revolution starting in England, and the political revolution in France (see Chapter 2). At least since the beginning of the twentieth century, large parts of populations in many European countries enjoyed a state of welfare in the context of increased life expectancy and widening life chances, including improved opportunities of education and employment. This was the time when the concept of the 'social state' emerged. National governments started to invest in the development of comprehensive social security programmes, such as health-care insurance, pension funds, and unemployment benefits. While coverage by social security measures was initially restricted to the economically active part of populations, these programmes were successively extended to cover the country's whole population. However, large differences in the extent of coverage and the timing of this process are observed across countries. By proposing a typology of welfare state regimes researchers aimed to interpret these differences. According to a classical approach, three types of welfare regimes were distinguished (Esping-Andersen 1990; see Chapter 9). The 'conservative-corporatist' regime provides social security benefits according to insurance contributions derived from employees' salaries, thus privileging those in paid work and their families, where employers contribute to these costs. The generosity of public spending is limited, requiring compensation of certain costs by private payments. Germany is an instructive example of this regime. An even stronger limitation of public spending is observed in the 'liberal' regime, where the state supports vulnerable groups, but relies largely on the investments of an active labour force in private insurance and pension systems. The United Kingdom may serve as an example. Distinct from these two types, the 'social-democratic' regime distributes tax-based welfare services to all citizens according to need, thus minimizing poverty and financial loss in case of illness or unemployment. This system is well developed in Scandinavian countries, but its functioning relies on an economy with extensive labour market participation. The typology of the three welfare state regimes was modified more recently to take additional country differences into account that became apparent from Southern and Eastern Europe. In the former case, family-based social security measures played a more important role, whereas Eastern countries developed heterogenous policies after the breakdown of communist rule.

As a particular strength, the 'welfare state regime' approach allows identification of different priorities between countries in assigning responsibility to public vs private stakeholders when coping with basic social security needs. Yet, a limitation with this generalized approach is that it is not possible to disentangle the differential significance of single components within a country's framework of social security programmes, an important prerequisite for analysing population health effects. For instance, educational policies may be rather similar across these regimes, while labour policies vary strongly, offering full protection to jobless people in one regime while leaving them exposed to poverty risk in another. Therefore, welfare research concerned with health effects increasingly relied on country-specific indicators of distinct components of national labour and social policies (Dahl and van der Wel 2013). These indicators use available information on the amount of expenditure for a specific policy, or they rely on institutional regulations, such as eligibility criteria for access to benefits (Lunau et al. 2020a). By this inductive approach, cross-national comparisons between European countries enable the analysis of differences in investments into distinct policies and their associations with working, living, and health conditions of the country's population. The next section presents several examples of such cross-national analyses, demonstrating a significant role of national welfare policies for quality of life across Europe.

Europe was not only advancing welfare measures at the level of single states, but—with the establishment of the European Union—it developed its own supranational framework of social and labour policies. Twenty-eight countries—now twenty-seven after the British exit—formed a political and economic union founded upon numerous treaties. This union was developed along three basic 'pillars', one regulating economic, social, and environmental policies, one establishing a common foreign and security policy, and one dealing with supranational police and jurisdiction. Concerning occupational health, the first 'pillar' is of crucial significance as a common social policy was developed, regulated by legislation, guidelines, and concerted practices. This policy focuses on the three goals of promoting equal opportunities and access to the labour market, strengthening fair working conditions, and ensuring social protection and inclusion. By a series of binding directives released by the European Commission, these goals were successively implemented in the member states. The Safety and

Health Work Directive enacted in 1989 is one example. Based on this legislation a 'European Union (EU) strategic framework on health and safety at work 2021–2027' was launched (for detailed information, see 'Useful websites'). This recent initiative proposes measures and means to adapt to the new world of work, to strengthen the prevention of work-related diseases and accidents, and to prepare for tackling future health threats. Member states are supported in these efforts by financial resources (EU funds) and by research and counselling activities. In this way, a supranational framework supplements and deepens national social and labour policies of member states of the European Union, providing a robust policy background for the development of sustainable and healthy work (Abrahamsson 2021).

11.1.2.1 Links between national policies and psychosocial work environments

Empirical analyses of links between labour and social policies and the quality of psychosocial work environments rely on three crucial preconditions. Firstly, comparable data on reliably assessed indicators of psychosocial work environments across several countries are required. This requirement can be met by relying on cross-country analyses applying measures of main models of stressful work in their study design. In fact, in the European context, this was mainly accomplished with regard to the demand-control (DC) and the effort-reward imbalance (ERI) models of stressful work. For instance, several reports on associations between stressful work and cardiovascular health listed in Chapter 6 used these models in cross-country studies (Dragano et al. 2017; Kivimäki et al. 2012). Fortunately, two large-scale cross-national European studies including a longitudinal dimension and focusing on working populations were established within the past two or three decades and included some indicators of these two models in their study design. These are the Survey of Health, Aging and Retirement in Europe, and the European Working Conditions Survey:

- Survey of Health, Aging and Retirement in Europe (SHARE) (Börsch-Supan et al. 2011):
  Since 2004, a longitudinal survey of aging populations beyond age 50 was conducted in eleven European countries, with repeated data waves every two years. The number of countries was extended in later waves (e.g. 15 in 2010/11), and in the third wave (2008/9), a retrospective assessment of work-related life course experience was

included (SHARELIFE). This unique cross-national cohort contains a broad spectrum of socio-economic, socio-cultural, and health-related data, based on high-quality standards of social survey research. It was developed in close collaboration with the English Longitudinal Study of Ageing (ELSA) (Marmot et al. 2003). Information on links between national policies and quality of work represent a small fraction only (and a limited time period) of this comprehensive multi-disciplinary study (for detailed information on SHARE see 'Useful websites').

• European Working Conditions Survey (EWCS) (Eurofound 2022): Developed, conducted, and analysed by Eurofound, this repeated survey collects standardized individual data on working conditions from representative random samples of working populations in several European countries. Started in 1990, waves are repeated every five years. From 2005, twenty-seven countries are included. Unlike SHARE, this is not a cohort study. Therefore, it contains non-repeated individual data, whereas at the level of populations (e.g. countries) repeated data are available. The country sample size was about a thousand in each wave. Again, this is a very comprehensive dataset, where the focus on national policies and psychosocial work environments reflects a small fraction only (for detailed information on EWCS see 'Useful websites').

In both surveys, abbreviated measures of the DC and ERI models of stressful psychosocial work were included. SHARE initially assessed the component of control by using two items, the component of effort by using two items, and the component of reward by using five items. Likert-scaled items were derived from the original scales. Scale scores were composed, and a ratio of effort and reward was constructed to quantify imbalance at individual level (Lunau et al. 2015). In SHARELIFE, a list of sixteen items was applied to assess retrospectively the quality of working life. Eleven items measured demand/effort, control, reward, and social support at work. Five further items assessed the overall satisfaction with work. Information was either used as a binary summary index or as variables representing the single theoretical dimensions (Wahrendorf and Siegrist 2014). In EWCS, proxy measures were constructed from a broader set of items, representing control by ten items, effort by four items, and reward by five items (Rigó et al. 2022).

As a second precondition, comparable indicators of national labour and social policies had to be available for integration into these studies. As the data concerned countries rather than individuals, they could be derived from established administrative databases and inserted in secondary data analysis. In both surveys, selected indicators of active (ALMPs) and passive, protective labour market policies (PLMPs) were used, mainly derived from OECD or EUROSTAT databases (for a related description in EWCS, see Lunau et al. 2020b; for a detailed description in SHARE, see Wahrendorf and Siegrist 2014). Having cross-sectional data on indicators of psychosocial work environment and on national labour policies, enables the analysis of associations between the two measures. Additionally, some datasets (e.g. EWCS) can be categorized as comparative longitudinal datasets including repeated cross-sectional observations on countries. This allows the use of multilevel statistical analysis. Including higher-group units into the analysis of comparative longitudinal individual-level survey data is an appropriate way to reflect the hierarchical structure of information. Accordingly, in multilevel linear models individuals (level 1) are clustered in country-years, while countries are observed in several consecutive years (level 2), and country-years are clustered in countries (level 3) (Rigó et al. 2022).

The first results from the two studies meeting these preconditions are derived from SHARELIFE. In 2008/9, 11,181 retired female and male participants from thirteen European countries assessed the stressfulness of their psychosocial work environment retrospectively, based on the list of sixteen items mentioned, and additional relevant sociodemographic and biographical data were collected. As a core research question, the impact of proximal factors (adverse childhood circumstances; disadvantaged access to labour market) vs distal factors (integrative and protective labour policies) on stressful work was analysed. This outcome variable was defined by a sum score of the sixteen items, ranging from 0 (no stress) to 48 (high stress) (Wahrendorf and Siegrist 2014). To measure national policies, two indices developed by OECD were integrated in the analysis, a compensation and an integration index. Each index listed the availability and quality of ten respective programmes for each country, varying from a score of 0 (poorest policy) to 50 (best policy). In a series of multilevel linear models, the effect sizes of proximal vs distal factors on stressful work were estimated. In the final model, a highly significant regression coefficient of the variable measuring integration policies was observed, explaining a large amount of the between-country variation. To visualize this latter observation, mean scores of stressful work per country were plotted against the two policy indices. The results are displayed in Figure 11.1. Associations are less pronounced in case of the compensation index ($R^2 = 24.2$) than in case of the integration index ($R^2 = 66.5$). Poor integration policies go along with high

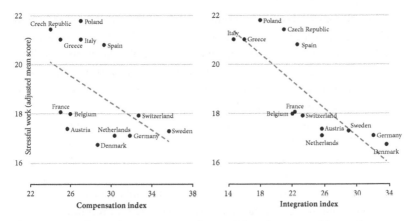

Figure 11.1 Adjusted mean scores of stressful work among older male and female employees (N = 11,181) and policy indices. Mean scores of stressful work are adjusted for sex, age, retirement age, periods of disability, job absence due to disability, childhood circumstances (occupational position of main breadwinner, number of books, housing conditions and overcrowding), and labour market disadvantage (occupational position in main job, involuntary job loss (late off) and plant closure) and period of unemployment.

Source: Reproduced with permission from Wahrendorf, M., and Siegrist, J. (2014), 'Proximal and distal determinants of stressful work: framework and analysis of retrospective European data', *BMC Public Health*, 14, 849. [Figure 3, p. 9] (Creative Commons Attribution 4.0 International License, https://creativecommons.org/licenses/by/4.0/).

work stress levels (in countries like Italy, Greece, Poland). Conversely, high integration investments are associated with poor work stress (in countries like Denmark, Germany, Sweden) (Wahrendorf and Siegrist 2014).

In a further study, based on SHARE data from the fourth wave (2010/11) and supplemented by comparable data from the ELSA study, associations of stressful psychosocial work with policy indicators were again investigated. This analysis included sixteen European countries and put a special focus on social inequalities of stressful work (Lunau et al. 2015). In this multilevel analysis, two single components of integrative national policies (coverage of training on the job; level of public spending on return to work) and two components of protective policies (financial replacement rate after job loss; total expenditures of disability pensions and unemployment benefits) were used. Work stress was assessed by the short scales of effort, reward, and control. Three findings are of interest in this context. Firstly, higher levels of education (as indicator of socioeconomic position) were associated with lower levels of work stress. As a second result, mean levels of stressful work were lower in countries with high investments in labour and social policies, specifically in case of integrative policies. Thirdly, the steepness of educational differences in stressful work was attenuated in these countries. This was obvious for both work stress models (results not shown; Lunau et al. 2015).

Yet, longitudinal information is required, and two reports derived from EWCS data may contribute to a more robust conclusion. The first report is based on three consecutive data waves from 2005 to 2015 obtained from over 60,000 employed persons recruited from twenty-seven European countries. To estimate longitudinal and cross-country policy effects on stressful work, as measured by abbreviated scales of the two work stress models, three-way multilevel models (individuals, country-years, country) were analysed (Lunau et al. 2020b). In addition to between-country effects, where mean policy scores across all years for each country were used, within-country effects variations of policy scores over time were simultaneously estimated. This enabled a test of whether changes in policy levels over time were related to changes in work stress in respective countries. In these analyses, integrative and protective national policies were measured by the OECD indicators mentioned above. The findings demonstrated that an increase in integrative policies over time was related to a decrease of work stress in terms of effort-reward imbalance within countries (results not shown; Lunau et al. 2020b).

The second study, based on a more comprehensive analysis of EWCS data containing information of five-year waves from 1995 to 2015 on 74,159 participants' occupational position, work stress (DC or job strain model), and covariates, explored longitudinal associations of work stress along occupational positions with labour and social policies derived from fifteen European countries (Rigó et al. 2022). In this analysis, policies were classified according to the country's own agenda, as expressed by the sum of active and passive labour market expenditures over time. Along the tertiles of level of spending, three groups were defined: countries with low policy investments (e.g. Greece), middle investments (e.g. Germany), and high investments (e.g. Sweden). In addition to confirming the expected social gradient of stressful work, the results of a three-way multilevel analysis with individuals nested within country-years nested within countries demonstrated a marked increase of job strain over time among all occupational groups in countries with low policy investments. The increase was particularly steep in the group of most disadvantaged workers (manual low-skilled). In countries with middle or high policy investments, no increase of work stress over time was observed (see Figure 11.2) (Rigó et al. 2022).

To summarize, these cross-country findings from Europe support the hypothesis that a higher level of investment into active labour market policies goes along with a lower level of stressful psychosocial work environment within the country's workforce. However, continued social inequalities point to priorities in preventive efforts.

Undoubtedly, well-established labour and social policies exert positive effects on workers' health and well-being by multiple pathways. Whether psychosocial working conditions improved by labour and social policies result in direct benefits for workers' health has not been demonstrated by the above findings. One can postulate such positive effects (Dragano et al. 2011; Lunau et al. 2013), but more robust evidence will be needed. Perhaps, the case of unemployment offers a promising view. Intervention studies demonstrated that measures of subsidiary employment and job search assistance were associated with improved mental health, in particular if combined with psychological support for self-efficacy and self-esteem (Puig-Barrachina et al. 2020; Rose 2019). Even short-term support, such as provision of a national job retention scheme, as applied during the COVID-19 crisis, resulted in tangible effects on employees' mental health (Wels et al. 2022).

In conclusion, investments in national labour and social policies exert beneficial effects on people's quality of work. By multiple pathways, they strengthen health and well-being, and they reduce human suffering. These beneficial effects of modern welfare states have universal significance. The only reason to focus our analysis on recent developments in European countries relates to the availability of new knowledge on the impact of these policies on psychosocial work environments, derived from cross-national investigations. This evidence underlines the need of extending health-promoting activities among employed populations beyond the level of company-based workplace interventions. If embedded in—and reinforced by—national labour and social policies these activities are likely to produce extended and sustainable beneficial effects.

11.1.3 Contributions of international organizations

The strongest impact of labour and social policies on occupational health occurs at the national level. Nevertheless, there are several supranational

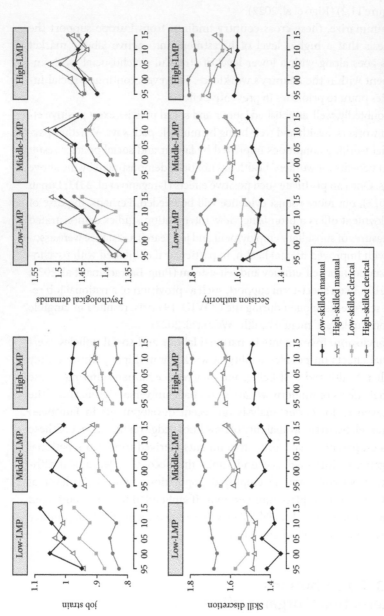

Figure 11.2 Predicted values of job strain by occupational categories and amount of labour market policy spending (N = 74,159). EWCS data 1995–2015 from fifteen European countries. Multilevel regression analysis with covariates. LMP, labour market policy.

Source: Reproduced with permission from Rigó, M., Dragano, N., Wahrendorf, M., et al. (2022), 'Long-term trends in psychosocial working conditions in Europe – the role of labor market policies', *Eur J Public Health*, 32 (3), 384–91. [Extract from Figure 1, p. 388]; (Creative Commons Attribution 4.0 International License, https://creativecommons.org/licenses/by/4.0/).

organizations with relevance to occupational health, acting either as inter-governmental organizations with a legal mandate or as nongovernmental organizations. Core organizations are briefly described in Box 11.1. Their aims vary considerably, with a spectrum reaching from binding conventions on basic rights and standards of occupational safety and health to the dissemination of guidelines and the provision of administrative databases or scientific research evidence.

Other organizations, such as the International Monetary Fund, the World Trade Organization, and the World Bank, deal with matters of relevance for occupational health but do not include the topic in their core business. With the launch of the Sustainable Development Goals initiative (and specifically goal number eight on promoting decent work), the United Nations (UN) put some priority on occupational health (see Chapter 10).

In terms of preventive activities through strengthening occupational safety and health, the conventions released by ILO have by far the strongest supranational impact (International Labour Organization 2019). They are embedded in a larger framework of human rights, as declared in the 'Social Protection Floor Initiative' (International Labour Organization 2013). Yet, so far, many member states resisted ratifying conventions, thus limiting the enforcement of labour standards. In addition, relevant parts of the global workforce are not represented in this organization, either due to informal and precarious employment conditions, including self-employment, or due to declining impact of trade unions (Håkansta 2020; International Labour Organization 2022). Unlike the ILO, WHO does not enforce laws, but rather releases resolutions, recommendations, and guidelines to their member states. For instance, in influential reports, such as the report of the Commission on Social Determinants of Health, it recommends full and fair employment and decent work as priorities of national policy agendas, and it calls for application of occupational health and safety programmes to all workers (World Health Organization 2008). In another comprehensive report, WHO offers guidelines on mental health at work, designed for organizational interventions, for training of managers and workers, and for people with mental health conditions returning to work (World Health Organization 2022). At the level of regional offices, WHO prepared several reviews on social determinants of health, containing sections with recommendations on the reduction of health inequalities through action on employment and working conditions (e.g. World Health Organization 2014). Recommendations and guidelines are also released by OECD. The report on disability and work (OECD 2010) and the guidelines on measuring

Box 11.1 Core international organizations with relevance to occupational health

- International Labour Organization (ILO):
  As a specialized agency of the United Nations (UN), it has a mandate to tackle universal labour and social policy concerns in member states. Its unique organizational structure consists of three ruling bodies, governments, employers' and employees' organizations. It aims at implementing international labour standards and at strengthening occupational safety and health at regional levels. Moreover, ILO continuously publishes influential reports and collaborates with other international organizations.
- World Health Organization (WHO):
  A truly intergovernmental agency of the UN with 193 countries as member states deals with public health on a global scale. In addition to a headquarter in Geneva, Switzerland, it operates through several regional offices. Occupational health is not a central topic but a cross-cutting issue with links mainly to mental health, communicable diseases (COVID-19), and health inequalities. With a large number of worldwide collaborating centres, the WHO advances scientific evidence on determinants of health, prevention, and health care. Recently, a significant collaboration between WHO and ILO has been initiated (see text).
- Organisation for Economic Co-Operation and Development (OECD):
  As an international nongovernmental organization, OECD contributes to policy developments in favour of social and economic progress and availability of sustainable solutions for global challenges. With 38 member states from high-income countries, it focuses on international standard-setting and the provision of expert knowledge through influential reports and policy advice.
- International Commission of Occupational Health (ICOH):
  This is an international professional organization of occupational health experts, their professional associations, and national health and safety institutes that aims to advance and disseminate scientific evidence on work-related diseases, their prevalence, determinants, and prevention.

- International Social Security Association (ISSA):
  Similar to ICOH, this large international organization is concerned with the administration of social security among its member organizations, with a special interest in safety at work and the prevention of injuries. To this end, it develops guidelines and provides services and advice (for detailed information on these organizations, see Håkansta 2020).

the quality of the work environment (OECD 2017) are examples. An interesting recent initiative termed 'Vision Zero' was developed in the frame of International Social Security Association (ISSA) in collaboration with ILO. This large campaign aims to reduce severe accidents and occupational diseases by raising awareness, developing competencies, and capacity building. To this end, enhanced cooperation among professional stakeholders and integration of prevention into social security systems are proposed, based on an explicit culture of prevention shared by leaders and employees acting in participatory ways. This campaign is currently running in more than eighty countries (Björnberg et al. 2022).

Developing scientific evidence on work-related diseases and their prevention is a further important task of international organizations. In 2016, WHO and ILO agreed to establish a scientific cooperation by producing a unified methodology to estimate the work-related burden of disease, using available databases. In 2021, a first report from this collaboration was published (World Health Organization and International Labour Organization 2021). In this methodological approach every major known occupational risk factor was linked to the specific disease resulting from relevant exposure. To this end, the population-attributable fraction of disease was estimated for each risk factor, based on evidence from epidemiological cohort studies. Here, the Global Burden of Disease study provided essential input (GBD 2017 Risk Factor Collaborators 2018). These fractions estimate to what extent the number of deaths or disability-adjusted life years is potentially reduced by removing the occupational risk factor of a specific disease. The analysis was initially focused on carcinogenic hazards and other material occupational risk factors. Asbestos and particulate matters, gases and fumes contributed most to avoidable deaths. In addition, occupational ergonomic factors, injuries, and noise were studied, and they were particularly relevant for the burden of disability-adjusted life years. In the second step of analysis, a new occupational risk factor, long working hours, was considered. The main relevant health outcomes used were stroke and ischaemic heart disease (IHD). With this second step, for the first time, an exposure reflecting material and psychosocial occupational risks was included. Working fifty-five hours or more per week was defined as risk condition, and the hypothesis was tested whether exposure to long working hours was associated with elevate morbidity and mortality risks of these cardiovascular diseases. The results demonstrated that almost nine per cent of the global workforce included were exposed to this excess working time. The population attributable fractions for death were 3.7 per cent for IHD and 9.3 per cent for stroke. In absolute numbers, more than 300,000 deaths from IHD and almost 400,000 deaths from stroke would theoretically be avoided by reducing excess working time to the standard level (35–40 hours per week). Men were at higher risk than women, and those working in the south-east Asian region were most affected (Pega et al. 2021).

These findings have important policy implications. At country level, the ILO convention on limitation of working time (standard: 48 hours per week) should be implemented. So far, fewer than a third of member states have ratified this convention (World Health Organization and International Labour Organization 2021). At the level of companies and organizations, employers, occupational health and safety professionals, and human resource managers are asked to implement appropriate working time conditions and to monitor them. This is an important component within organization-level workplace health promotion measures (see Chapter 10). Working time control is just one of the many aims of occupational health promotion that demonstrates how important it is to extend organization-level activities by policy measures at the national and international level.

11.2 The Global South as a future challenge

This book admittedly offers a selective view of psychosocial occupational health as its substance is derived from research that was mainly conducted in high-income-countries in the Global North over the past several decades. These countries were also pioneering in promoting occupational safety and health measures, in developing labour and social policies, and in improving working and employment conditions during a process of transformation from industrial into post-industrial, service-oriented economies. Neglecting the Global South is therefore a major limitation of this contribution that deserves a further discussion on the final pages.

Before addressing this problem, a few reflections on some further limitations of our analysis may be instructive for readers. As mentioned earlier on, the theoretical basis of psychosocial occupational health research deserves some expansion to unravel new developments in labour markets, technology, and the significance of work for society. Currently dominating concepts were developed during the second half of the twentieth century, a time before the extension of microelectronic revolution, the increase of non-standard employment, and the outbreak of a new pandemic (see Chapter 3). In part, these contextual features may explain the priority put on the world of work, thus neglecting its embeddedness in cross-over and spill-over processes between the two spheres of work and family or private life (Allen and Eby 2016; Shockley et al. 2018; Westman 2001). An extended frame of analysis is also required with regard to the time dimension. Importantly, a life-course perspective on work and health is now increasingly applied in this area of research, considering pre-employment resources and vulnerabilities, bi-directional associations of work and health during more varied and flexible employment histories, and long-term effects on ageing (Hoffmann 2023; Wahrendorf et al. 2023). At the level of transfer of scientific evidence to practices and policies, our attention to opportunities of a pro-active role of researchers and main professional groups involved in occupational health may not have been broad enough (Chapter 10). There are important initiatives of reducing the gap between scientific evidence and real-world practices through innovative training programmes in higher education curricula and in continued education initiatives, in addition to publicizing new knowledge to relevant stakeholders and audiences through different media. As an example, a European network of fourteen national institutes of occupational safety and health (PEROSH) offers webinars on sustainable work. Moreover, this network collaborates on joint research projects dealing with healthy work, and it plays a role in advising authorities and governments on topics covering their expertise (for detailed information, see 'Useful websites'). At the global level, the International Commission of Occupational Health (ICOH) has a similar mission. Yet, so far, activities related to psychosocial occupational health remain scarce. Initiatives should have an even wider scope, given the continued challenge of substantial social inequalities in work and health. For instance, a Health Equity Network has recently been established in the United Kingdom. This is a professional network that aims to support public and private organizations, including businesses, to promote and coordinate their actions on reducing social inequalities in health (for detailed information, see 'Useful websites'). It is hoped that more such efforts can be documented and discussed in the near future.

Dealing with the complexity of problems of occupational health in the Global South is a difficult task. First of all, in general, morbidity and mortality rates are higher, and life expectancy is lower than in high-income countries (GBD 2017 Risk Factor Collaborators 2018). Health-care systems are often unable to adequately deal with this high burden, due to lack of resources and restricted developments. This also holds true for urgent need in case of rehabilitation (Bright et al. 2018). Secondly, as already mentioned (Chapter 2), employment conditions are more precarious, given high rates of informal employment, in-work poverty, and unemployment. High levels of hazardous and stressful working conditions are not mitigated by protective regulations and by appropriate provision of occupational safety and health services. For example, the largest contribution to cardiovascular disease-related death and disability due to long working hours was reported from developing countries in Asia, where legally binding prescriptions of working time limitations were poorly developed (Pega et al. 2021). A third challenge concerns severe shortcomings in securing civil rights and antidiscrimination policies, and in offering opportunities of return to work with chronic disease or disability in Low and Middle-Income countries (LMICs). For instance, working-aged people with acquired spinal cord injury remain excluded from the labour market due to a lack of rehabilitation care (Bickenbach et al. 2013). Similarly, return to work following the manifestation of chronic disease is less often provided because a trained workforce and specialized institutions of medical and vocational rehabilitation are not available. A report on global availability of cardiac rehabilitation concluded that sixty-eight per cent of the seventy-five high-income countries studied offered cardiac rehabilitation. This percentage was twenty-eight per cent in 103 middle-income countries, and it was as low as eight per cent in the 36 low-income countries. Taken together, around twenty-three per cent of middle- or low-income countries provided cardiac rehabilitation, while eighty per cent of globally reported cardiovascular deaths occurred in these countries (Pesah et al. 2019; Turk-Adawi et al. 2014). A thoughtful perspective paper on deficits of rehabilitation among people with stroke and other disabling chronic diseases in LMICs pointed to major obstacles against access and delivery of rehabilitation services, and illustrated the potential benefits of upscaling these services (Prynn and Kuper

2019). Although the shortage of medical and vocational rehabilitation services and professionals in LMICs has been widely documented (Kamenov et al. 2019), policy efforts of improvement at national, regional, and global level remain scarce. The list of such examples could be extended to many more health conditions, thus illustrating the imbalance between working populations' health-care needs and available resources in less developed countries.

At a broader scope, many countries in the Global South are particularly vulnerable to three main critical global developments. The first one concerns the recent COVID-19 pandemic with its dramatic consequences for population health, economic loss, and threats to working and employment conditions (see Chapter 1). As the majority of the world's population is living in LMICs, this is the region where this critical global development will have its strongest impact. With the COVID-19 outbreak, this became already a concerning reality. Children, women, and men in LMICs were far more seriously hit by the pandemic than people in more privileged regions of the world. A higher level of suffering was reported at all levels, that is, the rate and severity of infection, the death rate attributable to COVID-19, access to vaccination and treatment, poverty rate, amount of job loss and long-term unemployment, and coverage by some measures of social security (International Labour Organization 2020, 2022). In addition, the burden of poor mental health in the context of this pandemic was particularly worrying (Kola et al. 2021). Within working-age populations, some high-risk groups became extremely vulnerable by this outbreak. Migrant workers from Asia and the Pacific are one such group. As temporary, low-skilled workers hired by labour markets in rapidly developing countries, they suddenly lost jobs and income with the massive lockdowns, and as the large majority were not covered by any social security system, a humanitarian crisis occurred. According to a report 'the economic recession caused by the COVID-19 pandemic threatens the job security and well-being of over 91 million international migrants from Asia and the Pacific' (Asian Development Bank Institute et al. 2021, p. 37). In consequence, the pandemic has worsened poverty and income inequality in the Global South, compared to the pre-pandemic period, and it has nullified the slight economic progress that became visible in several parts of the developing world since the 1990s.

Widening income inequalities on a global scale define a second challenge. Again, discrepancies between a poor disadvantaged majority and a highly privileged minority are largest in developing countries. Of particular concern, working poverty, indicating the proportion of employed population below the internationally defined poverty line, was about forty per cent in low-income countries, compared to about ten per cent in lower-middle income countries, and less than one per cent in upper- and high- income countries (for detailed information collected by ILO, see 'Useful websites'). These two developments are not independent, but they tend to mutually reinforce each other. If aggravated by the instability of financial markets and elevated risks of economic recession, they seriously threaten collective human progress. According to a recent report, the United Nations' Human Development Index, measuring life expectancy, education, and gross national income per capita for 191 countries, has fallen back globally in 2020/ 2021 to the level reached in 2016, thus losing recent advances of human welfare to a worrying extent (United Nations Development Programme 2023).

As a third critical development, people living in LMICs are exposed to the devastating consequences of climate change far more often than people living in developed parts of the world. Countries most affected by drivers such as rising temperature or extreme temperatures, drying of vegetation, rising sea levels with risk of coastal floating, and extreme weather events include Pakistan, Bangladesh, Philippines, Viet-Nam, India, and China (Hijioka et al. 2014). Suffering from food insecurity, water shortage, job loss, poverty, and precarious living conditions are causes of involuntary migration among considerable parts of exposed populations in these countries. Increasing awareness of far-reaching impacts of climate change on employment opportunities and on the health and well-being of working populations contributed to the implementation of national and supranational efforts towards reducing global warming and related threats (e.g. Munro et al. 2020). Within occupational health research, global climate change has now been defined as a prioritized topic of concern (Sorensen et al. 2021).

Against this background of critical global developments, opportunities for stable and decent work and employment are extremely limited in LMICs. A majority of workers continues to be employed in the informal economy, lacking statutory regulation, social security benefits, and access to occupational safety and health services and measures. A global report estimates that some sixty per cent of the worldwide workforce is engaged in informal employment, and that almost one third is obliged to work on their own account, often in subsistence activities pursued because of lack of formal job availability (International Labour Organization 2019). Under these conditions, basic labour standards are often absent, while discrimination/violence and exposure to hazardous and stressful working conditions are widespread (Benach et al. 2007; Takala 2020). At the same time, efforts to strengthen global occupational health are still poorly developed, compared to international action programmes of fighting communicable diseases. Although priorities were clearly identified and targeted recommendations were prepared (e.g. Lucchini and London 2014; World Health Organization 2008), implementation activities remained scarce. One such priority concerns the development of Occupational Health and Safety (OHS) services and professionals in LMICs. In these countries, access to OHS services is restricted to the small fraction of formally employed workers, and integrated settings of care and rehabilitation are largely absent. A report on the availability of OHS services and professionals in four countries in Southern Africa (Zimbabwe, Zambia, South Africa, and Botswana) illustrates the case (Moyo et al. 2015). Despite differences in economic development and in adoption of international standards of worker protection, they all suffer from the absence of a comprehensive system of OHS services available to the entire workforce, and from specialized clinics for treatment and rehabilitation of patients with occupational diseases and injuries. Moreover, there is a substantial shortage of occupational health professionals, with poor training and career opportunities. In terms of personnel, services are mainly delivered by occupational nurses, as only a few dozens of specialized occupational physicians are available in these countries (Moyo et al. 2015).

In view of these urgent needs and fundamental gaps in development one may ask whether psychosocial occupational health deserves special priority on the agenda of work-related health promotion in developing and emerging economies (Houtman et al. 2007). As one answer to the question, we may look at population-attributable fractions of work-stress related diseases. In Chapter 6, updated estimates on elevated risks of ischaemic heart disease, depression, and some other chronic diseases due to exposure to adverse psychosocial work environments were demonstrated. In combination with data on exposure prevalence, attributable fractions can be calculated from these relative risks, indicating the proportion of incident events of a specific disease that can theoretically be attributed to the exposure of a psychosocial work stressor, such as demand/control or effort/reward. Despite some uncertainties related to the statistical assumptions underlying these estimates and despite variations in the prevalence of exposure and its effect size, several recently conducted calculations resulted in preliminary estimates of the size of such attributable fractions. As indicated in Chapter 6, attributable fractions of psychosocial work-related stress in case of depression were estimated to amount up to twenty per cent (Pena-Gralle

2022). Assuming a causal link underlying the association, and estimating the worldwide incidence of depression as high as twenty-five million cases (Liu et al. 2020), some five million cases of incident depression could theoretically be avoided by preventing psychosocial stress at work. Despite its questionable assumptions the figure may point to potential benefits of occupational prevention efforts in the Global South.

A second answer to the question of priority of psychosocial occupational health on the agenda of work-related health promotion in developing and emerging economies points to a more fundamental fact: in times of economic globalization and increasing worldwide interdependence, a process of rapid transformation of traditional working and employment conditions in these countries has been initiated. It is characterized by adaptation to, and implementation of, structures and modalities of producing goods and delivering services that dominate high-income countries. Industrialization; expansion of the service, information, and communication sectors of employment; impact of transnational corporations; trade liberalization; and growing transnational labour migration are the main manifestations of a pervasive process of transformation occurring in economically less developed countries (see Chapter 2). Accordingly, more and more work environments, most obviously in rapidly developing countries, will be similar to those prevailing in modern Western societies. With a decline of jobs requiring heavy physical effort and exposure to material hazards, and with an increase in tasks defined by mental and emotional demands psychosocial aspects of work and employment gain momentum in these regions, where new, educated, and skilled generations enter the labour market, prepared for dealing with complex and mentally demanding jobs. This far-reaching transformation has been accelerated by new threats emanating from the global COVID-19 pandemic. In a masterly review, Susan E. Peters and colleagues identified relevant drivers of new working conditions enhanced by the pandemic, such as widespread application of technological innovations (especially automation), the expansion of remote work, a growth of delivery economy, and forced redistribution of jobs across sectors (Peters et al. 2022). The dramatic losses of life among workers exposed to viral infection and the indirect, stress-mediated mental health effects caused by the disruptions of work and employment raised awareness and promoted preventive efforts among employers, safety and health professionals, and other stakeholders with responsibility for safety and health at work. While these developments favour the process of transformation and adaption of work and employment in less developed countries, they also widen social inequalities between more privileged parts of the workforce and those in low-skilled, low-wage occupations.

To summarize, dominant features of work and employment of high-income countries are likely to expand in less-developed regions of the world, and this large-scale transformation will reveal a critical role for psychosocial occupational health in these new contexts. Coordinated original research activities on psychosocial occupational health on site are expected to emerge in order to monitor, evaluate, and support this process. Fortunately, promising research activities have already been inaugurated, in particular in the Asia Pacific region (Dollard et al. 2014; Shimazu et al. 2016) and in Latin America (Pujol-Cols and Lazzaro-Salazar 2021). It is hoped that knowledge derived from new research can help to prevent or at least reduce the negative health consequences of exposures to adverse psychosocial work environments that afflicted—and continue to afflict—working populations in the modern Western world. We hope that the evidence presented and discussed in this book can provide a convincing learning experience for the Global South and for all those who are committed to promote healthy work at a global scale.

11.3 Summary

In this final chapter, the intervention perspective of healthy work was extended beyond the meso-level context of enterprises and businesses to include national labour and social policies as well as programmes of international organizations. Strong investments in these policies go along with improved psychosocial work environments, as documented in cross-national studies in Europe. While a major source of evidence discussed in this book is derived from economically developed countries, essential gaps of knowledge related to less developed regions are observed. Promoting occupational health research, including its psychosocial dimensions, strengthening occupational health and safety services, and implementing international standards of decent work in combination with comprehensive labour and social policies in the Global South are therefore priorities for the near future.

11.4 Relevant questions

- Some results reported in this chapter document an association between the extent of implemented national labour market policies and the quality of the psychosocial work environment among employed people in respective countries. How would you interpret this association? And can you, based on your interpretation, propose a recommendation for practice and policy?
- Work- and health-promoting legal standards and guidelines released from international organizations often fail to be incorporated at national level, most often in low- and middle- income countries. What are the main reasons for these failures?
- In the final part of this chapter, some challenges of developing health-conducive occupational conditions in regions of the Global South were proposed. In your view, what additional challenges deserve attention in priority-setting of future policy agendas?

Recommended reading

❖ Björnberg, K., Belin, M., Hansson, S. O., et al. (eds.) (2022), *The vision zero handbook. Theory, technology and management for a zero casualty policy.* Cham: Springer.

❖ International Labour Organization (2020), *ILO monitor: COVID-19 and the world of work* 6th edn. Geneva: ILO.

❖ Lunau, T., Rigó, M., and Dragano, N. (2020), 'From national labor and social policies to individual work stressors'. In T. Theorell (ed.), *Handbook of socio-economic determinants of occupational health: from macro-level to micro-level evidence.* Cham: Springer, 131–48.

❖ Peters, S. E., Dennerlein, J. T., Wagner, G. R., et al. (2022), 'Work and worker health in the post-pandemic world: a public health perspective', *Lancet Public Health,* 7 (2), e188–e94.

❖ Shimazu, A., Bin Nordin, R., Dollard, M. F., et al. (eds.) (2016), *Psychosocial factors at work in the Asia Pacific. From theory to practice.* Dordrecht: Springer.

❖ World Health Organization, and International Labour Organization (2021), 'WHO/ILO joint estimate of the work-related burden of disease and injury. 2000-2016', (Geneva: WHO, ILO).

Useful websites

❖ European Commission, EU strategic framework on health and safety at work 2021-2027 https://ec.europa.eu/social/main.jsp?catId=151&langId=en

❖ SHARE https://share-eric.eu/
❖ EWCS https://www.eurofound.europa.eu/surveys/european-working-con ditions-surveys-ewcs
❖ Institute of Health Equity https://www.instituteofhealthequity.org/
❖ International Labour Organization: ILOSTAT 2021 https://ilosts.ilo.org./data
❖ PEROSH https://www.perosh.eu

References

Abrahamsson, K. (2021), 'Sustainable work in transition: policy background, concepts and research areas', *Eur J Workplace Innovation*, 6 (1-2), 19–46.

Allen, T. D., and Eby, L. T. (eds.) (2016), *The Oxford handbook of work and family*. Oxford: Oxford University Press.

Asian Development Bank Institute, OECD, and International Labour Organization (2021), *Labor migration in Asia. Impact of the COVID-19 crisis and the post-pandemic future*. Tokyo: Asian Development Bank Institute.

Benach, J., Muntaner, C., and Santana, V. (2007), 'Employment conditions and health inequalities. Final report to the WHO Commission on Social Determinants of Health (CSDH)', (Geneva: WHO).

Bickenbach, J., Officer, A., Shakespeare, T., et al. (eds.) (2013), *International perspectives on spinal cord injury*. Geneva: World Health Organization.

Björnberg, K., Belin, M., Hansson, S. O., et al. (eds.) (2022), *The vision zero handbook: theory, technology and management for a zero casualty policy*. Cham: Springer.

Börsch-Supan, A., Brandt, M., Hank, K., et al. (2011), *The individual and the welfare state: life histories in Europe*. Heidelberg: Springer.

Bright, T., Wallace, S., and Kuper, H. (2018), 'A systematic review of access to re-habilitation for people with disabilities in Low- and middle-income countries', *Int J Environ Res Public Health*, 15 (10), 2165.

Dahl, E., and van der Wel, K. A. (2013), 'Educational inequalities in health in European welfare states: a social expenditure approach', *Soc Sci Med*, 81, 60–9.

Dahl, E., and van der Wel, K. A. (2020), 'Policies of reducing the burden of occupational hazards and disability pensions'. In U. Bültmann and J. Siegrist (eds.), *Handbook of disability, work and health*. Cham: Springer, 85–104.

Diderichsen, F. (2020), 'Investing in integrative active labour market policies'. In U. Bültmann and J. Siegrist (eds.), *Handbook of disability, work and health*. Cham: Springer, 661–74.

Dollard, M. F., Shimazu, A., Bin Nordin, R., et al. (eds.) (2014), *Psychosocial factors at work in the Asia Pacific*. Dordrecht: Springer.

Dragano, N., Siegrist, J., and Wahrendorf, M. (2011), 'Welfare regimes, labour policies and unhealthy psychosocial working conditions: a comparative study with 9917 older employees from 12 European countries', *J Epidemiol Community Health*, 65 (9), 793–9.

Dragano, N., Siegrist, J., Nyberg, S. T., et al. (2017), 'Effort-reward imbalance at work and incident coronary heart disease: a multicohort study of 90,164 individuals', *Epidemiology*, 28 (4), 619–26.

Esping-Andersen, G. (1990), *The three worlds of welfare capitalism*. Oxford: Policy Press.

Eurofound (2022), *European Working Conditions Survey Integrated Data File, 1991–2015. [data collection]* 8th edn.: UK Data Service. SN: 7363.

GBD 2017 Risk Factor Collaborators (2018), 'Global, regional, and national comparative risk assessment of 84 behavioural, environmental and occupational, and metabolic risks or clusters of risks for 195 countries and territories, 1990–2017: a systematic analysis for the Global Burden of Disease Study 2017', *Lancet*, 392 (10159), 1923–94.

Håkansta, C. (2020), 'International organizations as drivers of change in occupational health'. In T. Theorell (ed.), *Handbook of socioeconomic determinants of occupational health: from macro-level to micro-level evidence*. Cham: Springer, 149–65.

Hijioka, Y., Lin, E., Pereira, J. J., et al. (2014), 'Asia'. In V. R. Barros, C. B. Field, D. J. Dokken, et al. (eds.), *Climate change 2014: impacts, adaptation, and vulnerability. Part B: regional aspects. Contribution of Working Group II to the Fifth Assessment Report of the Intergovernmental Panel on Climate Change*. Cambridge: Cambridge University Press, 1327–70.

Hoffmann, R. (ed.), (2023), *Handbook of health inequalities across the life course*. Cheltenham: Edgward Elgar.

Houtman, I., Jettinghof, K., and Cedillo, L. (2007), *Raising awareness of stress at work in developing countries: advice to employers and worker representatives*. Geneva: WHO.

International Labour Organization (2013), *World of work report*. Geneva: ILO.

International Labour Organization (2019), *Safety and health at the heart of the future of work*. Geneva: ILO.

International Labour Organization (2020), *ILO monitor: COVID-19 and the world of work* 6th ed. Geneva: ILO.

International Labour Organization (2022), *World employment and social outlook – trends 2022*. Geneva: ILO.

Kamenov, K., Mills, J. A., Chatterji, S., et al. (2019), 'Needs and unmet needs for rehabilitation services: a scoping review', *Disabil Rehabil*, 41 (10), 1227–37.

Kivimäki, M., Nyberg, S. T., Batty, G. D., et al. (2012), 'Job strain as a risk factor for coronary heart disease: a collaborative meta-analysis of individual participant data', *Lancet*, 380 (9852), 14917.

Kola, L., Kohrt, B. A., Hanlon, C., et al. (2021), 'COVID-19 mental health impact and responses in low-income and middle-income countries: reimagining global mental health', *Lancet Psychiatry*, 8 (6), 535–50.

Liu, Q., He, H., Yang, J., et al. (2020), 'Changes in the global burden of depression from 1990 to 2017: findings from the Global Burden of Disease study', *J Psychiatr Res*, 126, 134–40.

Lucchini, R. G., and London, L. (2014), 'Global occupational health: current challenges and the need for urgent action', *Ann Glob Health*, 80 (4), 251–6.

Lunau, T., Rigó, M., and Dragano, N. (2020a), 'From national labor and social policies to individual work stressors'. In T. Theorell (ed.), *Handbook of socioeconomic determinants of occupational health: from macro-level to micro-level evidence.* Cham: Springer, 131–48.

Lunau, T., Wahrendorf, M., Dragano, N., et al. (2013), 'Work stress and depressive symptoms in older employees: impact of national labour and social policies', *BMC Public Health*, 13, 1086.

Lunau, T., Siegrist, J., Dragano, N., et al. (2015), 'The association between education and work stress: does the policy context matter?', *PLoS One*, 10 (3), e0121573.

Lunau, T., Wahrendorf, M., Dragano, N., et al. (2020b), 'Associations between change in labour market policies and work stressors: a comparative longitudinal survey data analysis from 27 European countries', *BMC Public Health*, 20 (1), 1377.

Marmot, M. G., Banks, J., Blundell, R., et al. (eds.) (2003), *Health, wealth, and lifestyles of the older population in England: the 2002 English Longitudinal Study of Aging.* London: Institute for Fiscal Studies.

Moyo, D., Zungu, M., Kgalamono, S., et al. (2015), 'Review of occupational health and safety organization in expanding economies: the case of Southern Africa', *Ann Glob Health*, 81 (4), 495–502.

Munro, A., Boyce, T., and Marmot, M. G. (2020), *Sustainable health equity: achieving a net-zero UK.* London: Institute of Health Equity.

OECD (2010), *Sickness, disability and work: breaking the barriers. A synthesis of findings across OECD countries.* Paris: OECD.

OECD (2017), *OECD guidelines on measuring the quality of the working environment.* Paris: OECD.

Pega, F., Nafradi, B., Momen, N. C., et al. (2021), 'Global, regional, and national burdens of ischemic heart disease and stroke attributable to exposure to long working hours for 194 countries, 2000–2016: a systematic analysis from the WHO/ILO Joint Estimates of the Work-related Burden of Disease and Injury', *Environ Int*, 154, 106595.

Pena-Gralle, A. P. B. (2022), 'Inégalités socioéconomiques, contraintes psychosociales aú travail et données administratives sur la depression: résultats du PROspective Québec. Dissertation', (Université Laval, Québec, Canada). https://corpus.ulaval.ca/server/api/core/bitstreams/5bbde76c-e9a7-450e-8be8-8ddc73ca4bce/content.

Pesah, E., Turk-Adawi, K., Supervia, M., et al. (2019), 'Cardiac rehabilitation delivery in low/middle-income countries', *Heart*, 105 (23), 1806–12.

Peters, S. E., Dennerlein, J. T., Wagner, G. R., et al. (2022), 'Work and worker health in the post-pandemic world: a public health perspective', *Lancet Public Health*, 7 (2), e188–e94.

Prynn, J. E., and Kuper, H. (2019), 'Perspectives on disability and non-communicable diseases in low- and middle-income countries, with a focus on stroke and dementia', *Int J Environ Res Public Health*, 16 (18), 3488. doi:10.3390/ijerph16183488

Puig-Barrachina, V., Giro, P., Artazcoz, L., et al. (2020), 'The impact of active labour market policies on health outcomes: a scoping review', *Eur J Public Health*, 30 (1), 36–42.

Pujol-Cols, L., and Lazzaro-Salazar, M. (2021), 'Diez años de investigación sobre riesgos psicosociales, salud y desempeño en América Latina: una revisión sistemática integradora y agenda de investigación. [Ten years of research on psychosocial risks, health, and performance in Latin America: a comprehensive systematic review and research agenda]', *J Work Organiz Pychol*, 37 (3), 187–202.

Rigó, M., Dragano, N., Wahrendorf, M., et al. (2022), 'Long-term trends in psychosocial working conditions in Europe—the role of labor market policies', *Eur J Public Health*, 32 (3), 384–91.

Rose, D. (2019), 'The impact of active labour market policies on the well-being of the unemployed', *J Eur Soc Policy*, 29 (3), 396–410.

Shimazu, A., Bin Nordin, R., Dollard, M. F., et al. (eds.) (2016), *Psychosocial factors at work in the Asia Pacific: from theory to practice*. Dordrecht: Springer.

Shockley, K. M., Shen, W., and Johnson, R. C. (eds.) (2018), *The Cambridge handbook of the global work-family interface*. Cambridge: Cambridge University Press.

Sorensen, C. J., Cook-Shimanek, M., and Newman, L. S. (2021), 'Climate change and worker health: implications for clinical practice'. In J. LaDou and R. J. Harrison (eds.), *Current diagnosis and treatment: occupational and environmental medicine*, 6e. New York, NY: McGraw Hill, 783–800; Chapter 49. https://accessmedicine.mhmedical.com/content.aspx?bookid=3065&sectionid=255657919

Takala, J. (2020), 'Burden of injury due to occupational exposures'. In U. Bültmann and J. Siegrist (eds.), *Handbook of disability, work and health*. Cham: Springer, 105–26.

Turk-Adawi, K., Sarrafzadegan, N., and Grace, S. L. (2014), 'Global availability of cardiac rehabilitation', *Nat Rev Cardiol*, 11 (10), 586–96.

UN General Assembly (2007), 'Convention on the Rights of Persons with Disabilities: resolution / adopted by the General Assembly, 24 January 2007, A/RES/61/106', https://www.refworld.org/docid/45f973632.html, accessed 20 March 2023.

United Nations Development Programme (2023), 'Human development report 2021/2022. Uncertain times, unsettled lives: shaping our future in a transforming world ', http://report.hdr.undp.org, accessed 23 March 2023.

Wahrendorf, M., and Siegrist, J. (2014), 'Proximal and distal determinants of stressful work: framework and analysis of retrospective European data', *BMC Public Health*, 14, 849.

Wahrendorf, M., Chandola, T., and Descatha, A. (eds.) (2023), *Handbook of life course occupational health*. Cham: Springer.

Wels, J., Booth, C., Wielgoszewska, B., et al. (2022), 'Mental and social wellbeing and the UK coronavirus job retention scheme: evidence from nine longitudinal studies', *Soc Sci Med*, 308, 115226.

Westman, M. (2001), 'Stress and strain crossover', *Hum Relat*, 54 (6), 717–51.

World Health Organization (2008), 'Closing the gap in a generation: health equity though action on the social determinants of health. Final report of the Commission on Social Determinants of Health.', (Geneva: WHO).

World Health Organization (2014), 'Review of social determinants and the health divide in the WHO European region: final report ', (2nd ed.; Copenhagen: WHO, Regional Office for Europe).

World Health Organization (2022), *WHO guidelines on mental health at work*. Geneva: WHO.

World Health Organization, and International Labour Organization (2021), 'WHO/ ILO joint estimate of the work-related burden of disease and injury. 2000–2016', (Geneva: WHO, ILO).

Index

For the benefit of digital users, indexed terms that span two pages (e.g., 52–53) may, on occasion, appear on only one of those pages.

Tables, figures, and boxes are indicated by *t*, *f*, and *b* following the page number